APPLIED KINESIOLOGY

APPLIED KINESIOLOGY
Revised Edition

A Training Manual and Reference Book
of Basic Principles and Practices

Robert Frost, PhD

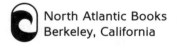

North Atlantic Books
Berkeley, California

Published by
North Atlantic Books
Berkeley, California

Cover design by Jasmine Hromjak
Cover art © iStockphoto.com/agsandrew
Book design by Jan Camp
Photography by Andreas Werda, Lukas von Saint-George
Illustrations by Tatjana Schuba
Printed in the United States of America

Applied Kinesiology, Revised Edition: A Training Manual and Reference Book of Basic Principles and Practices is sponsored and published by the Society for the Study of Native Arts and Sciences (dba North Atlantic Books), an educational nonprofit based in Berkeley, California, that collaborates with partners to develop cross-cultural perspectives, nurture holistic views of art, science, the humanities, and healing, and seed personal and global transformation by publishing work on the relationship of body, spirit, and nature.

North Atlantic Books' publications are available through most bookstores. For further information, visit our website at www.northatlanticbooks.com or call 800-733-3000.

MEDICAL DISCLAIMER: The following information is intended for general information purposes only. Individuals should always see their health care provider before administering any suggestions made in this book. Any application of the material set forth in the following pages is at the reader's discretion and is his or her sole responsibility.

Library of Congress Cataloging-in-Publication Data

Frost, Robert, 1950–
  Applied kinesiology: a training manual and reference book of basic principles and practices / Robert Frost.—Rev. ed.
     p.; cm.
  Includes bibliographical references and index.
  ISBN 978-1-58394-612-1 (pbk.)—ISBN 978-1-58394-629-9 (ebk.)
  I. Title.
  [DNLM: 1. Kinesiology, Applied—methods. 2. Musculoskeletal Physiological Phenomena. 3. Physical Therapy Modalities. WB 890]
  RZ999
  612.7'6—dc23
                          2013015174

2 3 4 5 6 7 UNITED 19 18 17 16

Printed on recycled paper

TABLE OF CONTENTS

Chapter 7
STRUCTURE 233

FOREWORD

Applied Kinesiology had a simple beginning in 1964, based on the concept that muscle weakness is involved in most muscle spasms and, indeed, is primary.

Applied Kinesiology is based on the fact that body language never lies. The opportunity of understanding body language is enhanced by the ability to use muscles as indicators for body language. The original method of testing muscles and determining their function, first brought to my attention by Kendall, Kendall, and Wadsworth, remains the prime diagnostic device.

Once muscle weakness has been ascertained, a variety of therapeutic options is available, too numerous to enumerate here. The opportunity to use the body as an instrument of laboratory analysis is unparalleled in modern therapeutics because the response of the body is unerring; if one approaches the problem correctly, making the proper and adequate diagnosis and treatment, the response is adequate and satisfactory both to the doctor and to the patient.

The name of the game, to quote a phrase, is to get people better. The body heals itself in a sure, sensible, practical, reasonable, and observable manner. "The healer within" can be approached from without. Man possesses a potential for recovery through the innate intelligence or the physiological homeostasis of the human structure. The recovery potential with which he is endowed merely waits for the hand and the heart and the mind of a trained individual to bring it into manifestation, allowing health to come forth; this is man's natural heritage.

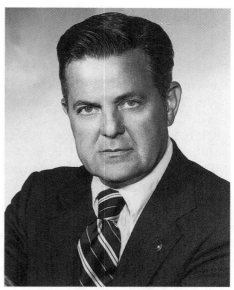

DR. GEORGE J. GOODHEART, JR.

This benefits mankind individually and collectively. It benefits the doctor who has rendered the service, and it allows the force which created the structure to operate unimpeded. This benefit can be performed with knowledge, with physiological facts, with predictable certainty. It should be done, it can be done, and this book offers a means and a measure of how it can be done. My appreciation to the author and his staff for the excellent job he has performed in advancing these principles, and my best wishes are extended to all who read this manual.

—George J. Goodheart, Jr., DC, FICC
Diplomate, ICAK

ACKNOWLEDGMENTS

First of all, I would like to give a heartfelt thanks to the founder of Applied Kinesiology, George Goodheart, DC. His insights and research are the reason this field exists at all.

Next, I am indebted to the excellent texts of David Walther, DC, David Leaf, DC, and Wolfgang Gerz, MD. These were my most-used references for the writing of this book. Dr. Gerz was also kind enough to read the text, answer questions by phone and fax, provide various diagrams, and to help with specific questions including the correct translations of Applied Kinesiology terminology (*Fachbegriffe*) for the German edition. His critical reading of this text, corrections and suggestions greatly assisted its accuracy and completeness.

My deepest thanks go out also to my personal teachers of kinesiology: John Grahme, Andres Bernard, Richard Harnack, Jimmy Scott, Gordon Stokes, Daniel Whiteside, John Thie, Frank Mahoney, Dominique Monette, Richard Utt, Sheldon Deal, Joan and Bruce Dewe, John Varun Maguire, Hap and Elizabeth Barhydt, Irene Yaychuk Arabei, and Andrew Verity. Their dedication and personal love of kinesiology constitute an ongoing inspiration. A special thanks to Irene Yaychuk Arabei and Andrew Verity for the personal balancing sessions that helped me rid myself of various health and personal problems, making the writing of this book and the achievement of other life goals possible.

Parts of this text were derived from my doctoral thesis. While I was writing that thesis, my father played the role of the interested but uninformed student of kinesiology. Through his continual questioning, I rewrote and rewrote until a beginner could understand what I meant. Through the magic of electronic mail (between California and Switzerland/Germany), he assisted me in clarifying this text as well. He taught me to seek unity, coherence, and emphasis in my writing. I hear his guiding words whenever I write. Thanks to you, Joe Frost.

A special thanks to Tatjana Schuba (*Heilpraktikerin*, acupuncturist, fitness trainer, designer). Her design and precision craftsmanship produced the various anatomical and other graphic drawings. During the initial writing of this book, Tatjana sat next to me and translated the text into German. Through her extensive knowledge of anatomy and physiology, the text achieved scientific accuracy. In particular the parts about the nervous system, neurophysiology, hormones, and the meridian system have, through her research and reworking of my text, achieved greater precision. Writing together made the work fun and stimulated us both to keep at it for long hours. Through her questioning of exactly what I meant to say, many unclear sections of the text were rewritten and greatly improved.

I also want to thank Kaitlyn Vera, CPT, the model in chapters 7–9, as well as Michael Lebowitz who allowed me to summarize his latest protocol of systemic corrections for dealing with difficult patients.

INTRODUCTION

This book is for those who want a detailed introduction to Applied Kinesiology (AK) as it is performed by qualified chiropractors, medical doctors and health professionals. The goal of this book is to present the principles and basic practices of AK in their original form as developed by George Goodheart, but in a manner and a format which may be understood even by the reader with no prior medical training. Standard medical terminology as used in AK is adhered to in this text. However, since most every specific term or concept is defined and logically presented, even the complete beginner should be able to follow and understand the ideas. Since I especially wish to present these concepts using the vocabulary common to occupational groups with medical background, I utilize the following terminology which is also typical in AK literature: The "examiner" tests the "patient," "diagnoses" and provides corrective "treatments."

At the beginning of the first chapter, I present short definitions of traditional kinesiology (biomechanics), Applied Kinesiology and muscle testing so that the reader may more easily understand these topics. Then a short history of Applied Kinesiology, its methods and techniques is provided. In order to describe how living beings move (the original meaning of kinesiology or biomechanics), I describe the anatomy and physiology of muscles and related structures. Since muscles are driven by nerves, sections on neurophysiology and nerve receptors are included. The stress concept of Hans Selye and how this relates to muscular dysfunction follows. Since many of the phenomena of Applied Kinesiology cannot be adequately described within the limitations of the old Newtonian cause-and-effect scientific model, this is contrasted with the new worldviews provided by quantum and chaos theories. Biological medicine, which uses quantum and chaos theories to provide a basis for a holistic model of healing, and which often uses Applied Kinesiology for diagnostic purposes, is then described at length. There follows a section on how to use the concepts of biological medicine to improve and maintain optimal health.

For those with some experience in muscle testing, the main portion of this book will provide the theoretical background necessary to deeply understand and to explain to others how muscle testing is performed and how muscle strengthening techniques function. The testing and strengthening of thirty-three muscles are illustrated and carefully described. The muscle strengthening techniques discussed in this text include Goodheart's original origin-insertion technique, neurolymphatic reflex point massage, neurovascular reflex point holding, appropriate nutrition, and manipulation of the neuromuscular spindle cells and Golgi tendon organs. The detailed explanations of how these techniques are performed in AK will enable the "apprentice" muscle-tester to use muscle testing and strengthening techniques with improved precision and effectiveness. The advanced AK diagnostic and treatment techniques explained in this book include therapy localization, challenge, nutritional and other substance testing, individual activation of the right and left halves of the brain, repeated muscle testing, muscle stretch response, and reactive muscles. Use of these techniques will produce much greater ability to locate and correct the energy imbalances that affect health and optimal functioning. These basic and advanced AK techniques are described in a step-by-step format I designed for easy application in a therapeutic session. A selection of case histories using this format is presented to help the reader bridge the gap from theory to practice. Most anatomical and other specific terms used in this text are defined in the glossary.

The AK techniques in this book should give the student a thorough theoretical grounding in muscle testing and its application. However, nothing can replace "hands-on" experience. It is highly advisable to seek training with a health professional experienced with AK techniques before attempting to perform them. Readers who already have experience in muscle testing will find the techniques that are new for them described in enough detail here that they will be able to put them directly into use. It is hoped that this text will also whet their appetite for more. For all those who have the required prior training in a health profession, it is recommended that they acquire training under the guidance of a qualified teacher of Applied Kinesiology.

Sports trainers and physical therapists of all sorts will learn useful techniques from this book and thereby be better able to help their clients. Mastery of the practical techniques in this text should give any health professional who practices them the ability to help patients dispel health problems, improve posture and coordination, increase endurance, eliminate pains, increase the recuperative powers and many other salutary effects.

Applied Kinesiology was created in the 1960s by the American chiropractor, Dr. George Goodheart. It has been further developed by other chiropractors and by medical doctors. The requirements for the highest accreditation, the "diplomate" of Goodheart's International College of Applied Kinesiology (ICAK), are high indeed. To join the organization, or take training courses, you must already be a chiropractor, medical doctor, or other health professional with a four year medical training and the legal right to diagnose. Then you must have at least 300 hours of accredited instruction in AK, publish two AK research papers and practice AK for two years. Finally, you must pass intensive written, oral and practical examinations. The ICAK diplomates have tremendous training, knowl-

edge, and experience behind them. But due to the stringent and extensive requirements for accreditation, there are not many of them, and the successful work they do is not yet very widely known.

In the German branch (ICAK-D), membership and specially designed AK training programs are available for accredited practitioners of all state-recognized health professions including Heilpraktiker, Krankengymnasten, Physiotherapeuten and Psychologen. A special branch of ICAK-D, the International Medical Society for Applied Kinesiology (IMAK), exists to serve the interests of medical doctors and dentists, offering an exclusive AK training program for them. Germany, Austria and Switzerland are the first countries where the medical community is beginning to take serious interest in AK. In fact, there are more medical doctors who use AK techniques in the German- speaking countries than in the rest of the world combined.

In an of itself, AK is not a profession. Therefore, in the world of AK, there are no "applied kinesiologists." As mentioned, to study AK one must already be a chiropractor, medical doctor, or at least a state-approved therapist. For simplicity in this book, qualified therapists who use AK will be referred to as "examiners" or "therapists who use AK."

John Thie (chiropractor and first president of Goodheart's International College of Applied Kinesiology) gave some of his patients AK techniques for self-application as "homework." He saw that the patients who did this homework had better and swifter results than those who didn't. Excited by these practical results, he then urged Dr. Goodheart to write a popular book about his discoveries in AK. Dr. Goodheart gave the job back to Dr. Thie. First with the help of Mary Marks, and then with both research and writing assistance from Richard Duree and Gordon Stokes, Dr. Thie wrote the now famous *Touch for Health* book, first published in 1973. This was designed for use by lay persons. The only requirements were that the chosen techniques be easy to learn, would (even in simplified form) be able to do a lot of good and, even if done incorrectly, would cause no harm.

It is an excellent system for mothers to help improve the health and performance of their children. As far as it goes, the system works very well. In fact, it works so well, that many people use it professionally as a therapy system. This was a great surprise to its founders. No one ever intended that Touch for Health become a professional system of healing. Through its widespread popularity, Touch for Health has greatly increased the awareness of Applied Kinesiology. More than two million people world-wide have been introduced to kinesiology muscle testing techniques through Touch for Health. The many "kinesiologies" that have been developed from the root of Touch for Health are today referred to as belonging to the field of "Specialized Kinesiology."

In many countries such as Germany, Touch for Health was being taught long before Goodheart's Applied Kinesiology became known at large. And many of the practitioners of Touch for Health and related kinesiologies called their work "Angewandte Kinesiologie," the German translation of Applied Kinesiology. At that time there were few therapists using Applied Kinesiology and there seemed to be no reason not to translate from English and use the term themselves. This can be compared with California calling its sparkling wines "champagne." The French complained bitterly but to no avail. Although no one denies that Champagne is a province in France, the French had not internationally patented the word "champagne." Similarly, Goodheart never patented the term "Applied Kinesiology." One unfortunate consequence is that many therapists believe that Touch for Health and Applied Kinesiology are identical. And seeing that Touch for Health is for lay persons, they do not pursue studies in Applied Kinesiology. In order to avoid further confusion, Goodheart's original work, even in foreign language texts, is now called "Applied Kinesiology" with no translation of the term.

The simplified techniques of Touch for Health do not go as far or do as much good as can be achieved by the original and more complicated techniques of AK. For example, Touch for Health advises, as a muscle strengthening technique, that the neurovascular points be gently held. AK teaches that neurovascular points be not only held, but gently tugged in various directions, until the direction that produces maximum pulsation is detected. Then the points are held in this exact direction for 20 seconds longer. Just holding the points will often strengthen the muscle test. Careful experimentation has revealed that the best effects upon the associated organ and bodily areas are only achieved with the precise application taught in AK (and explained in this book).

In most systems of Specialized Kinesiology, there is a conspicuous absence of descriptive detail of the anatomy and physiology involved. And an explanation of how the techniques function is also lacking. This is to be expected, because Touch for Health was designed for lay persons. For those who began with Touch for Health and/or other branches of Specialized Kinesiology and are now ready for more detailed knowledge and precision, this book will provide a bridge toward the deeper understandings and applications of the original techniques of Applied Kinesiology. It is hoped that this book will demonstrate the professional level of knowledge, the wide range of application and the practical usefulness of the techniques of AK and thereby attract more health professionals to study AK.

The English version of this book has been in print for eleven years. I am proud now to present the revised edition.

—Robert Frost, PhD
June 2013

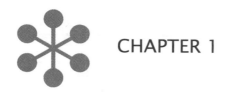

CHAPTER 1

From BioMechanics
To Applied Kinesiology

KINESIOLOGY (from the Greek *kinesis,* movement) began in antiquity as the study of human and animal movement. Over the course of many centuries, this original, traditional form of kinesiology *(biomechanics)* has produced a broad body of knowledge of how nerves stimulate muscles to act upon bones in order to produce posture and movement. Like physiotherapy, kinesiology is a therapeutic profession with a long history. Medical muscle testing existed in biomechanics long before the emergence of Applied Kinesiology.

The biomechanic principles of kinesiology (such as the application of the minimal force necessary to produce maximal result) have been successfully applied to a wide variety of ergonomic problems of industry, sports, and medicine. The application of biomechanics in industry has resulted in the design of tools, chairs, work stations, etc., that are "user friendly." It has stimulated the development of ergonomic work techniques (e.g., how to lift heavy objects without endangering the body) that result in fewer injuries and yield greater productivity. Athletes work with kinesiologists to learn how to more efficiently and successfully perform the movements required by their sports. And biomechanic principles have many applications in the various fields of medicine including the designing of artificial joints and the development of more effective rehabilitation methods.

The research and developments of biomechanics or "traditional" kinesiology can be traced back over

thousands of years and continue into the present. By contrast, Applied Kinesiology (shortened in this book to AK) began in 1964 with the research of the American chiropractor, George J. Goodheart, Jr., DC. His extraordinary powers of observation, his curiosity, his drive to research the causes of what he observed and the resulting discoveries have been the source of most of the diagnostic techniques used today in this relatively new discipline.

Various kinds of health professionals schooled in AK use standard medical muscle tests of biomechanics to directly assess the functional integrity of the nervous system and the muscles. Muscle testing is described at length later in this book. As a preliminary introduction, a brief description of muscle testing as performed in AK is given below:

How Muscles Are Tested
in Applied Kinesiology

1. Most muscles are attached through their tendons at both ends to bones that meet in a moveable joint. When muscles contract, they shorten. This shortening pulls one of the attached bones toward the other.

2. To prepare for the muscle test, one bends the joint over which the muscle is attached. This shortens the muscle, bringing it into a position of contraction. The examiner places his hand in a position to resist the further contraction of the muscle.

3. The patient initiates the test by steadily contracting the muscle from zero force up to the maximum force of contraction against the examiner's unmoving hand. During this short period, the examiner provides an equal and opposite, steadily increasing resistance to maintain the starting position of the muscle test. When the patient has willfully contracted his or her muscle as much as possible, the examiner applies a bit more force. The whole test procedure should not last longer than 2–3 seconds. If the patient can maintain the original test position against this small extra force without movement, the muscle "tested strong." If not, it "tested weak."

4. In the first part of the muscle test, one is testing the determination and ability of the patient to strongly contract the muscle. In the second part of the muscle test, one is also testing the ability of the patient's nervous system, "on its own," to provide a little more contraction than the patient can willfully provide. By this technique, one is actually assessing the functional integrity of the complete circuit of the muscle and the portion of the nervous system involved with that muscle. This initial muscle test is performed "in the clear," i.e., with no extra stimulus of any kind. The muscle is contracted as strongly as the patient is consciously able. In the second part of the muscle test, the question asked is: After the patient has completely contracted the muscle, and the examiner then applies additional pressure, can her nervous system finely coordinate the muscle to contract just a bit more than he or she is consciously able to do?

5. AK uses not only muscle testing "in the clear" as described above, but also "indicator" muscle testing. In this type of muscle testing, a muscle that previously tested strong in the clear is used as an indicator for testing some other stimulus. The extra stimulus can be provided by touching an area of the patient's body that is "disturbed" or dysfunctional because of injury, infection, etc. If this is done while repeating the test of a previously strong-testing indicator muscle, such stimulus may cause that muscle to test weak. The stimulus provided by the patient touching himself or herself is referred to as "therapy localization."

In practice, many examiners touch the patient to therapy-localize, which is often easier, faster, and usually produces the same results. However, on occasion, when the examiner touches the patient, the results of therapy localization are different than when the patient touches the same area of the body. Therefore it is recommended that the patient touch herself for therapy localization. When the patient is presented with some other kind of stimulus besides touch, or performs some kind of activity and the effect is then measured with muscle testing, this is called "challenge."

Much of the fascination of Applied Kinesiology lies in the fact that most factors influencing health may be tested using an indicator muscle and therapy localization or challenge. As will be described later, health professionals familiar with AK techniques use standard muscle testing "in the clear" and indicator muscle testing of various stimuli to evaluate the structural, mental/emotional, and biochemical functions of the human organism.

Applied Kinesiology is primarily a diagnostic technique. Although extensive methods for the evaluation (diagnosis) of dysfunction were developed early within the field of AK, most of the treatments used in AK have been gathered from other (sometimes quite foreign) areas of healing. Besides its well-developed diagnostic techniques, the practical advantage of AK is that one can determine which of many possible therapy methods will be the most effective for the individual problems of specific patients. In this way, before applying any therapeutic technique, the examiner can determine the relative effectiveness and thus choose accurately from a wide variety of treatments.

The diagnostic techniques of AK allow one to determine which body system is disturbed and which treatment modalities are best suited to the correction of the disturbance. Interventions of all sorts (structural, chemical, nutritional, mental, electromagnetic, etc.) may be individually tested in advance to assess their worth in treating a specific problem. After treatment, the same techniques can be applied to determine whether the treatment was appropriate, correctly applied, and effective.

The Development of Traditional Kinesiology or Biomechanics

Beginning with the ideas of Aristotle (384–322 BC), who is often called the "father of biology," the study of movement (the original kinesiology) has for centuries centered upon anatomy and mechanics. Leonardo da Vinci (1452–1519) is especially well known for studies of human structure and function. These make him one of the best known pioneers of the study of movement, or kinesiology.

Mechanics is the branch of physical science that deals with energy and forces and their effect upon bodies. The central interest of the early kinesiologists was the mechanical consideration of how muscles act upon bones and joints to produce posture and movement. Eventually, in the modern age, representing the bones as levers, the joints as fulcrums, and the muscles as springs provided a simple model of body mechanics for mathematical calculations. Although idealized, such models do provide useful insights into human and other animal movement. Kinesiology was originally defined as the study of the structures and their functions that produce animal and human movement. Today this study is called biomechanics, and it is sometimes referred to as "traditional" kinesiology.

After the spectacular contributions of Leonardo da Vinci in the fifteenth century, traditional kinesiology made little progress for more than two hundred years. When Luigi Galvani made his discovery (1780) that muscular contraction is produced by electrical impulses, the development of kinesiology began again. Galvani applied a small electrical voltage to a frog's leg, which produced a twitch contraction in the mus-

cles of the leg. From this he correctly concluded that muscular contraction is initiated by electrical impulses. Until his time, a muscle was considered to have a will of its own. This thinking is still to be observed in certain phrases such as "the biceps act to bring the wrist toward the shoulder." Galvani's experiment demonstrated that muscular contraction, and thus movement of the body, is the result of electrical stimulation of the muscles. With the further discovery that electrical impulses were, in the living animal, provided by nerves under central nervous system (brain and spinal cord) control, the study of the function of nerves and the central nervous system *(neurophysiology)* automatically came to be included in the study of movement (kinesiology). Neurophysiology will be discussed at greater length in the following chapter. First we will continue with the historical development of kinesiology.

A Short History of Applied Kinesiology

Applied Kinesiology grew out of Dr. George J. Goodheart's analysis of his day-to-day chiropractic practice. Accepted chiropractic procedures served him well in his practice, most of the time. However, he was keenly disturbed by his lack of techniques to adequately diagnose the occasional set of paradoxical (or just plain puzzling) symptoms. And without adequate diagnosis, he was at a loss to devise effective treatments. When stumped by a patient's unusual symptoms and diagnostic results, Goodheart continually asked himself the age-old query of the scientist-researcher: "Why is this?"

In his search for explanations that might lead him to effective corrective procedures, Goodheart carefully considered the anatomy and physiology involved in his patients' problems. This knowledge often led him directly to possible interventions. Examples of new methods he deduced include his theory and treatment of reactive muscles and his effective treatment for sustained muscle use. (Both of these methods are described in detail later in this text.)

Goodheart explored beyond the boundaries of his formal chiropractic training to consider the concepts of other innovative healers and scientists. He studied the traditional knowledge and research findings of many other healing systems (Chinese acupuncture, lymphatic drainage, nutrition, neurology, etc.) and then found ways to incorporate them into Applied Kinesiology. He experimented with many alternative treatment modes such as Chapman's reflexes, Bennett's reflexes, synchronization of pulses in reflex points, etc. When a puzzling diagnostic situation could not be solved with the techniques he already knew, he experimented, even with highly unusual measures. Out of his uniquely open-minded search for procedures came most of the techniques used in Applied Kinesiology today.

In 1964, Goodheart made the discovery that marks the birth of Applied Kinesiology. As a chiropractor, he assumed that correcting structural imbalances in the body (postural problems, false alignment of bones, etc.) will reduce or eliminate most health problems. Structural balance, optimal postural alignment of the parts of the body, is the goal of chiropractic. But structural balance cannot be obtained when muscles are overly tense or too limp.

For several months, Goodheart unsuccessfully treated a patient whose presenting symptom was one shoulder blade that stuck out away from his back. He remembered reading in Kendall and Kendall's classic, *Muscles: Testing and Function*, about a muscle that pulled the shoulder blade down upon the back. He used the muscle testing technique described by Kendall and Kendall to test this muscle, the serratus anticus (often called the anterior serratus). It tested weak only on the side where the shoulder blade protruded. The serratus muscle is called "serrated" like a saw because of its "toothed" shape (see illustration on page 207). It connects the upper eight or nine ribs to the inner vertebral side of the scapula, the shoulder blade. The muscle was not less developed on the weak-testing side and Goodheart found no other reason for the one-sided test weakness. Exploring the weak-testing muscle with his fingers revealed painful

little lumps (nodules) where the tendons of serratus anticus attach to the ribs. When he firmly rubbed one of these nodules, it disappeared. As an experiment, he firmly massaged all of these nodules and upon retesting found an immediate increase in the "test strength" of the muscle. Encouraged by this discovery, Goodheart used Kendall and Kendall's book to teach himself how to muscle-test many other muscles as well. This was the first discovery of Applied Kinesiology and the beginning point of ongoing and very fruitful research.

This surprising discovery that a weak-testing muscle may be made to test strong through the massage of its extreme ends where its tendons attach to bone is referred to in Applied Kinesiology today as the "origin-insertion technique." This technique worked often enough in establishing muscular balance (and thus structural balance also) that many chiropractors began to use manual muscle testing to assess structural balance, the goal of chiropractic. When the origin-insertion massage strengthened weak-testing muscles, many other health problems often disappeared without further treatment. This provided more confirmation of the basic chiropractic premise that structural balance affects all aspects of health.

However, the origin-insertion technique often failed to strengthen weak-testing muscles and reestablish muscular balance. Muscle-building exercises didn't help either. Such exercises, specifically designed to strengthen the weak-testing muscle, often did increase the mass of the muscle and its weight-bearing strength, but it still "muscle-tested" weak. Factors other than pure physical strength were at work that needed to be unearthed. Goodheart's further research revealed that muscular imbalances may be the result of problems not just in the origin-insertion area of the muscle itself, but also in any of the areas represented by the three sides of the chiropractic "triad of health"— that is, dysfunction could be the result of structural, chemical, and/or mental problems.

The interaction of the three sides of the triad of health is an important and very useful principle in Applied Kinesiology evaluation. Some examples of how one side of the triad may affect another side are well known. For example, certain foods or chemicals may cause mental disturbances. Fear (mental) causes the release of adrenaline (chemical), which increases the tension in skeletal muscles (structural) in preparation for fight or flight. Tension in the neck (structural) may cause severe headaches and depression (mental). Emotional problems (mental) may cause

Allergy / Psyche

Toxicity / Stress

Orthomolecular Medicine / Homeopathy (High Potency)

Homeopathy / Bach Flower Remedies

Allopathy / Electromagnetic Therapies

Nutrition

Herbs / Esoteric

Chemical / Mental

Structural

Chiropractic, Cranial Osteopathy, Stomatognathic System, Muscle Techniques, Acupuncture, Reflex Points

THE TRIAD OF HEALTH

over-acidity in the stomach (chemical) which may result in a painful stomach that causes the patient to bend forward and down (structural).

The various healing professions each tend to specialize in only one side of the triad of health. *Structural* therapeutics include chiropractic, massage, osteopathy, surgery, and dentistry. *Chemical* therapeutics include nutrition and medication. *Mental* therapeutics include counseling and psychology. Specialists in one of these systems are rarely well-trained in dealing with problems involving the other sides of the triad of health. With patients, specialists naturally use the concepts and techniques with which they are experienced. However, counseling is not likely to relieve a

headache if the cause is primarily nutritional. To pictorially illustrate this point, if the only tool one has is a hammer, the whole world looks like nails. What all of these specialists need are better techniques for diagnosing the causes of the problems of their patients and determining which treatments are likely to be successful.

When a health problem exists for an extended period of time (becomes chronic), all three sides of the triad of health usually become involved. And the problem that brings a patient to a therapist is often not the primary problem, but rather a reaction on another side of the triad.

As long as the primary problem is not diagnosed and treated, the same symptoms will return or other secondary problems may emerge.

Goodheart recognized that in order to most effectively help his patients, he needed to extend his field of inquiry. From his chiropractic training, he was aware of the need to be able to evaluate and treat problems on all three sides of the triad of health. To do so, he investigated the capacity of the muscle testing technique to comprehensively test all three sides. Extensive investigation convinced him that muscle testing worked well in the assessment of all of the factors affecting health. He found that:

a) Specific health problems may cause specific muscles to test weak.

b) The muscle that tests weak due to a health problem can be used as an indicator to determine possible treatments.

c) Treatments making the muscle test strong may positively influence the health problem.

Considering that Goodheart was already fully trained in chiropractic, his flexibility of thought is amazing. After all, like any professional, he was already focused upon the limiting concepts of his specialized field of knowledge. With uninhibited enthusiasm, Goodheart evaluated a wide variety of therapeutic approaches in his attempts to achieve the chiropractic goal of structural balance. He thoroughly researched any procedure that resulted in the strengthening of a weak-testing muscle.

Sometimes, patients with the same symptoms require very different therapies. Many of the most successful interventions that Goodheart studied had been previously developed but were seldom used due to a lack of diagnostic techniques that could identify when a specific intervention would be helpful. The use of muscle testing provided him with the needed diagnostic tool to choose among the many possible interventions for each disturbance. Since muscle testing uses the patient's body itself as the instrument for performing diagnostics, it provides a direct method for studying the effects upon the body of just about any kind of healing modality. Goodheart found muscle testing to be the most direct method to locate the treatment best suited to the needs of each particular patient.

For use in his own practice and for the benefit of other practitioners, Goodheart gathered, adapted, developed, and codified many techniques useful in the strengthening of weak-testing muscles. The greater portion of the techniques known and used in AK today stem from his research.

Goodheart's research is remarkable for its intuitive conceptual leaps. For example, he first determined that a correct treatment measure almost always swiftly returns a weak-testing muscle to testing strong. He then intuitively jumped to the proposition that muscle testing conversely might be used to test for the effectiveness of any treatment after it has been applied. Further careful research proved the inspiration to be true. He established the rule that by using muscle testing after the treatment, one can determine whether the applied treatment has been effective. Health professionals using AK today stand on the shoulders of the giants like Goodheart that have gone before. From this perspective, we can mistakenly feel that such intuitive jumps are actually obvious. The challenge is to be such a giant and to discover some of the similar "jumps" of realization still waiting to be made in this young field of research.

A Short Discussion of the Anatomy and Physiology of Muscles

In order to understand the depth of Goodheart's work, a very short discussion of the anatomy and physiology of muscles is included here. Definitions of the words used will also be discussed briefly. These topics will be discussed at greater length in later sections of the book.

Many muscles work in functional pairs (agonist-antagonist), with one contracting to open a joint (moving the attached bones apart) and the other contracting to close the same joint (moving the attached bones together). The biceps and triceps form a clear example of two such opposing muscles. Contraction of the biceps brings the wrist toward the shoulder, closing the elbow joint. Contraction of the triceps brings the wrist away from the shoulder, straightening the arm and opening the elbow joint. A more complex example is provided by the upper trapezius muscles, one function of which is to elevate the shoulders, and the latissimus dorsi muscles which, among other functions, pull the shoulders down.

Muscle tone is defined as the level of continual contraction while the muscle is at rest, meaning not actively contracting. In medical terminology, when a muscle has too much tone, and feels hard by palpation (examination through touch), it is said to be *hypertonic*. When a muscle has optimal tone, it is said to be *normotonic*. When a muscle has too little tone and feels somewhat limp, it is *hypotonic*. When a muscle has no tone, it is *atonic* (flaccid or limp). In AK, these same medical terms have slightly different meanings: A *normotonic* muscle tests strong and can be weakened by specific methods. A *hypertonic* muscle tests strong but cannot be weakened. The term *hypotonic* is found in the literature and refers to a weak-testing muscle.

A hypertonic muscle, by palpation, feels hard and usually muscle-tests very strong. Sheldon Deal (through the work of his patient, Richard Utt) was

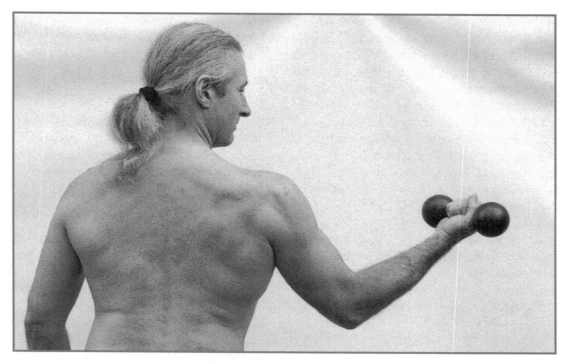

AGONIST-ANTAGONIST MUSCLE PAIRS:
BICEPS-TRICEPS, LATISSIMUS DORSI-UPPER TRAPEZIUS

the first in AK to present a term to define a muscle that tests strong but cannot, by usual means, be made to test weak. He called the state of such a muscle "frozen." Others describe this state as "hypertonic" or "over-facilitated." Referring to the results of muscle testing, Goodheart stated that the muscle is "weak" or "strong." He also mentioned the existence of *hypertonic* muscles once by stating that "strong"-testing muscles can test "too strong." Unfortunately,

Goodheart never deeply explored the state of muscles that test "too strong," nor were his terms "weak" and "strong" really accurate descriptions. And he never "laid down the law" by choosing the precise nomenclature to be used by all in AK. Therefore various AK authorities use different vocabulary for the same items, which can lead to confusion for those studying the AK literature.

For simplicity and clarity in this book, the terms

Weak-Testing	Normotonic	Hypertonic	Author
Schwach	Normoton	Hyperton	(Wolfgang Gerz)
Weak	Strong	Too Strong	(George Goodheart)
Under-Facilitated	Normal-Facilitated	Over-Facilitated	(Joe Schaffer)
Hyporeaktive	Normoreaktive	Hyperreaktive	(Hans Garten)
Unlocked	Locked	Blocked	(Richard Utt)
Flaccid	Homeostasis	Frozen	(Sheldon Deal)

used for the response of a muscle in muscle testing will be "weak-testing," "normotonic," and "hypertonic." The medical term hypertonic will be referred to in this text as "palpatory hypertonic," an accurate description of a medically hypertonic muscle. Goodheart's term "weak" will be rendered here as "weak-testing." Goodheart's terminology of a muscle testing "strong" as used so far in this text will be now further differentiated into "normotonic" and "hypertonic." The table shows the various terms used by various authorities for these three basic possible reactions of a muscle when tested.

It is interesting to note the similarity of the terminology that the medical doctor, F. X. Mayr (Austria), used in the 1920s in the diagnosis of the various states of the intestinal tract in problems of digestion. He used the terms *Hypoton, Normoton* and *Hyperton* to describe the muscle tone of the intestines.

MEDICAL DEFINITIONS

Muscle tone: the continual tension in a muscle that occurs without any conscious effort.

Hypotonic: the medical term for a muscle that has too little tone and is soft to the touch.

Palpatory Normotonic: the state in which a muscle has a normal amount of tone and feels firm but not hard when touched.

Palpatory Hypertonic: the state in which a muscle has too much tone, feels hard and often is painful when touched.

AK DEFINITIONS

The three responses of a muscle when tested:

1. Weak-Testing: The muscle cannot contract sufficiently to prevent the bones to which it is attached from moving during the muscle test.

2. Normotonic: The muscle can contract sufficiently to prevent the bones to which it is attached from moving during the muscle test. And the muscle can be weakened by standard methods such as TL to its sedation point.

3. Hypertonic: The muscle tests strong but cannot be weakened, e.g., by touching the appropriate sedation point.

Challenge: applying some stimulus and measuring the effect it has upon the results of muscle testing.

Therapy Localization or TL: This is a special form of challenge in which the patient touches himself or herself upon an area where some problem is suspected. The effect is assessed with muscle testing.

Active: A point upon the body is active when touching it (TL) changes the results of a muscle test.

Sedation Point: Precise locations on the body are used in acupuncture to drain energy away from a particular meridian. In AK, therapy localization of the sedation point should cause the muscle(s) related to this meridian to test weak.

History of Applied Kinesiology
(continued)

Early in his research, Goodheart noticed that the opponent (antagonist) to a weak-testing muscle was often painfully over-contracted (palpatory hypertonic). Strengthening the weak-testing muscle alone often caused the overly tight antagonist muscle to relax and become less painful. For example, it is common for the upper trapezius muscle, which lifts the shoulder toward the head, to be overly tight and painful. In such cases, its agonist partner (the latissimus dorsi, which pulls the shoulder down) usually tests weak. Strengthening the latissimus dorsi through the techniques used in Applied Kinesiology often causes the trapezius to relax, allowing the shoulder to drop and thus relieving pain. Pressing on the trapezius before and after the strengthening of the latissimus dorsi will reveal that softening of the muscle tissue of the upper trapezius has occurred as well. The patient will also typically report that after such treatment, digital (finger) pressure on the trapezius causes less pain.

An unopposed muscle is known to contract and

shorten. For example, a muscle that is torn away from one of its attachments no longer has opposition and, as a result, bunches up in a cramp. Knowing this mechanism, Goodheart deduced that lack of adequate muscle tone in one muscle (as revealed by muscle testing) is often the cause of overly tense (hypertonic) opposing (antagonist) muscles. Direct treatment to relax an overly tense antagonist muscle through massage, heat, or other means does not affect the weak-testing muscle, which soon causes its treated antagonist to tense up again. For this reason, the results of massage or other treatment directed solely toward an overly tight muscle are often temporary. It is interesting to note that when such treatment is successful, it is so by causing the overly tight antagonist to also test weak like its agonist partner. Thus such treatment results in two pathologic muscles instead of just one. This theme is discussed in greater detail in the section on nerve receptors (page 21).

While gathering data from his daily work with patients, Goodheart observed identical organ or gland problems in various patients who had the same muscle weakness. He then began to make a list associating specific muscles with specific organs and glands. The first correspondence he discovered was that patients with stomach problems often had a weak-testing pectoralis major clavicular muscle (see illustration on page 175), the upper part of the breast muscle that brings the arm up and in (cranial and medial). Furthermore, he found that treatment which made a weak-testing muscle test strong usually improved the health condition of the gland and organ associated with that muscle. These correspondences form an important portion of the diagnostic techniques of Applied Kinesiology. When a particular muscle tests weak, the examiner knows to check the corresponding gland and organ. When a gland or organ is malfunctioning, the examiner may use any existing weakness in the corresponding muscles to identify the causes and to indicate a proper treatment, i.e., a treatment that strengthens the muscle (makes it normotonic). More than one type of treatment may need to be determined and applied before the vari-

ous causes of the presenting problem are corrected.

In the 1930s Frank Chapman, an osteopath, developed a system of reflex point massage to increase the lymphatic drainage of particular organs and glands and to positively affect specific health problems. In Chapman's system, these points were diagnosed by palpation. Chapman believed that swelling and tenderness in these points indicated the need for massage to these points to increase the lymphatic drainage in the corresponding bodily areas, organs, and glands. Goodheart experimented with the Chapman reflexes and found that many of them were capable of strengthening weak-testing muscles. The reflex point that Goodheart found to strengthen a weak-testing pectoralis major clavicular muscle is Chapman's "emotional reflex." Goodheart, through his own research with muscle testing, had already observed a correlation between weakness in the pectoralis major clavicular and stomach problems. And it is well known that emotional problems often adversely affect the stomach. Inspired by this similar research finding, he began in 1965 to correlate the other Chapman reflexes with weaknesses in specific muscles. As Chapman's reflexes are all associated with organs and glands, these correlations helped Goodheart complete his growing list of the correspondences of specific muscles with specific organs and glands. In Applied Kinesiology, the Chapman reflexes are called the *neurolymphatic reflexes* (page 100).

Also in the 1930s, the chiropractor Terrence Bennett found that when he touched certain points upon the skin, the flow of blood to specific organs increased. This increased flow favorably affected one or more bodily functions. Excited by the possibilities of his discovery, Dr. Bennett spent hundreds of hours touching various points on patients' skin and scalp, while observing the reactions of their organs under an x-ray fluoroscope. Tragically, this is reported to have led to his death by radiation poisoning. Through experimentation, Goodheart found out which of Bennett's reflex points can strengthen weak-testing muscles. Bennett's reflex points and the organ associations that Goodheart confirmed and tabulated are known in Applied Kinesiology as the *neurovascular reflexes* (pages 107). The points lie mostly in the skin of the face and scalp.

In 1969, Goodheart explored the mechanics of cranial motion (movement of the bones of the skull) and experimented with methods to affect it. From his studies and experiments, he defined the Applied Kinesiology concepts of cranial motion. From this he developed effective techniques for the diagnosis and correction of misalignments of the cranial bones (cranial faults).

He found that correcting cranial faults did make some weak-testing muscles test strong. And he found a few cranial faults that almost always caused a specific muscle to test weak (for example, weak-testing abdominals with a sagittal suture fault—the only cranial fault correction technique included in the Touch for Health system). In these cases, correcting the cranial fault strengthened the associated muscle. But such specific correlations were the exception. Most individual cranial faults produced different weak-testing muscles in different patients. His cranial studies, though important therapeutically, did not add a new dimension to his growing set of muscle-organ/gland correspondences.

In 1970, Goodheart researched and detected a direct correspondence between the muscle-organ/gland associations from his own research and the meridian-organ/gland associations found in acupuncture. In the ancient Chinese system of acupuncture, a known correspondence exists between the meridians (upon which the acupuncture points lie) and the organs and glands. Meridians are believed in Chinese medicine to be channels for *Chi* energy, or life force. When the energy in a meridian is deficient, the corresponding organs and glands are weakened and may become diseased or otherwise dysfunctional. Goodheart found that techniques to correct specific meridian imbalances positively affected the organs and glands associated with the meridian in the acupuncture system. More of interest, balancing the energy of a meridian strengthened the various weak-testing muscles associated with the same glands and organs

(in his research) as the meridian is associated with in the acupuncture system. He also discovered that through strengthening weak-testing muscles, he could affect the meridians. Now he had a system of muscle-organ/gland-meridian relationships. This provided both a confirmation and a great extension of his own research results. In fact, in AK today, the fourteen main meridians of Chinese medicine provide the basis for defining the systems of regulation of all the structures and functions of the human body. (Acupuncture, meridians, acupuncture points and Chi are defined and further discussed on page 111).

In 1971, Goodheart presented his discovery of the correlation between muscles, organs, and glands with the meridian system of Eastern medicine. He determined that lack of sufficient energy in a meridian can be associated with both muscle weaknesses and disturbances in the functions of specific organs and glands.

However, an excess of energy in a meridian can also disturb the function of its corresponding organ and gland without causing the associated muscle to weaken. Indeed, in such a case, the muscle may test hypertonic. The correlation of meridians with muscles, organs, and glands led to more complete diagnostic measures in Applied Kinesiology, including methods that test the existence of excess energy in a meridian and its associated muscle.

Chemicals, including nutritional compounds, medicines, and pollutants, have also been correlated with the muscle, organ, gland, and meridian groupings. The compounds known to affect a specific organ generally affect the associated muscle as well. The nutrition that affects specific muscles is included in the section on muscle tests (pages 153–231).

The correlations of muscles with organs/glands, and meridians provide the therapist who uses AK a framework within which to systematically research the causes of any health problem. However, at times an organ will be improperly functioning, but the associated muscle will test strong. In the beginning of Applied Kinesiology, such cases threw doubt upon the correlation of muscles with organs and glands.

One cause of such incongruent test results is the existence of hypertonic muscles. In other cases, the body can compensate for a problem, strengthening weak-testing muscles and thus hiding these correlations. This compensation may make the muscle test normotonic, but the underlying problem remains. Applied Kinesiology techniques, such as therapy localization of the various reflex points can reveal hidden problems (see page 121). The correlations of muscles with organs/glands, and meridians have been confirmed in thousands of tests. Seeming exceptions, when studied with techniques for detecting hidden problems, have led to a broader understanding of how the body compensates for imbalances. Research with such hidden problems has turned seeming exceptions into confirmations of Goodheart's correspondences between muscles, organs/glands and meridians.

Through careful research, Goodheart demonstrated that the relative test strength of a muscle may reflect the influence or the condition of one or more of five main systems in the body. These are the *nervous, lymphatic, vascular, cerebrospinal fluid, and meridian systems*. All of these systems are represented in the spaces between each vertebrae on both sides of the spinal column (the intervertebral foramina). Passing through each "foramen" are nerves, lymph vessels, veins and arteries. In an experiment, radioactive tracing chemicals injected into the cerebrospinal fluid were later detected in the spinal nerves that pass through the foramina. This demonstrated that cerebrospinal fluid is also present in the foramina.

That the acupuncture "associated points" are located along each side of the vertebral column near the foramina is not coincidental and is for the therapist quite useful. These paired points have a connection with each of the meridians. When the energy in a meridian is out of balance, its associated point may become tender and swollen, and the muscles in the area may tighten inappropriately. This swelling and muscular tension may cause the neighboring vertebra to move out of its natural position (to subluxate). When a vertebra is out of position, the nerves that enter and exit above and below this vertebra may become mechanically irritated, causing extensive disturbance to the function of the organs innervated by these irritated nerves. The concept that active meridian associated points may cause vertebral lesions provides a model for understanding the interrelatedness of chiropractic and meridian theories. Stimulating the associated point will increase the function of the meridian-related organ. The associated points appear to be closely related in function to the neurolymphatic points that are located in the same area.

Since all five main systems of the body are present in the area of the foramina, they are referred to as *the five factors of the intervertebral foramen* or IVF. An understanding of these five factors is very important to the examiner using AK because most of the treatments used in Applied Kinesiology can be identified as belonging to one of the above five systems.

In AK, imbalances due to disturbances on any side of the triad of health (structural, chemical, or mental) are approached through the five systems. Thus it was a logical choice that the symbol of a man standing in a triangle (the triad of health) with five points balanced around him in a circle (the five factors of the IVF) has become the logo of Applied Kinesiology.

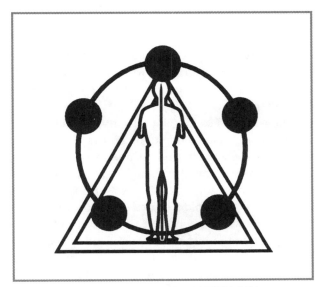

THE LOGO OF APPLIED KINESIOLOGY

Applied Kinesiology Today

In Applied Kinesiology, as in any science, phenomena are encountered for which no current explanation exists. But an attempt is always made to generate a hypothesis—a theory that if proved true would explain why a particular technique works. Such theories are very useful in that they generate new ideas and suggest new procedures to test. As knowledge grows, some of these theories must inevitably prove inaccurate and be discarded. Although disappointing to the originator, such discarding of a theory is no disgrace. Applied Kinesiology is a very young science. Theories underlying and attempting to explain its effectiveness will surely continue to evolve. To the extent that its procedures are successful in both diagnosing the underlying causes and locating effective treatments for many human difficulties, the techniques of AK will continue to grow in popularity and use, not only by chiropractors and medical doctors but also by many others involved in healing professions.

George Goodheart is to be honored for his outstandingly incisive powers of observation and deduction, and for his openness to the consideration of systems of healing that had not yet received official recognition. His pioneering contributions are an inspiration to those who continue research into this fascinating new field of Applied Kinesiology. Many follow in his footsteps, using Applied Kinesiology muscle testing to avidly experiment with both new methods and with procedures from a wide variety of the fields of healing.

In the late 1960s, Goodheart's first working group of twelve associates came to be known as the "dirty dozen." In 1974, the much-expanded group of mostly chiropractors founded the International College of Applied Kinesiology (ICAK). As various members suggested new techniques, criteria were developed to determine which techniques would be officially accepted into the ICAK system of Applied Kinesiology. In their deliberations, the group recognized that sometimes the practitioner of AK is dealing with very subtle energies; and that some practitioners can pro-

duce excellent therapeutic results with techniques that use these subtle energies and others cannot. It was decided that the only techniques to be officially accepted as ICAK techniques would be those that anyone with proper training could readily reproduce.

The ICAK meets twice each year. Diplomate members (health professionals who have taken the required training and passed all the ICAK exams) are expected to present new research. Their research reports are printed into large journals after each meeting (*The Collected Papers of the Members of the International College of Applied Kinesiology*). These journals (and Dr. Goodheart's prolific personal research writings) are only available to members. Furthermore, only chiropractors, psychologists and medical doctors may join the ICAK in America. It appears that the ICAK doesn't want to make its techniques available to anyone except members of ICAK. Most other professional organizations in the world have their research journals at every major library, but not the ICAK. Unfortunately, this reluctance to make their research journals generally available has resulted in many professionals concluding that AK is unscientific and not worthy of further consideration.

Although the journals are not generally available, two of the founding members have written monumental works, compiling the knowledge and accepted techniques of Applied Kinesiology. David Walther has performed a superhuman task of gathering most of the techniques of Applied Kinesiology into his series of books entitled *Applied Kinesiology*. Beginning with the basic concepts and describing in detail how to perform hundreds of the techniques known to Applied Kinesiology, his texts are likely the best source books for professionals who study and use AK, and they are generally available. However, some techniques are not described in enough detail to enable the student examiner to put them directly into practice. And a rather high level of prior knowledge of anatomy and physiology plus medical vocabulary is assumed. The most complete single book on Applied Kinesiology is Walther's *Applied Kinesiology Synopsis*.

David Leaf has produced an excellent workbook for the professional entitled *Applied Kinesiology Flowchart Manual*. However, this book assumes a more thorough understanding of the field than Walther's and is thus suited only for the therapist with extensive experience and understanding of AK.

The most complete work upon Applied Kinesiology currently available in the German language was written by Wolfgang Gerz, a German medical doctor who became so fascinated with Applied Kinesiology that he studied to became a diplomate of the International College of Applied Kinesiology. His own personal additions to the field plus his gatherings from the works of David Leaf and David Walther are to be found in his *Lehrbuch der Applied Kinesiology in der naturheilkundlichen Praxis*.

The book you are now reading was originally published in German and is often used for teaching the fundamentals of AK in German-speaking countries.

For detailed information about all references, see the bibliography.

AK in German-speaking countries is structured somewhat differently than in the U.S. Most state-recognized health professionals may join the ICAK-D, the German branch of the ICAK. In German-speaking countries, more medical doctors use AK than in all other countries combined. The ICAK-D and the IMAK (International Medical Society for AK), the ICAK group for medical doctors, publishes the *Medical Journal of Applied Kinesiology* which is generally available. Due to the efforts of the members of IMAK, Vienna (Zahnärztlicher Interressenverband Österreich-ZIV) has the first medical school program to formally include studies in Applied Kinesiology. Due to the efforts of ICAK-D and the IMAK, AK in German-speaking countries is being taught to and used by a great variety of health professionals.

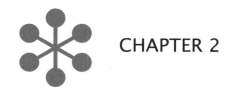 CHAPTER 2

Scientific Principles
of Applied Kinesiology

Anatomy and Physiology of the Muscles and Related Structures

Biology is the scientific study of life and living matter, including all of its forms and processes. *Anatomy* is a branch of biology that deals with the structure of organisms. *Physiology* is the branch of biology that deals with the functions and activities of living organisms and their parts such as organs, tissues, and cells. We will now consider in more detail the anatomy (the structures) and the physiology (the functions of these structures) involved in human movement.

Within each muscle is a huge number of tiny *contractile fibers* that contain filaments of the chemicals, actin and myosin. When the brain sends electrical signals through the *motor* (movement) *nerves* to the muscles, actin and myosin filaments slide together, shortening the muscle. This is the mechanism of muscular contraction. *Muscles* merge into strong connective-tissue *tendons* before attaching to *bones*. Tendon-like tissues that connect bones directly to bones are called *ligaments*. Ligaments are relatively unstretchable and thereby provide structural stability to joints. The shortening (contraction) of a muscle pulls upon the bones to which the muscle is attached at each end. In most cases, there is a joint (articulation) between the two bones to which the two ends of the muscle attach. Stabilization of the bones by muscular tension creates posture, the ability to hold a body position. Muscular contraction moves a bone

with respect to the adjoining bone around the joint connecting them. This is the basic mechanism of human movement. Representing the muscles as springs, the bones as levers, and the joints as fulcrums gives us an approximate model of the action of muscles.

There are *two types of muscle fibers*, the slow contracting and the fast contracting. These are also known as "slow twitch" and "fast twitch" fibers. Both types of fibers utilize a chemical substance, ATP (adenosine triphosphate), as their direct energy source. The splitting of ATP releases the energy used in muscular contraction. There is only a limited amount of ATP within muscles. When it is split, it must be quickly resynthesized to support further contraction of the muscle. The energy for this synthesis is won for the slow fibers from the oxidation of sugar and fat, and for the fast fibers by the splitting of sugar in the absence of oxygen.

The *slow fibers* are capable of long periods of contraction and thus provide endurance. They are found in the highest ratio in "tonic" or postural muscles, which must work for long periods of time without pause. They have a high concentration of myoglobin (muscle hemoglobin), which supplies them with the oxygen needed *(aerobic)* for their long-continuing contractions. The red-colored myoglobin has a six times greater affinity for oxygen than the hemoglobin (which carries the oxygen in the blood). So it is easy for the myoglobin to take the oxygen from the hemoglobin. It is the presence of oxygen-bearing myoglobin which gives the slow fibers their red color. The slow fibers utilize sugar (glucose) for fuel and can completely oxidize it to carbon dioxide and water. Twenty times more ATP is produced by the oxidation of glucose in the slow fibers than by the splitting of glucose in the fast fibers. The slow fibers can also use fatty acids for their fuel.

Fast fibers contain little or no myoglobin and are therefore white in color. They are thicker than the red slow fibers. They don't require oxygen *(anaerobic)*. The end product of the anaerobic splitting of glucose is lactic acid. When muscles contract strongly, lactic acid builds up in the muscle, and the muscle becomes more acidic, it hurts, and it fatigues (gradually fails to further contract). In order to dilute the lactic acid, extra water is retained in the muscle, which produces the swollen, "full" feeling of muscles after strong exercise.

To "refresh" the tired muscle and prepare it for further contraction, the lactic acid needs to be absorbed into the capillaries and carried out of the muscle through the veins. All activities that increase the circulation, including massage, hot baths, and gentle exercise of the same muscles the next day, can speed this process of elimination of lactic acid from fatigued muscles. Ice is often applied for a maximum of fifteen minutes to reduce the pain of sore muscles. Ice, while applied, reduces the circulation in a muscle. However, after the ice is removed, the circulation increases strongly and remains so for an extended period of time. For this reason, the application of ice is an excellent way to increase the circulation in selected areas of the body.

Since fast fibers use glucose much less efficiently than slow fibers, fast fibers run out of fuel and fatigue more quickly. However, the rate of contraction of fast fibers may be ten times faster than that of slow fibers. "Phasic" muscles which are required to contract quickly and precisely, such as the muscles that move the eyes (extraocular muscles), have a high ratio of fast fibers.

Every muscle has both fast and slow fibers. As would be expected, those having a higher ratio of slow fibers are more red in color. As an example, the lifestyle of the chicken requires it to make only occasional bursts of flight. Thus, its pectoralis muscles (the breast muscles used in flying) are white. The same muscles are dark red in a duck, which is typically "on the wing" for longer periods of time. Postural muscles (those that must work without pause) contain a higher percentage of slow fibers, giving them their ability to sustain continued contraction for long periods of time without tiring.

At birth, the rate of contraction of every muscle fiber is identical. In response to the type of nerve signal a muscle receives, it develops a greater ratio of either fast or slow fibers. This development consists of both the transformation of the muscle fibers present at birth and the creation of new muscle fibers. The basic pattern of nerve signaling to a muscle, and thus the resultant ratio of fibers developed, appears to be determined genetically. For decades, the Russians and Scandinavians have analyzed the ratio of red and white fibers in muscle samples from young potential athletes to determine the types of sports in which they are genetically predisposed to succeed. If there are proportionally more white fast fibers, they are guided to train for short "burst of energy" events like sprinting. If they have more slow red fibers, they train for endurance activities like the 5,000-meter dash. As a result of these techniques, many youths have been guided into sports in which they indeed become world class athletes.

Although the proportion of muscle fibers is partially determined by genetic predisposition, the ratio of fast and slow fibers is also adjusted by a change of use. Even in the adult, new requirements upon the muscle may change the proportion of fast and slow fibers. If incorrect posture places constant strain upon a muscle that is rich in fast fibers, some of the fast fibers will be transformed into slow fibers. Walking with a cast upon one leg, or limping to avoid pain, will place greater than normal stresses upon the muscles used. As this imbalanced use continues, the concentration of fast and slow fibers in the over-stressed muscles may be altered. This change of muscle fiber concentration may result in continuing patterns of misuse, even after the injury is healed.

If through athletic training, a muscle is called upon to make short bursts of intense activity, many slow fibers will be transformed into fast fibers. For example, the calf muscles of a sprinter develop a greater ratio of fast fibers. This principle of changing the ratio of muscle fibers is important in considering the effects (upon the muscles themselves) of faulty posture and use, or of specific activities required in work or sports.

The names of the two ends of a muscle (the origin and the insertion) are functionally defined. The *origin* of a muscle is attached (through its tendon) to the bone that does not move when the muscle contracts. The *insertion* of a muscle is attached to the bone that is moved toward the origin. So when a muscle contracts, its insertion moves toward its origin.

In some cases, either end of the muscle may be correctly called the origin, depending upon the activity of the muscle. For example, when the rectus femoris (one of the quadriceps, the four-headed muscle on the front of the thigh) lifts the leg (flexes the thigh on the hip), its origin is on the hip, which is stable in this motion. When the thigh is stabilized and the rectus femoris causes the body to bend forward (flexing the hip on the thigh), the hip attachment is its insertion, and its attachment to the knee becomes the origin.

At any one time, a muscle may have one of four functionally defined roles. It may be the main muscle involved in a movement *(prime mover or agonist)*. It may work with another muscle *(synergist)*, against a muscle *(antagonist)*, or hold bones in position to make other movements possible *(stabilizer)*.

Muscles contract in response to electrical signals sent through nerves from the central nervous system. Some active muscle contractions (such as the muscles used in walking and talking) are initiated by conscious decision and will. Other active muscle contractions, such as those of the stomach and intestines in the process of digestion, are effected by the central nervous system without any conscious involvement. Muscles also have a passive level of continuous contraction called *muscle tone.* As already mentioned, a *hypertonic* muscle has too much tone. A *hypotonic* muscle has too little tone. A *flaccid* muscle has very little or no tone at all. It is the balance of tone among groups of muscles pulling upon their bones throughout the body which creates posture and structural balance. When the level of tone in some muscles is too high (hypertonic) or too low (hypotonic), the structure of the body will become imbalanced, creating poor posture, malfunction of organs, and even mental problems. The level of tone in a muscle, its synergists, stabilizers, and antagonists is controlled, adjusted, and fine-tuned mainly by the activity of the nerve receptors within the muscle.

NEUROPHYSIOLOGY: THE NERVOUS SYSTEM

Of necessity, the following description of the brain and nervous system will be superficial and simplistic. There is not enough space in this book to do more than name the basic structures and define some of their functions. Only the aspects that concern the muscles will be considered in any depth.

The main organ of the nervous system is *the brain*. More complex than the most advanced computers in existence, the brain is beyond our ability to understand it. This is logical. After all, if the brain were simple enough for us to understand, we (who use the brain to think with) would not be intelligent enough to understand it. The brain's three distinct divisions have a structural relationship to the story of the evolution of all vertebrates (animals with a spinal column). Starting at the base of the skull where it meets the vertebral column and moving forward, we have the hindbrain (rhombencephalon), midbrain (mesencephalon), and forebrain (prosencephalon).

The most ancient evolutionary structure of the brain is the *hindbrain* which consists of the medulla oblongata, the pons and the cerebellum. These three together are often referred to collectively as the "brainstem." The *medulla oblongata* connects the rest of the brain with the spinal cord through a hole at the base of the skull. The medulla controls the rate of breathing, the rapidity of the heartbeat, and the blood pressure. Immediately above the medulla, the brainstem enlarges to form the pons and then continues onward as the midbrain. The *pons* is the signal bridge between the medulla and the middle brain. The neurotransmitter dopamine is produced in the middle brain. Dopamine has a direct effect upon muscle tone. In the absence of sufficient dopamine, various symptoms and syndromes may emerge including muscle spasticity, tremors and even psychic disturbances such as found in Parkinson's disease.

Wrapped around the brainstem and filling the back bottom of the cranium is the *cerebellum*. The cerebellum is largest part of the hindbrain and the second-largest part of the brain. It controls the coordination of body movements and muscle tone. The input to the cerebellum comes mainly from the muscle, tendon and joint receptors, the eyes, skin and labyrinthine of the inner ear. All this information about the position of the limbs and posture of the body is integrated within the cerebellum. Messages from the cerebral cortex can override and change the action of the cerebellum. Impulses, influenced by the cerebral cortex, are generated in the cerebellum and from there travel via the spinal cord to the muscles to maintain or change the positioning and posture of the body.

The *forebrain* is the most massive and recently evolved portion of the brain. It consists of two parts, the interbrain (diencephalon) and the cerebrum (telencephalon). The interbrain (often called the *midbrain*) includes the thalamus, hypothalamus and pineal gland plus the nerves connecting these to the cerebrum. The cerebrum consists of the two massive cerebral hemispheres, which are connected by a massive nerve bundle called the corpus callosum. A cross-section of the cerebrum reveals the thick grey *cerebral cortex* of nerve cells surrounding a white core of nerve fibers. All mental pictures and the patterns of bodily movement are stored within the cerebrum. The cerebrum gathers and processes the reports of sensory impressions (sight, sound, touch, etc.) and is the center of memory. Conscious thought and awareness appear to occur here. Today, the differing concepts of the functions of these "two halves of the brain" are the basis for much research and discussion in various medical and non-medical disciplines, including psychology.

Located in the interbrain (diencephalon) are the most important control centers for unconscious body function, the thalamus and the hypothalamus. The *thalamus* receives and transmits incoming nerve signals from the body and between most parts of the brain. Information from the cerebellum is processed in the thalamus, where it is prepared for becoming conscious. For this reason, the thalamus is called the "door of consciousness." It integrates the functions of the brain and is involved with drive, emotion, personality, and with the perception and interpretation of pain.

The *hypothalamus* is the main director of the autonomic nervous system which directs all the functions like digestion, secretion, metabolism, etc., that are not normally under the control of the will. The hypothalamus also controls instinctive responses like hunger, thirst, sex and self-preservation. The hypothalamus is located above and controls the functions of the pituitary gland, the "master gland" of the body. Indeed, directly or indirectly through controlling the pituitary, the hypothalamus controls all of the endocrine glands.

The brain and the spinal cord together form the *central nervous system* of the body. Attached to the base of the cranium is the spine or backbone, the vertebral column, consisting of a group of twenty-four separate bones (vertebrae) stacked vertically, one on top of another. Under these twenty-four are the sacrum and the coccyx (the tailbone), which form the lower end of the vertebral column. The vertebral column has a vertical hole passing through each vertebra, combining to form a tube. Passing from the hindbrain through and protected by this long tube is the *spinal cord,* the largest bundle of nerves in the body with the exception of the brain itself.

The central nervous system has two main jobs. The first one is to maintain structural integrity by keeping the internal environment of the body at a homeostasis, that is, at a constant level of temperature, pressure, balance of chemistry, etc. Its second job is to direct the body to respond (adapt) to the changing external environment.

Most of the physiological processes of the body are under the control of the central nervous system.

Many occur without any conscious awareness. The central nervous system has two main routes of communication with and control over the rest of the body: chemical and electrical.

Glands are organs that produce, store and release chemicals that produce an effect upon the physiology of the body. *Exocrine glands* deliver their produced chemicals (sweat, lubricating oils, odor producing chemicals, etc.) onto the inner or outer skin of the body (mucous membranes, intestinal lining, outer skin). *Endocrine glands* produce chemicals called hormones, released directly into the bloodstream. Chemical communication is effected by the central nervous system through the control of the release of those hormones into the bloodstream.

The hypothalamus produces two hormones, oxytocin and vasopressin (the anti-diuretic hormone, ADH). These are excreted from the posterior portion of the hypothalamus into the bloodstream. Oxytocin causes contraction of the musculature of the uterus in the birth process. When the uterus is producing adequate contractions, a nerve signal goes back to the hypothalamus, causing the release of oxytocin to cease. The suckling of the baby on the breast sends a nerve signal to the hypothalamus to produce more oxytocin, which also causes the contraction of the milk-producing glands and consequent excretion of milk from the breast.

Vasopressin, or ADH, has an effect upon the kidneys, which filter wastes out of the blood and deliver this "urine" to the bladder. Vasopressin causes the kidneys to reabsorb water, making urine more concentrated. This process conserves bodily water when water intake is low and/or loss through perspiration is high. In higher concentrations than required to affect the kidneys, vasopressin stimulates the contraction of the musculature around arteries and veins, which raises the blood pressure.

The *pituitary* gland is located behind the nose in a depression of the sphenoid bone above the roof of the mouth. This depression is referred to as the "Turkish saddle" because of its shape. In the Eastern mystical traditions, the pituitary is associated in location and function with the "third eye." It is the "opening of the third eye" which is supposed to proffer the supersensory ability to see, hear, feel and otherwise sense at a distance. These functions are called clairvoyance, clairaudience and clairsentience. In many countries, police use such "seers" to locate missing persons. A scientific explanation for these abilities does not yet exist.

Notwithstanding the metaphysical phenomena described above, the pituitary is considered to be the most important gland in the body and is often referred to as the "master gland." The posterior part of the pituitary consists mainly of nerve tissues. The anterior part consists of endocrine tissue that secretes at least ten different hormones into the bloodstream. It is the excretion of these pituitary hormones into the bloodstream which chemically signals the other glands to act. This is the most important function of the pituitary known to science today. It is likely that the pituitary gland and the hypothalamus which controls it have still more differentiated functions not yet elucidated by science.

Through the hypothalamus, the central nervous system controls the pituitary which, in turn, controls all other endocrine glands of the body. As the integrator of the functions of the endocrine and nervous systems, the hypothalamus has a central role in the control of the body's physiological functions.

Endocrine glands exist in the head, the neck and the trunk of the body. They include the thyroid, parathyroid, thymus, pancreas, ovaries, testes and adrenals. As noted above, release of their various hormones is controlled primarily by the prior release of hormones from the pituitary gland. Other organs such as the liver, lungs, kidneys and heart also produce hormones, though only in very small quantities.

Although some glands are controlled by nerves, the level of secretion of the various endocrine glands in general is *"feedback controlled."* For example, when the hypothalamus detects that the amount of estrogen in a woman's blood is not sufficient, it sends its estrogen "releasing hormone" (RH) directly to the pituitary gland. This transport occurs along the nerves that connect the hypothalamus and the pituitary. As a result, the pituitary releases its follicle stimulating hormone (FSH) into the bloodstream. When the follicle stimulating hormone reaches the ovaries, it stimulates them to produce and release estrogen into the blood. When the hypothalamus detects that the estrogen circulating in the blood has reached the desired level, it stops sending its releasing hormone. As a result, the pituitary stops producing FSH and the ovaries stop producing and releasing estrogen.

Hormone control is slow and is thus suited for body functions that occur slowly such as the menstrual cycle. The other main type of communication within the central nervous system (CNS) and between the CNS and the rest of the body is electrical. Electrical impulses travel along nerves from the muscles, skin, inner organs and glands to the CNS. The CNS processes these signals and generates new signals that return to the organs. In the next example, the CNS sends nerve signals to the adrenal glands much more rapidly than hormones could arrive there. In comparison with communication via hormones, "neural signaling" is much faster and more specific.

Situations such as the "fight or flight" reaction require an immediate release of hormones. More so in the distant past than now, an immediate reaction could mean the difference between life and death. In such situations, survival may depend upon the speed with which the body can prepare to "fight for its life" or "flee to save itself." The hormone adrenaline from the adrenal glands is needed for the body to swiftly prepare for such action. However, in a situation of danger, a chemical signal via the bloodstream to the adrenal glands to start producing and releasing adrenaline would be too slow. The adrenal glands can be activated by chemicals in the blood, including hormones. But they are more swiftly stimulated to release their hormones (particularly adrenaline) by electrical stimulation via the nerves.

Adrenaline in the blood causes many generalized effects throughout the body. Organs required for the fight or flight reaction experience increased blood circulation and increased activity. Organs not required receive less blood and slow their rate of activity. Thus adrenaline causes constriction of superficial capillaries, causing the skin to pale. Pupil dilation is increased

to let in more light. The heartbeat and respiration are increased. A generalized increase of the circulation and tension of all the voluntary muscles prepares the body for dynamic muscular activity. The activity of non-voluntary muscles such as those that move food through the intestines is reduced. Although some hormones have a specific effect upon only one particular gland, other hormones like adrenaline have a very general and widespread effect.

Nerve cells *(neurons)* consist of a cell body containing the nucleus and various long, thin extensions. Many short extending fibers called *dendrites* transmit impulses into the nerve cell body. One long extending fiber called the *axon* or nerve fiber transmits impulses out of the nerve cell body. The axon of one nerve meets and stimulates dendrites of other nerves or acts directly upon other kinds of cells.

Nerves are not directly connected with one another. Where an axon meets dendrites is a fluid-filled cavity called a *synapse*. When the electrical impulse from an axon meets the synapse, it causes a chemical reaction in the synapse. If the incoming impulse is strong enough, the chemical reaction in the synapse usually causes the next nerve to "fire," carrying the new electrical signal onward. However, when the same nerve circuit fires through the same synapse many times, the fluids in the synapse become exhausted. When that happens, the incoming nerve signal can no longer stimulate the following nerve to fire. The result is that the signal dies at the exhausted synapse.

We have all experienced mental exhaustion when we "just can't get our thoughts together." This statement is quite literally true on a neural level. We start a thought, but since the synaptic fluid is exhausted, the signal dissipates. The result in this case is that we forget what we were thinking. The underlying cause of this "forgetting" due to exhausted synapses is often a deficit of B vitamins, which are the main "precursors" of the synaptic fluids. A precursor is a chemical the body uses to make some other chemical that it needs. The body can store great amounts of B12 but can only partially store the other B vitamins, uses them up quickly under any kind of stress, and requires a new supply daily. When we take a good supply of B vitamins (which should be taken together with vitamin C), the synaptic fluids are renewed and mental exhaustion quickly disappears. As long as one has no sensitivity to yeast, a mixture of orange juice, some vitamin C powder, plus a few spoonfuls of brewer's yeast will supply the C and B vitamins needed. About twenty to thirty minutes after drinking this brew, the synaptic fluids will be renewed, mental exhaustion will disappear, and one will be mentally refreshed.

As mentioned, the largest nerve bundle in the body outside the brain is the spinal cord. When the spinal cord is transected (horizontally severed) and the cut surface observed, a white substance with the shape of a butterfly is seen embedded in a grey substance. The two "butterfly wings" that extend anteriorly are called the *ventral horns*. The two that extend posteriorly are called the *dorsal horns*. All of the outgoing motor or *efferent nerves* emerge from the ventral horns of the spinal cord. All of the incoming sensory or *afferent nerves* go into the dorsal horns. "Sensory" as used here does not refer to conscious awareness, only to the fact that the nervous system receives a signal. The white substance consists of the nerves that carry signals vertically through the spinal cord. These nerves connect various segments of the spinal cord and carry signals to and from the brain.

On both the right and the left side of two adjacent vertebrae in one "segment" of the spinal cord, an incoming (afferent) nerve brings sensory information from specific muscles and other organs to the central nervous system. From the same segment emerges an outgoing (efferent) nerve that directs the function of the same muscles and organs. The related bodily region is also referred to as a segment. The name of the segment, for example C7, in determined according to the location of the nerves entering into and emerging from the vertebral column. In our example, the nerves emerge and enter between the seventh cervical (neck) vertebra (C7) and the first thoracic (trunk) vertebra (T1).

The ventral side of the vertebral column is less exposed and more protected from injury than the dorsal side. Since the motor nerves emerge from the ventral side of the spinal cord, it would appear that evolution has given the motor nerves a higher priority for protection than the sensory nerves. Perhaps survival is better served by giving a higher priority to the brain and spinal cord being able to send the correct nerve signals out to the body than the ability to sense the incoming signals. Before the efferent and afferent nerves emerge from the "intervertebral" spaces and connect with the body, they join together into one paired nerve.

The speed of signals through nerves is very rapid. However, every synapse through which the signal must pass slows the overall speed significantly. Thus the overall speed of a nervous signal is determined by how far the signal must travel through the nerve(s) and the number of synapses through which it must pass. Some reactions must occur so fast that a pathway via the brain would be too slow. These kinds of signals, which take place between the body and the spinal cord and within the spinal cord itself with no involvement of the brain whatsoever, and the muscular reactions they produce are called *reflexes*. In simple reflexes such as the knee-jerk, the afferent (sensory) nerve from the knee tendon meets and stimulates, in one single synapse in the spinal cord, the efferent (motor) nerve that signals the rectus femoris muscle (page 196) to contract, causing the leg to swiftly extend. For a more complete description of the knee reflex, see page 24. Because the total distance traversed by the efferent and afferent nerves is short and because there is only one "interneuronal" synapse, such reflex reactions can occur very swiftly, possibly saving us from (further) injury.

THE NERVE RECEPTORS

As described in the last chapter, efferent nerves originate in the central nervous system and transmit signals to other parts of the central nervous system (CNS) and the body. The afferent nerves are stimulated by various types of nerve receptors to send signals into the CNS.

Mechanical receptors *(mechanoreceptors)* gather information about outside mechanical forces acting upon the body (sound, pressure, touch, movement, and gravity) and transmit this information to the central nervous system. The cochlea in the ear contains mechanoreceptors that transform external sound vibrations striking the eardrum into auditory nerve signals for the function of hearing. The brain uses input from receptors within the eye to orient the head upright (visual righting reflexes). The cochlea and visual receptors both respond to stimuli (light and sound) produced outside the organism.

Proprioceptors are a large group of nerve receptors that respond to stimuli produced within the organism. The central nervous system (mainly the cerebellum) compares signals from all types of proprioceptors to assess and regulate body integrity, movement, and positioning. There are three main groups of proprioceptors: ligament, joint, and skin proprioceptors; the neck and labyrinthine proprioceptors; and muscle proprioceptors. All measure the tensions acting upon body parts (through posture, motion, and acceleration) and produce correcting effects upon the function of the muscles.

The three main groups of proprioceptors are:

1. The proprioceptors in the ligaments, joints, and skin (Ruffini's end organs, Pacinian corpuscles, and free nerve endings)

These will not be discussed in this text.

2. The proprioceptors in the neck and the labyrinthine

The neck (especially the small muscles of the neck) contains an extremely high concentration of proprioceptors that are responsible for righting the head upon the neck and the neck upon the body. The labyrinthine is an organ within the inner ear that is responsible for the sense of equilibrium. It consists of a very compact hollow bone (the petrous bone) within which are the sensory organs of hearing and equilibrium. The labyrinthine is filled with a special lymph fluid. In its center is the vestibule, which contains the foramen ovale, a "window" in the hollow bone of the labyrinthine. The mechanical impulses that sound produces upon the eardrum are transmitted to the labyrinthine fluid through this window. As a result, the fluid moves through the vestibule into one end of the labyrinthine called the cochlea, which is shaped like a snail shell. In the cochlea, the moving fluid compresses sensitive cells that generate nerve signals. These nerve signals are transmitted to the brain. The processing of these signals in the brain results in the subjective awareness of sound.

At the other end of the labyrinthine are three semicircular canals, one oriented in each of the three dimensions. Like the whole of the labyrinthine, the semicircular canals are filled with lymph fluid. At the end of each one is an ampulla, a spherical cavity containing a fluid-filled sack lined with specialized hair cells. Nerves attached to these hairs measure the movement of the lymph fluid in the canals and thereby signal the nervous system as to the position and motion of the head in all three dimensions.

3. Muscle proprioceptors

Muscles perform two kinds of work: The active work of muscles is called *contraction*, which produces movement of the bodily parts. The passive work of muscles is called *muscle tone*, which is the state of tension in a muscle when it is at rest. Muscle tone is produced by the gamma motor neurons described in detail below.

The proprioceptors most involved with the work of muscles are the neuromuscular spindle cell receptors and the Golgi tendon organs. These muscle proprioceptors act directly upon human posture and movement. Neuromuscular spindle cell receptors monitor the *length* of a muscle. Golgi tendon organs monitor the *tension* in a muscle.

Neuromuscular Spindle Cells

Throughout the muscle, but concentrated in its "belly," are *neuromuscular spindle cells*. A neuromuscular spindle is 2–20 mm in length and is enclosed in a fluid-filled sheath of connective tissue. Within are 3–10 thin *intrafusal muscle fibers*. These lie parallel to the much larger *extrafusal muscle fibers* located outside the sheath. The extrafusal fibers make up the bulk of a muscle and are responsible for the

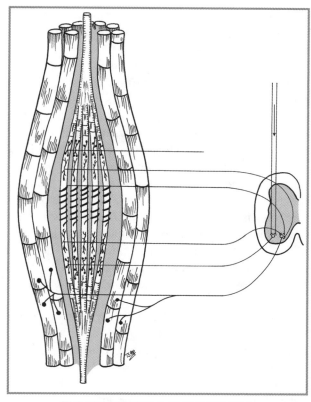

THE NEUROMUSCULAR SPINDLE CELL

The signal that a nerve conducts cannot be stronger or weaker. The nerve impulse always has the same strength. The intensity of a nerve signal is determined by how often the nerve "fires" per second.

Alpha motor neurons have their origin in the ventral horn of the gray matter of the spinal cord. When a nerve signal from type Ia afferent nerves reaches the spinal cord, the response returns to the muscle along the alpha motor neurons. There are two types of alpha motor neurons. "Tonic" alpha motor neurons innervate postural muscles that are active for extended periods of time. "Phasic" alpha motor neurons innervate phasic muscles that only contract for short periods of time. About 70% of the motor neurons going to the muscles are alpha motor neurons. These innervate the thick extrafusal muscle fibers that are responsible for the force of muscular contraction. The remaining 30% are the *gamma motor neurons*, which innervate the intrafusal muscle fibers. The intrafusal muscle fibers do not contribute to the strength of muscular contraction. Instead, gamma stimulation causes contraction of the intrafusal muscle fibers, which stretch the neuromuscular spindle. This process produces fine motor control, not raw force. The nerve impulses traveling through gamma motor neurons to the intrafusal muscle fibers originate in the cerebellum.

At each end of the neuromuscular spindle, the intrafusal muscle fibers attach to the muscle sheath and are thereby automatically lengthened or shortened with the rest of the muscle. In the middle of each intrafusal fiber is an area with no actin and myosin, which therefore does not contract. So when the gamma motor neurons stimulate the intrafusal muscle fibers to contract, the intrafusal muscle fibers pull toward each end and thus lengthen the central portion upon which the Ia nerve receptor fibers are wound.

Ia nerves are afferent nerves. They and their nerve receptors are called "primary" to distinguish them from the finer type II nerves. The primary Ia receptors of neuromuscular spindle cells are always sending signals into the spinal cord. When the central portion is

strength of contraction. Spiraling around the central portion of the intrafusal fibers are the neuromuscular spindle cell receptors. These stretch-sensing nerve receptors send their messages along the "primary" *type Ia afferent nerves* to the central nervous system. The efferent nerves that send the response of the CNS back to the muscle are the *alpha motor neurons* and *gamma motor neurons*.

As stated above, a neuron is one complete nerve cell. It consists of:

1. the cell body with its nucleus;

2. a long extension called the axon or nerve fiber;

3. many short branching extensions (dendrites) that connect the nerve via synapses with nerve receptors or other nerves, and

4. the synapse.

stretched, the output from the "primary" receptors is increased. Type Ia nerves are thick and the nerve signals travel through them swiftly. When the receptor area between the contractile portions of the intrafusal fibers is suddenly lengthened, it sends an especially intense signal (high number of nerve firings per second) through its type Ia nerves to the dorsal horn of the spinal cord. Only one synapse in the spinal cord needs to be stimulated before the speedy "monosynaptic" response is sent back to the same muscle to contract. This is the basis of reflex reactions such as the knee-jerk reflex. This type of response is called "monophasic" because it occurs once and immediately stops.

"Secondary" *type II afferent nerves* connect directly into the contractile portions of the intrafusal muscle fibers. Type II nerves are slender and slower than type Ia nerves. They are responsible for the second type of neuromuscular spindle response which, when stimulated, causes the muscle to raise its tension slowly and remain in a state of elevated tonus.

During the muscle test or any weight-bearing activity, there is both alpha and gamma efferent stimulation to the muscle. Alpha stimulation of the extrafusal fibers produces the force of contraction. Gamma stimulation of the intrafusal fibers stretches the central receptor area of the neuromuscular spindle cell. The receptor, which is always sending impulses, then sends a greater than normal impulse into the spinal cord and cerebellum. This is, in effect, an order for greater contraction in the muscle to meet the current demand. This results in a greater nerve signal being sent back through the alpha motor nerves to the extrafusal fibers of the muscle, increasing the force of contraction.

The neuromuscular spindle cells are responsible for signaling the nervous system to increase the tension in a muscle that is lacking adequate tone. As the examiner applies more force in the muscle test, the patient's neuromuscular spindle cells monitor the amount of force applied and signal the nervous system to produce the appropriate intensity of alpha nerve signal to contract the muscle enough to hold the limb

or other body part in position. Thus if the neuromuscular spindle cells in a muscle are not sending an adequate signal, the muscle will test weak.

The activity of the neuromuscular spindle cells excites its own muscle to contract. It further facilitates contraction of the muscle's synergists and its stabilizers. At the same time, the antagonists to the muscle are inhibited. As mentioned, the reflex excitation of the muscle itself occurs swiftly because only one single synapse in the spinal cord must be traversed between the neuromuscular spindle cell and the extrafusal muscles that provide the force of contraction. This allows the body to protect itself by very quickly jerking away from potentially damaging stimuli. The neural circuits that facilitate the synergists and stabilizers, and those that inhibit the antagonists, each have two synapses in the spinal cord to traverse and thus are somewhat slower.

It is the coupled activity of the alpha and gamma nerves in the neuromuscular spindle cells that makes muscular contraction smooth and coordinated. Postural or "tonic" muscles typically hold relatively high levels of tone for long periods of time. Such muscles have a high proportion of slow tonic fibers. The activity of such muscles does not require fine coordination. Therefore, tonic muscles have few neuromuscular spindle cells. "Phasic" muscles have a higher proportion of fast "phasic" fibers and far more neuromuscular spindle cells to provide for their faster, more intricate, finely coordinated movements.

Normally, the neuromuscular spindle cells continuously send signals to the nervous system concerning the length of the muscle. The length of a muscle may be manually adjusted by manipulation of the neuromuscular spindle cells. Pushing or pinching the neuromuscular spindle cells together (parallel to the length of the muscle) reduces the tension on the intrafusal muscle fibers. They then send signals of less intensity than normal through their Ia afferent nerves to the spinal cord. This temporarily reduces the level of alpha efferent nerve signaling, which results in less tension in the extrafusal fibers responsible for muscle strength. Thus, pinching the spindle cells together will

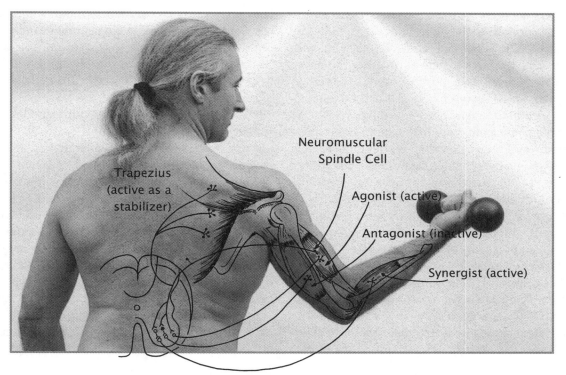

INHIBITION AND FACILITATION OF MUSCULAR CONTRACTION
THROUGH THE ACTIVITY OF THE NEUROMUSCULAR SPINDLE CELLS

cause a muscle to temporarily test weak. This may be used to determine whether a muscle is responding correctly (tests normotonic, see page 82).

Stretching and activating the neuromuscular spindle cells by pushing the two hands or fingers into the belly of a muscle and pulling apart stretches the intrafusal fibers, increasing their output to the spinal cord. As a result, more nerve impulses per second are sent through the alpha efferent nerves to the extrafusal fibers of the muscles, which then contract more strongly. Thus, pulling the neuromuscular cells apart increases the tension in a muscle.

It is believed that trauma, extreme contraction or stretching, or stretching performed too rapidly may cause the neuromuscular spindle cell to continuously send an impulse of inappropriate strength into the spinal cord. As a result, the muscle, its synergists, stabilizers and antagonists will all have inappropri-

ate levels of tension. This may disturb the posture, causing other muscles to contract in excess of their normal levels in order to support the incorrect posture. Their excess contraction will improperly inhibit their antagonists, etc. This chain of adaptations to an incorrectly functioning neuromuscular spindle cell is a common cause of neurological disorganization (page 84).

When a muscle (the agonist) acts, the action of its neuromuscular spindle cells causes its antagonist to be inhibited. When the antagonist to a muscle acts, the agonist is inhibited. This principle is call "reciprocal inhibition." Were both the agonist and antagonist to act simultaneously, they would be fighting against each other, which would be a waste of energy. Also, the two bones in the joint over which the two muscles act would be jammed together. Reciprocal inhibition occurs automatically at the level of the spinal cord where the synapses meet between the afferent nerve from the neuromuscular spindle cell and the efferent nerve that returns to the antagonist. However, higher brain centers can override this effect. A conscious decision can be made in the cerebral cortex to flex whole groups of agonists and their antagonists simultaneously. This is conveyed to the cerebellum and from there to the appropriate spinal segments and then on to the muscles. This is what occurs when a bodybuilder flexes most of his or her muscles at once to make an impressive pose.

It is normal that *while* a muscle is active, its antagonists are inhibited. An incorrectly functioning neuromuscular spindle cell may send impulses so overly strong that any activity of the muscle causes its antagonist(s) to *subsequently* test weak, even after the agonist has relaxed. This condition is called "reactive muscles." For a full discussion of this condition and its treatment, see page 131.

A dysfunctioning neuromuscular spindle cell will usually therapy-localize (TL). That is, if the muscle tests weak because of dysfunction of the neuromuscular spindle cell, touching the neuromuscular spindle cell will cause the muscle to test strong. Conversely, just about any normotonic indicator muscle will weaken when a dysfunctioning neuromuscular spindle cell is therapy-localized.

A dysfunctioning neuromuscular spindle cell is usually palpable as a hard lump. Locating it through therapy localization and palpation makes treatment more direct and easy to perform.

To strengthen a muscle that tests weak because of a dysfunctioning neuromuscular spindle cell, the examiner presses his fingers rather deeply into the muscle on each side of the neuromuscular spindle cell and then pulls his fingers apart from each other along the direction of the fibers of the muscle. This also can be used to "wake up" normally functioning muscles and thereby prepare them for strong contraction before or even during athletic competition.

To weaken a muscle that tests hypertonic (one that tests strong but cannot be weakened by usual means)

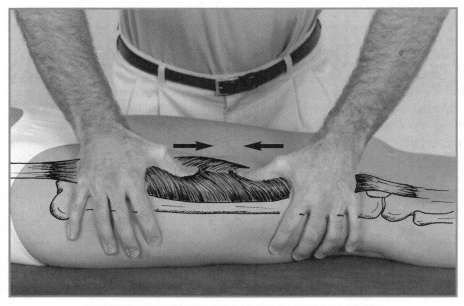

PRESSING THE NEUROMUSCULAR SPINDLE CELL TOGETHER
TO DECREASE TENSION IN A MUSCLE

because of a dysfunctioning neuromuscular spindle cell, the examiner presses his fingers into the muscle on each side of the problematic neuromuscular spindle cell and then repeatedly presses his fingers together along the line of the direction of muscular contraction (the line of the muscle fibers themselves). This effectively "pinches" the neuromuscular spindle cell together. This type of manipulation of the neuromuscular spindle cells can swiftly return full extension to shortened, tight muscles. It is not the most pleasant type of massage, but it is one of the most effective in promoting the relaxation of overly contracted muscles. For example, the application of this technique to a tight upper trapezius muscle between the neck and shoulder can swiftly reduce tension and pain in the muscle. This is assuming that the tension in the upper trapezius is primary and not caused only by its antagonist, the latissimus dorsi, having inadequate tone. Such treatment to the upper trapezius muscle may lengthen it so much that the shoulder sinks a few centimeters.

Treatment of neuromuscular spindle cells requires 1–7 kilograms of pressure. Sometimes even more pressure is required for the desired effect. Patients who have little tone in their muscles should be treated with less pressure. The pressure should be applied to a particular neuromuscular spindle cell several times. If the muscle is very wide and several neuromuscular spindle cells are involved, the treatment is repeated upon each active spindle cell, or simply across the whole width of the muscle. After adequate treatment, the neuromuscular spindle cells should no longer therapy-localize and the muscle should have the proper level of tension as measured by muscle testing.

If the same dysfunction of the neuromuscular spindle cell returns, or if there are neuromuscular spindle cell problems in many separate muscles, a nutritional correction is indicated. Goodheart recommends that the patient chew raw bone concentrate or raw bone nucleoprotein extract. Standard Process (see "Contact Addresses and Sources") supplies these nutrients. He suspects that the helpful factor in the

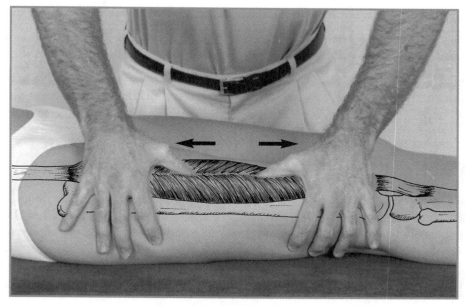

PULLING THE NEUROMUSCULAR SPINDLE CELL APART
TO INCREASE TENSION IN A MUSCLE

bone concentrate is phosphatase. As long as one has no allergy to the nightshade family of plants (potatoes, tomatoes, eggplant, and peppers), the phosphatase in raw potato also seems to work well for this purpose.

Correction of a Muscle that Tests Weak Due to Dysfunctioning Neuromuscular Spindle Cells

Indications of possible dysfunction of the neuromuscular spindle cells:

    a) The muscle has too little tone (is hypotonic).
    b) The muscle is palpatory hypertonic but tests weak.
    c) There are firm lumps in the belly of a muscle that hurt when pressed upon.
    d) The muscle contains neuromuscular spindle cells that therapy-localize.

Test:

1. Palpate the muscle for firm lumps. They will usually be in the belly of the muscle but may be located anywhere in the contractile fibers.

2. Touch (therapy-localize) the suspect area (on the lumps if any are palpated).

3. Test the muscle again while the suspect area is therapy-localized.

4. If the previously weak-testing muscle now tests strong, there are dysfunctioning neuromuscular spindle cells in the area therapy-localized.

Correction:

1. To raise the tone of a muscle that tests weak because it contains a dysfunctioning neuromuscular spindle cell, push the fingers (or sides of the hands) into the muscle on each side of it and pull the tissues apart along the direction of the muscle fibers. Do this several times with 1–7 kilos of pressure.

2. Retest the previously weak-testing muscle. It should now test strong. If not, return to test step 1, check for and correct other areas of dysfunction.

3. Therapy-localize the previously dysfunctioning neuromuscular spindle cell and retest the muscle. The muscle should again test strong. If not, repeat correction step 1.

4. Have the patient chew raw potato or raw bone concentrate at this time to lock in the correction.

Correction of a Muscle that is Hypertonic Due to a Dysfunctioning Neuromuscular Spindle Cell

Indications of possible dysfunction of the neuromuscular spindle cells:

    a) The muscle has too much tone (palpatory hypertonic) and is hard and painful.
    b) There are firm lumps in the belly of a muscle that hurt when pressed upon.
    c) Neuromuscular spindle cells therapy-localize.
    d) The existence of "primary muscles" (see "Reactive Muscles" page 131).

Test:

1. Palpate the muscle for firm lumps.

2. Therapy-localize the suspect area (on the lumps if any are palpated).

3. Test another normotonic indicator muscle while therapy localizing the suspect area.

4. If the previously normotonic indicator muscle now tests weak, there are dysfunctioning neuromuscular spindle cells in the area therapy-localized.

Correction:

1. To correct a muscle that is too tight because of dysfunctioning neuromuscular spindle cells, push the fingers (or sides of the hands) into the muscle on each side of the area that therapy-localized and push the tissues together (pinch the neuromuscular spindle cell together) along the direction of the muscle fibers. Do this several times with 1–7 kilos of pressure.

2. Therapy-localize the previously dysfunctioning neuromuscular spindle cell area and retest the

indicator muscle. The indicator muscle should now remain strong. If not, repeat correction step 1.

3. Test if the muscle that could not be weakened previously (hypertonic), now can be weakened (is normotonic).

4. Have the patient chew raw potato or raw bone concentrate to lock in the correction.

Golgi Tendon Organs

The treatment of the *Golgi tendon organs* can also be used to adjust the level of tension in a muscle. The Golgi tendon organs are proprioceptors located in the junction where muscles blend into tendons before attaching to bones. An average of 10–15 muscle fibers attach to each Golgi tendon organ. Golgi tendon organs have a function that is the opposite from that of the neuromuscular spindle cells: Neuromuscular spindle cells monitor the *length* of a muscle. Golgi tendon organs monitor the *tension* in a muscle.

When a muscle strongly contracts and thus quickly shortens, the neuromuscular spindle cells are shortened, but the Golgi tendon organs are stretched and activated. Neuromuscular spindle cells are *always* active and *increase* their output when a muscle is lengthened. Golgi tendon organs are passive until the muscle is quickly or extremely shortened (contracted). The activation of neuromuscular spindle cells increases the tension of (facilitates) the muscles in which they are found. This also facilitates the synergists and stabilizers while inhibiting the antagonists. The activation of Golgi tendon organs produces a decrease in the tension of (inhibits) the muscles in which they are found. Muscles that work together with the muscle containing the Golgi tendon organ (synergists and stabilizers) are also inhibited. The antagonists to the muscle are stimulated to increase in tone (facilitated).

The tendon receptors of the Golgi tendon organs are connected to a large type I afferent nerve, just like the neuromuscular spindle cells. To prevent confusion, the tendon receptor nerves are called *Ib afferent nerves* (to differentiate them from the Ia nerves attached to the neuromuscular spindle cells). Ib nerves go to the spinal cord where they meet and have an effect upon the alpha motor nerves that return to the muscle. Ib nerves also pass their signal through the spinal cord on to the cerebellum, which is highly involved with posture, balance and the integration of the movements of all parts of the body.

Many muscles are functionally strong enough to overstretch and thereby strain their own fibers or even pull their tendon away from its attachment to bone. Rapid or extreme stretching of the Golgi tendon organ results in a lowering of muscular tension, lengthening the muscle containing the Golgi tendon organ. Golgi tendon organs produce a greater output signal, and thus a greater inhibiting effect, when the muscle containing them is strongly contracted. This inhibiting effect of the Golgi tendon organ serves to prevent damage to the muscle fibers, the tendons, the attachment of the tendons to the bones, and to the bones themselves that could be caused by extreme tension in the muscles.

When the Golgi tendon organ signaling is strong enough, it turns the alpha motor neurons off. Then little or no signal to contract passes through the alpha motor nerves back to the muscle, which abruptly relaxes. This phenomenon can be seen in arm wrestling where the loser's arm typically gives out and goes down very suddenly. The protective mechanism of the Golgi tendon organs can be overridden by conscious decision and practice. Thus weight-lifters and arm wrestlers seeking to achieve maximum contraction may consciously prevent the Golgi tendon organs from inhibiting the muscle's contraction, even to the point of damaging the muscles, tendons or bones. It is postulated that in such cases, higher brain centers in the cerebrum send messages to the cerebellum and from the cerebellum on through the spinal cord to the segment level where the Ib afferent nerves form a junction with and affect the alpha efferent nerves. The end result is that the inhibiting effect of the Golgi tendon organs is itself inhibited and prevented from affecting the alpha motor neuron signaling.

The level of tension in a muscle (muscle tone) and its response to muscle testing can be directly affected by manipulation of the Golgi tendon organs. This can be demonstrated in a normally functioning muscle, as long as the location of the Golgi tendon organs can be correctly determined. In a normally functioning muscle, the Golgi tendon organs will not therapy-localize. This means that therapy localization cannot be used to determine their location. However, there is an easy way to locate the Golgi tendon organs, especially in a muscle with a narrow tendon. Activating the Golgi tendon organ by pulling either or both of the tendinous ends of a muscle toward the bone where the tendon attaches will cause a normotonic muscle containing this Golgi tendon organ to subsequently test weak. The effect will last from twenty seconds to several minutes. It may take a few tries to locate the exact position of the Golgi tendon organ.

In a muscle that tests weak due to a dysfunction of the Golgi tendon organ, the affected Golgi tendon organ will usually therapy-localize. Touching it will strengthen the weak-testing muscle itself and will also weaken most normotonic indicator muscles. Usually, there will be a lump in the junction between the tendon and the muscle that can be easily felt. Pulling this lump parallel to the fibers of the muscle toward the belly of the muscle several times should cause the muscle to return to testing normotonic.

Less often, a muscle may be hypertonic due to an overactive Golgi tendon organ. This can cause the muscle to become a primary muscle and cause other muscles to be reactive to it (see "Reactive Muscles," page 131). In this case, the Golgi tendon organ needs to be pulled away from the belly of the muscle.

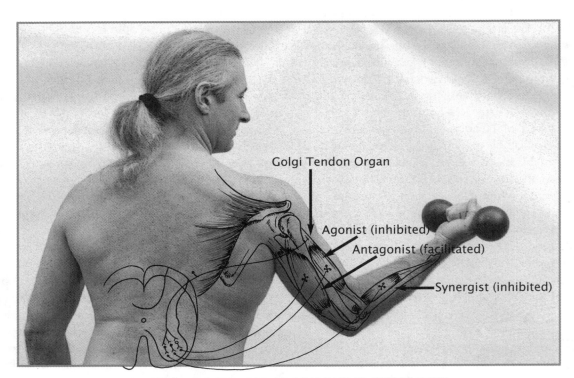

Golgi Tendon Organ

Agonist (inhibited)

Antagonist (facilitated)

Synergist (inhibited)

INHIBITION AND FACILITATION OF MUSCULAR CONTRACTION
THROUGH THE ACTIVITY OF THE GOLGI TENDON ORGAN

The Golgi tendon organs at both ends of the muscle should be evaluated. Either or both may be involved in a dysfunction. As with neuromuscular spindle cells, adjusting the signaling levels of Golgi tendon organs requires a pressure of about one to seven kilograms. The pushing or pulling motions should be repeated several times. Manual muscle testing before and after the treatment will reveal if the manipulation has been effective.

As with neuromuscular spindle cells, if the same dysfunction of the Golgi tendon organ returns, or if there are Golgi tendon organ problems in many separate muscles, a nutritional correction may be needed. Raw bone concentrate or raw bone nucleoprotein extract contain phosphatase, which Goodheart believes to be useful for problems with proprioceptors. For those who don't want to chew raw bone concentrate, as long as they have no adverse reaction to the nightshade family of plants, phosphatase can be obtained from raw potato. These same recommendations apply for the treatment of neuromuscular spindle cells.

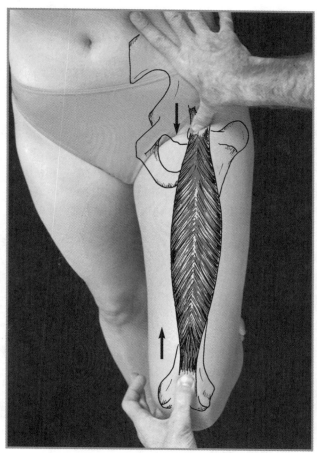

PUSHING THE GOLGI TENDON ORGANS TOGETHER TO INCREASE THE TENSION IN A MUSCLE

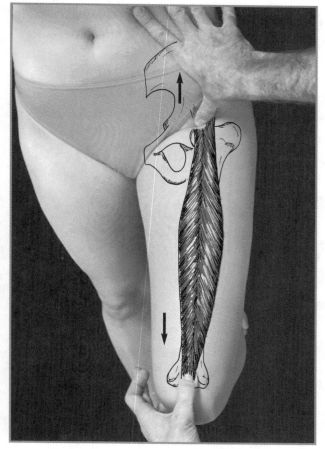

PULLING THE GOLGI TENDON ORGANS APART TO DECREASE THE TENSION IN A MUSCLE

Correction of a Muscle that Tests Weak
Due to Dysfunctioning Golgi Tendon Organs

Suspect dysfunctioning Golgi tendon organs when:

a) The muscle tests weak and cannot be strengthened with normal methods.

b) The muscle starts out testing strong and then, during strong contraction, suddenly becomes completely weak.

c) A lump which is tender to the touch is present at the junction of the muscle and its tendon.

Test:

1. Therapy-localize the junction of the muscle and its tendon on one end and retest the muscle.

2. Therapy-localize the junction of the muscle and its tendon on the other end of the muscle and retest the muscle.

3. If the muscle tested strong with therapy localization on one or both of its ends, it has a dysfunctioning Golgi tendon organ at that one end or both ends.

Correction:

1. Press the fingers into the muscle on the tendon side of the dysfunctioning Golgi tendon organ and pull it toward the belly of the muscle along the direction of the fibers of the muscle. Do this several times with 1–7 kilos of pressure.

Confirm the correction:

2. Retest the muscle. If the treatment was successful, it should now test strong and any previously tender lump in the Golgi tendon organ should be less tender.

3. Have the patient chew some raw potato or raw bone concentrate to lock in the correction.

Correction of a Muscle that Tests Hypertonic Due to
Dysfunctioning Golgi Tendon Organs (rare)

Suspect dysfunctioning Golgi tendon organs when:

a) The muscle tests hypertonic, and/or is hard and painful (palpatory hypertonic) but the neuromuscular spindle cells are not found to be responsible for the hypertonic state.

b) The muscle is a primary muscle but the neuromuscular spindle cells are not found to be responsible for the reactive condition.

Test:

1. Therapy-localize the junction of the muscle and its tendon on one end and test a previously nor-motonic indicator muscle (not the muscle itself).

2. Therapy-localize on the junction of the muscle and its tendon at the other end of the muscle and retest a previously normotonic indicator muscle.

3. If the indicator muscle tested weak with therapy localization on one or both of the ends of the suspect muscle, it has a dysfunctioning Golgi tendon organ at that one end or both ends.

Correction:

1. Press the fingers into the muscle on the muscle belly side of the dysfunctioning Golgi tendon organ and pull it toward the bone, away from the belly of the muscle, along the direction of the fibers of the muscle. Do this several times with 1–7 kilos of pressure.

Confirm the correction:

2. Retest the muscle. If the treatment was successful, the muscle should now test normotonic, be less hard, less painful and/or cause no further weakening of previously reactive muscles.

3. Have the patient chew some raw potato or raw bone concentrate to lock in the correction.

Good Posture and the Central Nervous System

If the muscle proprioceptors are out of adjustment and improperly signaling, they send false messages through the afferent sensory nerves into the central nervous system (spinal cord and cerebellum). When the CNS responds correctly to incorrect incoming signals, incorrect outgoing signals will be sent to the muscles through the efferent motor nerves. As a result, some muscles will be palpatory hypertonic (too tense) while others will be hypotonic (too relaxed). This results in poor structural alignment of the body (incorrect posture) and uncoordinated movements.

The central nervous system has been compared to a computer. If the input signals are incorrect, the output will also be incorrect. In the computer world, this principle is stated, "Garbage in, garbage out." Although this formula fits the central nervous system well, all in all the CNS cannot be accurately compared to a computer but rather to an "action-reaction pattern." This is in harmony with modern communication theories, especially that of Huberto Maturana and Franzisco Varela as presented in their book, *Der Baum der Erkenntnis (The Tree of Knowing)*. This book treats the principles of systems theory as they are currently presented in the areas of sociology, psychotherapy and medicine. Concerning the comparison of the central nervous system to a computer, Maturana and Varela write:

"It would be a mistake to look upon the nervous system as a simple input-output device. That would mean by definition that in the organization of the system there must be inputs and outputs like there is in a computer or a machine. These definitions would be fitting in the case of a man-made machine whose most important characteristic is our interaction with it.

However, the nervous system (or the organism) is not created by anyone. The nervous system is the result of a phylogenetic drift of biological entities centered on their own dynamic conditions. It is therefore fitting to look upon the nervous system as an entity that is defined by its internal relations, within which the interactions work only as modulations of its structural dynamic; as a unity that is operationally closed.

In other words: The nervous system receives no information—like one often says. More correctly, it brings forth a world within which it determines the representation of the perturbations of the environment and which alterations these release within the organism. The popular metaphor of the brain as a computer is not only misleading, it rather is simply false." (Maturana/Varela, 1987, p. 185, translation by the author).

This quote sounds complicated. Summarized and simplified, it means that the central nervous system does not only react to incoming information, it defines how this information is represented to itself. This, in turn, leads to internal processing of the information and consequent signaling to and control of other parts of the body. You might compare this to the differing reactions of various people to the same stimulus. Each person's representation (interpretation) of the stimulus is determined individually. Therefore each person's reaction is also individual.

Signaling levels from Golgi tendon organs and from neuromuscular spindle cells are responsible for the quality of our posture and patterns of motion, and for most of the subjective sense of posture and movement. Poor posture may cause some discomfort, but unless it becomes extreme, we simply ignore it. After all, our poor posture is a habit of long standing. And habits, even bad ones, come to feel correct with enough repetition.

When someone with poor posture is ordered to sit or stand straight, he does so by tightening the antagonists to his already overly tense and shortened muscles. The posture thus produced looks straighter but is twice as tight! The shortened, tense agonists are still tight. Their antagonists are now also tight, fighting against the tight agonists. The result is a jamming together of the joints, which often results in more discomfort than experienced before the attempt.

Being told not to slouch and to stand straight does not create lasting postural change because proprioceptor signaling has not been changed. The result of the attempt to attain better posture is that the old tensions are at least partially retained. They are not released but only counteracted with additional new tensions. Furthermore, the new posture feels wrong and the old poor posture still feels more comfortable. In such a case, one soon returns to the old posture (often with a sense of relief) as soon as one tires of the attempt … or as soon as the person who ordered,

"Stand straight!" is no longer looking.

Typical patterns of poor posture (poor structural alignment) include collapsing the front of the torso downward, lifting the shoulders, putting the head forward of the line of gravity, and pulling the head back upon the neck. Clearly, when the alignment of the body moves away from the line of gravity, muscles must contract to support it or the body will fall over. Continually holding such posture requires certain muscles to be excessively contracted. This inhibits their antagonists. Other muscles less designed for the task must tighten excessively to take over the job of the inhibited antagonists. This increasingly complicated chain of inappropriate tensions can produce discomfort, neurological disorganization, and eventually organic illnesses in the organs associated with the involved muscles.

AK muscle correction techniques have the goal of breaking the chain of compensations described above through precisely adjusting the signaling of the neuromuscular spindle cells and the Golgi tendon organs. The central nervous system receives this more accurate input and responds with more accurate output, which is sent back to the muscles. When each muscle then has balanced, optimal tone, the result is better structural alignment. The balanced muscular tone in the agonists and antagonists brings the vertebral column more into alignment with the line of gravity. Then the weight of the body passes through the bones of the vertebral column, pelvis and legs with less effort in the muscles. This results in better posture, better coordination and smoother, more graceful movement. This explains the observed improvement of posture and body use after an Applied Kinesiology muscle testing and correction session.

The Golgi tendon organ and neuromuscular spindle cell manipulation techniques described above are used to balance muscular tone by adjusting the signal levels produced by these proprioceptors. Through such treatment, the body's sense of its own balance and orientation changes, making the new postural tension levels in the muscles feel correct. Pain is lessened and the patient has better posture and use with no conscious effort at all.

As described above, the neuromuscular spindle cells and the Golgi tendon organs have functionally opposite, yet often simultaneous activities. Their reciprocal effect upon muscular tone makes human movement coordinated and graceful. For example, when one flexes the arm, as the biceps nears complete contraction, the shortening of its length deactivates its neuromuscular spindle cells and the increased tension activates its Golgi tendon organs.

At the same time, the triceps is extended, which lengthens its neuromuscular spindle cells. The result is an inhibition of the biceps and a facilitation of its antagonist, the triceps (reciprocal inhibition). Thus the speed of contraction automatically slows as the joint nears complete flexion. Without this reciprocal mechanism, our movements would be jerky and produce excess strain upon the tissues. A similar effect is observed when braking in a car. Were the driver to press firmly and continuously upon the brake until the car completely stopped, all in the car would be thrown sharply forward during the last few seconds of stopping. Instead, as the car nears a complete halt, a good driver slowly lifts his foot from the brake to slow down the process of deceleration. The effect of the muscle proprioceptors is similar to slowing down movements as a joint approaches complete flexion or complete extension.

As mentioned, muscles, even when inactive, have a continuous level of tension called *muscle tone*. When a muscle has too little tone, its antagonists react by tightening and shortening. This tightening of the antagonist may cause a further reduction of tension in the agonist. This result then causes the antagonist to tighten even more. In such cases, this reciprocal inhibition and facilitation (produced by the effects of the neuromuscular spindle cells and Golgi tendon organs) can result in a self-perpetuating problem. When a patient visits a massage therapist with such a problem, the therapist typically massages the overly-tight muscle. This sounds logical. After all, it is the tight muscle that hurts. But since the cause of the original problem (too little tone in the agonist) was not addressed, such corrections are short lived. The excess tension in the antagonist soon returns.

To illustrate this problem, Goodheart used the image of a swing-door. When the springs on each side have equal tension, the door sits balanced in the middle. When one spring (the "agonist") gets stretched out, it no longer has as much tension. In this case, the door gets pulled to the other side where the other spring (the "antagonist") has comparatively greater tension. Stretching out this spring too would bring the door back into the middle, but then both springs would be stretched out and their tone decreased below normal (weakened). This is not a desirable solution. What is desired is a return of the normal tension in the already weakened spring, the agonist. In this swing-door example, this could be effected by replacing the stretched spring with a new one of normal tension. Then the door would be back to its proper balance.

The side with the shortened spring corresponds in our example to the overly tight antagonist. It is short and tight for a reason, namely because its agonist partner has too little muscle tone. In our swing-door example, the antagonist spring hasn't changed its level of tension at all. By comparison to its stretched-out partner, it appeared tighter. Muscles go even further than this. When an agonist muscle has too little tone, its antagonist partner not only by comparison has more tone, it actively tightens by increasing its level of existing tone. The logical first step to solve this imbalance of tension must be the raising of the muscle tone in the agonist. This often causes an immediate relaxation of the antagonist.

For example, low back pain is often caused by excess tension in the sacrospinalis muscles of the low back, which are active in holding the trunk upright. Raising the level of tone in the abdominal muscles inhibits their antagonist, sacrospinalis. This lengthens the sacrospinalis, which lessens the curve of the lumbar spine and often relieves the pain immediately. If, however, contraction of the antagonist again causes the agonist to subsequently test weak, the tone of the antagonist will also need to be directly reduced with the treatment for reactive muscles (see page 131).

When the level of tone in a muscle and its antagonist is equal, the structure will be in balance.

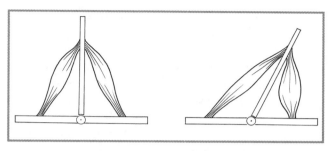

MUSCULAR BALANCE   THE SWING-DOOR

If the tone in a muscle is insufficient, the opponent tightens due to lack of opposition.

If proper treatment to the Golgi tendon organs and neuromuscular spindle cells is given soon after an injury, the maladapted responses typically caused by such trauma can be avoided. Such techniques may be helpful in treating sports injuries, allowing the athlete to quickly return to active participation. However, care must be observed to give the damaged muscle time to heal even though pain has been relieved and the range of motion restored by the use of these methods.

The correct application of muscle proprioceptor manipulation can relieve pain, increase the range of motion, balance muscle tone, improve posture and make all movements more efficient and graceful.

Stress Research and Applied Kinesiology

Hans Selye, a Vienna-born Hungarian who lived later in Canada, spent his life studying stress—what it is and its effects upon living beings. He not only coined the word "stress" but also the term "fight-or-flight response." He wrote more than 1700 papers and 39 books on the subject. He earned three doctorates (MD, PhD, DSc) plus 43 honorary doctorates. He not only carried out scholarly research but also made his the practical ideas of his work available to everyday people.

In 1936, Selye defined stress as *"the nonspecific response of the body to any demand."* So defined, stress is not simply a psychological phenomena but also includes all processes of response or adaptation. It encompasses all physical and psychological reactions to the demands placed upon the individual by both his internal and his external environments. Without stress, life is not possible. Stress is normal and cannot be avoided. Selye indicated this by further dividing stress into *eustress* and *distress*. Eustress is produced by doing what we like to do and what is good for us. Distress is elicited by those activities that we do not like to do but must (Gerz, 1996, pp. 30–33; Heine 1997, pp. 201–209; Selye, 1952).

The Three-Phase Reaction to Stress

Selye found out that every living being has a three-phase reaction to stress, which he called the *generalized adaptation syndrome* (GAS) as follows:

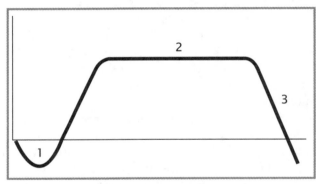

THREE-PHASE STRESS REACTION
ACCORDING TO SELYE

1. Alarm reaction:

In this first phase, the reaction of the body to stress is an "alarm reaction" in which the ability to respond temporarily decreases. This is a kind of shock reaction that is usually of short duration.

2. State of resistance:

If stress continues, extra cortisone and adrenaline are produced and released increasing the body's ability to adapt to the stress and improve performance of the activities required by the stressor. This adaptation to the stressor consists, for example, in a sharpening of the senses, an increase in the precision of motor control of the body, increased wakefulness and alertness, and a high metabolic rate. This results in increased performance of activities carried out at this time.

If the stress still does not stop, the quantity of these chemicals in the bloodstream increases until the body reaches its peak of ability to react to the stress. Selye calls this maximal adaptation the "state of resistance." This keeps the organism able to react swiftly and powerfully. This is a wise reaction of the body that promotes survival in conditions of extended stress. How long the body can support this process is individual.

3. State of exhaustion:

When this state of resistance continues too long, there comes what Selye calls the "state of exhaustion." When more or less completely exhausted, the body cannot produce the extra chemicals and energy for further resistance. The reserves are used up. In common parlance, this is referred to as "burn out." In this state, rest, therapy, good nutrition and a change of lifestyle are desperately needed for the body (and mind) to be relieved from stress and to recover from this exhausted state.

Selye found the following symptoms to be typically associated with stress:
 – recurring infections
 – allergies and hay fever
 – stomach and other digestive symptoms
 – insomnia, irritability, lack of energy, unusual mental symptoms
 – lack of concentration, confusion of thought
 – chronic fatigue, depressive tendencies
 – trembling, nervous tics, stuttering
 – teeth grinding at night, leading to a greater sensitivity to sweet/sour, hot/cold, perhaps problems with the temporomandibular joint (TMJ)
 – diarrhea
 – migraine, premenstrual syndrome
 – neck and back pain
 – too great or too small an appetite
 – a strong or even addictive desire for nicotine, alcohol, coffee or other stimulants/drugs

– recurring minor injuries or chronic aches and pains which, in spite of good treatment, refuse to go away

Note that this list includes the most frequent complaints of most patients everywhere today. This indicates how widespread the problem of stress is.

According to Selye, any animal responds to prolonged stress with hypertonicity of the skeletal muscles. This casts light upon the problem of hypertonic muscles, which is receiving increased attention in AK today. In fact, it is fascinating that Selye's concept of the three stages of stress has such a direct relation to all three states of reaction of a muscle in muscle testing: weak-testing, normotonic, and hypertonic.

Normotonic

A normotonic muscle is the ideal state in which both negative and positive stimuli are recognized and reacted to in a natural manner.

Weak-testing as a response to a stimulus -> Alarm reaction

A normotonic indicator muscle may test weak in response to TL to a scar or challenge by the oral presentation of an allergen. This can be compared to Selye's alarm reaction of the body in response to a new stress.

Hypertonic -> State of resistance

A single hypertonic muscle usually indicates a malfunction of a proprioceptor that can usually be corrected by proprioceptor manipulation.

A bilateral hypertonic muscle indicates that the corresponding muscle-organ-meridian circuit is stressed and is in a stress-adaptation phase.

General hypertonicity of muscles indicates that the whole system is in a massive stress-adaptation phase and working "overtime" to deal with the stress. In this phase, Selye says that rest and recuperation are the most needed treatment factors.

It is important that the patient correct the problem at this stage before a general state of exhaustion sets in. Natural healing techniques needed at this stage include clearing the body of toxins and focal infec-

tions, and obtaining exercise, fresh air, water, needed nutrients, and a change of lifestyle that includes less emotional stress.

Weak-testing muscles (without TL or challenge) -> State of exhaustion

An individual weak-testing muscle indicates that the body's ability to adapt to a stress has been exhausted, but only in the one specific regulating circuit related to the muscle tested.

If the general hypertonicity condition continues too long, the result will be a general weakness of most or all muscles. This corresponds to Selye's state of exhaustion. In this stage, the body can no longer adapt to the stress and is "giving up the fight." Typically with patients in this stage, it is difficult or impossible to find a single muscle that can be strengthened and used as an indicator muscle. The same steps listed for general hypertonicity are required at this stage, but they need to be applied more carefully and regularly. Most of all, such patients need rest, quiet, water, warmth, positive energy and a supporting environment of caring family or friends. This problem and its treatment are considered in detail in the section "General Hypertonicity," page 93).

Gerz compares the response of muscles to Selye's three states of stress as follows:

1. A previously strong-testing muscle tests weak = The stimulus that made the muscle test weak is greater than the ability of the body to adapt to it.

2. The normotonic muscle stays normotonic = The adaptation mechanism of the body, with respect to the stimulus, is adequate.

3. The normotonic muscle becomes hypertonic = The stimulus creates an alarm reaction in the body, which is expressed as a pathological increase of muscular tension. This can only take place at the cost of a "pre-damage"—the memory of a previous stress adaptation. In principle, this is what occurs in the reaction of the immune system to an allergen. For the body to have an allergic reaction,

it must have been previously exposed to the substance. It "learns" to react in an allergic manner. Hypertonic reaction is also a "learned response." In reaction to various kinds and amounts of stress, the body learns to tighten muscles.

4. A weak-testing muscle becomes normotonic = The stimulus (challenge) has a positive effect that enables the body able to improve its neuromuscular reaction.

5. A weak-testing muscle remains weak-testing = The challenge was not recognized by the body as significantly positive.

6. A weak-testing muscle becomes hypertonic = The body reacts to the challenge with an extreme alarm reaction. This is also a learned response to stress as in #3 above. (Gerz, 1996, p. 33).

In experiments with animals, Selye found that enough stress of any kind led to death. Three particular organs, the stomach, the thymus, and the adrenals, were always affected by extreme stress and usually in the same way each time.

1. The stomach became inflamed and developed ulcers.

2. The thymus shrunk in size and function.

3. The adrenal glands were filled with fat and their function reduced.

4. Other organs were affected by specific stressors, but these three were always affected by stress of any kind.

Although stress appears to produce similar symptoms in humans, there is still some controversy as to what extent these animal findings parallel the human reaction to stress. Human medicine widely recognizes the connection between stress and the stomach. And the thymus is well known as the main organ of the immune system (whose response to stress is common knowledge). Less attention is given to the extremely common problem of functional weakness of the adrenal glands. For that reason, this problem will be considered more completely here.

Typical problems associated with adrenal weakness include allergies, states of fear, arthritis, chronic tiredness, colitis, exhaustion, hormonal dysfunction, hypoglycemia (low blood sugar), dysfunction of the immune system, learning difficulties, excess weight, and ulcers of the duodenum. Besides laboratory tests for the detection of these conditions, there are also five simple tests for adrenal weakness:

1. The examiner compares blood pressure readings, first while the patient is lying, then while he is standing. When standing, the adrenal glands should release extra noradrenalin to elevate the blood pressure, ideally about 8 mm Hg (mercury). This keeps the blood from pooling in the abdomen and legs. If the lying blood pressure remains unchanged when the patient stands, or especially if it sinks, very likely the adrenal glands are weakened and are not producing and releasing enough noradrenaline. In medicine, this reaction is called the "Ragland sign."

2. A further test for adrenal weakness involves determining the pupil reaction to light. Light in the eyes should cause the pupils to contract. When the adrenal glands are weakened, the body loses sodium and the intercellular potassium increases. This extra potassium interferes with the function of the pupil sphincter muscles, which then are unable to adequately contract. If the pupils widen immediately when a light is shined upon the eyes or fail to contract even after about thirty seconds, an adrenal weakness is indicated.

3. The region where the last rib meets the sacrospinalis muscle is an adrenal reflex area. Pain in this area indicates possible problems with the adrenal glands. This response is known as "Rogoff's sign."

4. In AK, the sartorius muscle is associated with the adrenal glands. When the sartorius muscle tests weak, which it often does when the adrenal glands are not functioning properly, the ilium subluxates posteriorly. This "posterior ilium" is a classic sign of adrenal weakness.

5. The anterior neurolymphatic reflex points for sartorius (5 cm superior and 2.5 cm lateral to the navel) are approximately over the adrenal glands and are used in AK to therapy-localize the adrenal glands. A weak sartorius muscle or an active TL to these points provides an ideal starting point to determine measures that might help strengthen the weakened adrenal glands. For a complete discussion of this issue, the reader is directed to the relevant literature, especially Gerz, *Applied Kinesiology*; Schmitt, *Common Glandular Dysfunctions in the General Practice,* and Goodheart, *You'll Be Better.*

The stress-related degeneration of these three organs, the stomach, thymus and adrenal glands, occurs in the second and third stage of the "Generalized Adaptation Syndrome" (GAS). The important point here is that stress of any type, if intense and constant enough, will lead to damage and degeneration of these three organs and eventually to death.

Selye's research led him to the conclusion that to promote health, the best attitude and lifestyle for all living beings is "altruistic egotism" (Selye, 1974). He coined this phrase as an alternative to the nearly impossible recommendation of Jesus to "love thy neighbor as thyself." For Selye, altruistic egotism implies that being benevolent to others promotes self-preservation. This means that the best way to be assured that others will help you when you need them is to help them when they need you.

Simplified and summarized, Selye believed that one should arrange one's life to have as much eustress and as little distress as possible. His further recommendations include:

- Find your own natural stress level.
- Learn the difference between eustress and distress.
- Precisely analyze your problems.
- Don't force and overexert yourself. Rather learn to know and follow your own need for rest and relaxation.
- Avoid table salt. It makes the negative effects of stress worse. Instead use potassium chloride (KCl).
- Clear out all hidden infections such as in teeth,

impacted colon, sinuses. Selye noted that these are a cause of continual stress for the body, even when no noticeable symptoms exist.
- Avoid one-sided stresses. The body wants to balance one kind of stress like hard physical work with another kind of stress like reading or making music.
- Observe your stress quotient with relation to your specific stress and general stress. When there is too much specific stress, one needs to get involved in other kinds of activities. When there is too much general stress, one needs rest and relaxation in a quiet non-stressing environment.

Selye's research indicates that stress weakens the immune system whose job it is to recognize and fight against undesirable substances in the body. Since immune system weakness is the root of many of today's most prevalent and difficult medical problems, a deeper consideration of Selye's concepts by medical doctors and other health professionals is indicated.

Applied Kinesiology is an excellent instrument for diagnosis in the field of immunology. With the techniques of AK, the examiner can assess the state of the immune system and the reactions of the immune system to various kinds of stimuli. Muscle testing the body of the patient with the challenge techniques provides the perfect tool for revealing both the individually problematic stress factors and the specific treatments best suited to the patient. Seen in this light, Applied Kinesiology is a kind of "applied immunology" or "applied stressology."

A Change in Worldview: From Newtonian Physics to Quantum Mechanics and Chaos Theory

Modern medicine is in a time of great upheaval. The paradigms that were useful in solving the problem of infectious diseases in the past do not provide adequate solutions for the many chronic and degenerative diseases prevalent today. It appears that a new way of thinking, a new way of looking at health and disease is required. The modern scientific concepts of quantum mechanics and chaos theory provide the needed new viewpoint. Although these new theories have been demonstrated to more accurately represent reality than the worldviews of the past, in the field of medicine as in other areas of society, there is resistance to accepting and applying new ideas.

However, a diverse group of medical doctors, researchers and biologists has embraced these new concepts and is using them to develop a new medical viewpoint. With this new medical "Weltanschauung," they have already had ground-breaking success in providing new understandings and solutions to many of the medical problems of today. "Biological medicine" is the generic term used to describe this new conceptual field. Unlike classical medicine, biological medicine no longer follows the Newtonian "cause and effect" way of thinking. Classical medicine seeks single causes of illness and fights them. By contrast, the doctor using biological medicine draws together and analyzes all the possible factors that could be causing the health problem and attempts to positively influence them. Alternative medicine can thus be seen as an aspect of biological medicine. The therapy methods of biological medicine can be classified as follows (after Heine, 1997).

Phytotherapy (therapy using plant products):
1. Homeopathy
2. Traditional Chinese medicine
3. Physiotherapy

Therapy with the goal of specifically affecting the system of ground regulation (Pischinger):
1. Acupuncture
2. Neural therapy
3. Bioresonance

Therapy to stimulate the system of ground regulation in a general way:
1. Nutrition
2. Kneipp techniques (external application of water)
3. Anthroposophic medicine
4. Alternating activity and rest with the goal of strengthening the powers of recuperation

5. Music and art therapy
6. Psychotherapy; therapy that uses talking as the medium in general

Detoxification and elimination techniques
1. Purging and vomiting
2. Bloodletting
3. Sweating methods (exercise, sauna, etc.)
4. Stimulation/irritation of the skin
5. Diuretic (water-removing) interventions

The techniques of classical medicine (surgery, chemotherapy, pharmacology, the use of artificial organs, hormone and other biochemical substitution) seek to fight the apparent, superficial cause of illness. With such methods, the body has a more or less passive role. When treatment is effective, the body is said to have been "freed" from the illness. All these methods are oriented toward illness.

By contrast, the therapy procedures of biological medicine give the body an active role—for example, in eliminating toxins. They help support and stimulate the self-healing processes. Special attention is given to the re-establishment of the natural biological processes (sleep and waking rhythm, body temperature, digestion, etc.). These methods strengthen the powers of recuperation and the resistance to illness. Biological medicine is oriented toward promoting and maintaining health.

In order to understand this new medical ideology, the old "classical" worldviews prevalent in medicine will be reviewed here and contrasted with the new concepts of quantum and chaos theories (reviewed in detail later in this chapter, page 43).

TRADITIONAL WORLDVIEWS

It appears that man's concept of reality, his concept of himself and his immediate environment, is inextricably tied to the currently accepted concepts of the nature of the cosmos, in which he exists. Everything he thinks occurs within the framework of the currently believed facts of nature as defined by the popular thinkers and scientists of his time. In modern times, the physicists are most responsible for our definitions of reality. In earlier times, reality was defined by the metaphysicians and the religious scholars.

Until the time of the Renaissance, when scientific inquiry and the growth of secular values blossomed, man existed within an earth-centered, three-level, natural universe. Generally, his concept involved a heaven above the earth, man on the flat surface, and hell below. Believing this concept of reality, sea explorers had a real fear of sailing off the edge of the earth, which would not only mean their certain death but also their consequent eternal damnation.

Prior to the Renaissance, scientific thinking was not based upon the concept of cause and effect as we understand it today but rather upon Aristotelian logic. Aristotle (384–322 B.C.) defined four kinds of causes. If a chair is created, its builder is the efficient cause, the structure that makes it a chair is its formal cause, the matter that has been made into the chair is its material cause and the need it was made to fulfill (namely, for sitting upon) is its purposeful cause. Thus, in Aristotle's natural philosophy, all things were considered to have a kind of inherent purpose. According to this line of reasoning, the cause of rain falling was believed to be the plants and animals below that require it to live and grow. The purpose is the cause. The church chose to make Aristotle's ideas accepted dogma. This came about in part because his idea of purposeful cause was easily adapted to justify church dogma. Thus God created the world so that animals and humans could live here. And woman was created to serve man. The church claimed the ultimate authority to declare the purposeful causes of all things.

Aristotle believed that when one is familiar with a subject, its governing principles become evident to the faculty of reason. For example, Aristotle stated that a body with twice the weight, when lifted and released in the air, would fall twice as fast. This was logical and therefore considered true. In Aristotle's time, it was not yet common to test the veracity of a logically deduced idea. Familiarity with the topic plus reason were considered adequate tools for the determination of truth.

With the spread of Christianity, the (Catholic) church attained increasing influence upon scientific thinking and research. The church adopted Aristotle's concepts, such as those about weight and gravity and declared them to be correct. The church was placed in a position of great consternation and embarrassment when Galileo Galilei (1564–1642) made his famous experiment (~1604) of dropping iron balls of various weights from the tower of Pisa. All the balls fell at the same rate! The mainly Catholic witnesses were put into a true moral conflict. They could not believe their eyes or they would become heretics, and likely subjected to torture by the Inquisition. Even worse, they would most certainly be excluded from paradise and suffer eternal damnation. So, they chose not to believe their eyes, and to consider that what they saw was unreal.

In his *De revolutionibus orbium caelestium libri VI (Six books about the revolutions of the heavenly spheres,* 1543) Nicolaus Copernicus was the first to publicly question the idea of the geocentric cosmology accepted since the time of Aristotle. The Danish astronomer, Tycho Brahe (1546–1601), produced the most accurate measurements of the planets ever obtained without a telescope. In 1572 he observed a new star in the constellation of Cassiopeia. In 1573, he published his first work, proving that the observed object was a star beyond the moon's orbit. This revealed a flaw in the Aristotelian worldview of the immutability of the heavens. Although Brahe, unlike his colleague Johannes Kepler (1571–1630), did not believe in the heliocentric theories of Copernicus, he invited Kepler in 1600 to stay with him in Prague where Brahe was the astronomer and mathematician at the court of Emperor Rudolph II. Brahe was impressed with Kepler's work. One year later, Brahe died and Kepler inherited his scientific legacy, including Brahe's planetary observations. Kepler studied these and proved that the orbit of Mars is an ellipse with the sun as one of its foci. This became Kepler's first law of planetary motion. His second law concerned planetary velocity, and his third law defined a relationship between the orbital periods and the distances of the planets from the sun. His work clearly demonstrated that the planets orbit around the sun. His belief that the sun governs planetary velocity formed the foundation for Isaac Newton's theory of universal gravitation.

In 1609, Galileo learned of the newly invented Dutch telescope and in the same year constructed one with 20-power magnification and turned it upon the heavens. There he saw mountains upon the moon, the starry nature of the Milky Way, and some kind of "planets" orbiting Jupiter. His discoveries again ran against accepted church dogma. He argued for freedom of inquiry, stating that sensory evidence and mathematical proofs should not be subject to interpretations of scripture. The church had another idea in these matters and declared him a heretic, imprisoned him (soon commuted to house arrest) and banned all of his books in Italy. However, outside Italy, his ideas were pursued eagerly.

Isaac Newton (1643–1727) is often revered as the greatest scientific genius of all. During his first two years at Trinity College at Cambridge (1661–1662), students were only allowed to learn the philosophy of Aristotle. However, during his third year, some freedom of choice was instituted and Newton studied mechanics, algebra, analytical geometry and Copernican astronomy. When the plague closed the University in 1665, he returned home to Lincolnshire, England, where he swiftly made revolutionary advances in physics, optics, mathematics and astronomy.

Newton reasoned that planetary orbits are the result of two forces: a centrifugal force which drives the body away from the center, and a centripetal force which draws the body toward the center. He imagined that the force of the earth's gravity extended to the moon, providing the centripetal force. Using Kepler's third law of planetary motion, he deduced that the force of gravity between any two bodies must decrease with the inverse square of the distance. Thus if the distance between the bodies is doubled, the force of gravitation is one-fourth as much. If the distance is tripled, the force is one-ninth as much. Newton was the first to mathematically prove that if a body obeys Kepler's second law, which states that a line connecting a planet to the sun sweeps over equal areas in equal times, then the force of gravity must obey the inverse square law. Newton published his

Philosophiae naturalis principia mathematica (The Mathematical Principles of Natural Philosophy or "Principia") in 1687. The *Principia* is universally recognized as the greatest scientific book ever written.

Using his law of gravitation and the laws of motion, Newton was able to explain a wide variety of phenomena including the eccentric orbits of comets, the tides, the effect of the sun's gravitation in producing variations in the orbit of the moon, the motion of projectiles, falling bodies and pendula. Thus the Newtonian law of gravitation and system of mechanics was able to explain, within the accuracy of existing measurements, most of the observed phenomena of nature. The divergent works of Copernicus, Galileo and Kepler were united into one coherent whole. The Copernican worldview of heliocentricity at last had a firm physical and mathematical basis. Thus Newton completed the scientific revolution of his times and formed the content of modern science. By looking out into and analyzing the motions of the planets of our solar system and starry universe beyond, a new worldview was created which is still influential today.

As the concepts of Newtonian mechanics prevailed and became the accepted scientific belief, the model of the three-level universe was no longer convincing and lost its validity. Gradually the general populace came to accept the principles of Newtonian physics, which established that rather than being the center of the universe, the earth is but a mere speck in the total order of things. In this new worldview, the earth is just one planet rotating around our sun. And our sun is only one of a seemingly endless number of other stars in our universe. The whole worldview of reality changed. And with it, the power of the church over the minds of humanity decreased greatly. Freedom of thought and scientific inquiry, requested by Galileo but denied him, became the ideal of the new age.

Perhaps most importantly, Newton experimentally demonstrated the relationship between cause and effect and postulated this concept to be the basic defining principle of the universe. Today this principle is seldom questioned. It is, for us, a priori—

unquestionably true. In fact, it is quite difficult for us to conceive of any other way of thinking. In the still-prevalent Newtonian thinking of our times, the universe is considered by many to be absolutely ordered and all phenomena defined by clear, logical, mathematical laws. Anything that does not appear to follow these laws is considered to be illusion and unreality. Chaos and uncertainty were not only ruled out, as long as Newtonian thinking ruled, they were not even conceived of as possible. As a new worldview becomes popular, even the uneducated often wonder how prior generations could have been so narrow-minded as to accept the old concept of reality.

QUANTUM AND CHAOS THEORIES

In very recent times, physicists looking within the atom found both a firm natural order and a totally unanticipated chaos and uncertainty. In order to express and work with these new ideas mathematically, scientists developed the uncertainty principle coupled with the science of quantum mechanics and chaos theory. Curiously, as the new conception of the nature of the universe began to emerge, reality again was defined a new type of three-level universe. The first layer consists of those aspects of our everyday world that may be accurately described by Newtonian physics. The third level consists of all objects and phenomena that are best described by chaos theory. Located between these two levels is the area of relative uncertainty (determined chaos) within which all the phenomena of life exist. Within this new and still emerging worldview, it is believed that life cannot exist either in rigid form or in chaos. Life can only exist within defined limits, between strict rules of structure and utter chaos.

With this new definition of reality, our worldview has once again drastically changed. In this new light, people are beginning to review their assumptions, concepts, and even their prejudices. Many find it hard to give up the comfortable certainty of Newtonian mechanics, but forward thinkers everywhere are adopting and adapting to the new concepts. Expres-

sion of the new worldview may be seen in various sciences, art and music. Chaos theory has even been successfully applied in predicting trends in the fields of economics and business. With the framework of these new concepts, repeatable but previously unexplainable phenomena in the field of alternative medicine are receiving a strong theoretical basis. It took several centuries after the Renaissance before the established dogmas gave way and the new concepts of Newtonian physics were generally accepted. Today, it may take decades before the general consensus of the established medical profession, which is still greatly dominated by the Newtonian concepts of cause and effect, accepts those facets of alternative medicine that are now being explained and proved in the light of quantum and chaos theories.

In the AK literature, one can see that explanations of muscle testing have been limited to the most widely accepted medical concepts of physiology and neurophysiology. However, within the generally accepted medical model, many of the observed phenomena of AK simply cannot be explained. Bioresonance and multi-resonance therapy systems such as electroacupuncture (Voll) are used by some in AK. Examiners using AK often test subtle energy substances such as homeopathic remedies, Bach Flower Remedies and gemstones held in the hand. An explanation of how the above methods could function does not exist within the models of classical medicine. Explanations and verifications, however, are now being developed in terms of quantum mechanics and chaos theory.

For both diagnosis and treatment, examiners using AK often utilize systems of reflex that have no, or only tenuous, basis in conventional anatomy. Examples of such reflex systems include neurolymphatic reflexes, neurovascular reflexes, hand and foot reflexes (reflexology), cranial stress receptors, the meridian system, and ear acupuncture. Jochen Gleditsch in his book, *Mundakupunktur*, has demonstrated that such reflex areas exist all over the body. According to his research, one can affect any chosen part of the body by stimulating reflex points located more or less upon every other part of the body. In all of these systems, remote areas are stimulated to produce an effect in a target organ or group of organs. Although attempts and some progress have been made, all efforts to explain these phenomena using the models of classical medicine have had limited success.

In this difficult situation, and as outlined above, a review of the evolution in mathematics and physics over the past century may provide a path-finder for understanding the new thinking in medicine. During that time, most of the hallowed Newtonian concepts gave way to Einsteinian theories, and particularly to quantum mechanics and chaos theory. In order to provide an explanation of the peculiar, very useful, and hitherto unexplainable AK phenomena, classic scientific and especially medical thinking will now be contrasted with quantum mechanics and chaos theory.

A Comparison Between Traditional and Modern Models of Reality

Classical linear cause-and-effect thinking developed during the Renaissance and ascended to its peak in Newtonian mechanics. The "one disease-one cure" concept still dominant in medicine today is a reflection of this thinking. In the classical scientific model (and also in classical medicine), a separation between the observer and the observed phenomena is assumed. In this model, it is believed that separate objects act one upon one another without any influence being caused by the act of observation. The basic premise of this viewpoint is that one object can cause an effect upon another object, fully independent of the observer.

In modern quantum theory, it has been determined that independent observers (those who have no effect upon that which is observed) do not exist. That which is sought, and the act of seeking itself, have an influence upon what is found. In physics, the validity of this principle was clearly demonstrated by the wave-particle duality of electrons. It was not known if electrons were waves or particles. In an experiment to detect waves, electrons behaved like waves. In another

experiment to detect particles, electrons behaved like particles. So which are they? These experiments demonstrated that electrons appear to be what the experimenter is looking for and measuring! The act of observation, more than any inherent reality, determines how they appear. A philosophical expression of this idea is reflected in the popular saying, "If you are looking for trouble, you will probably find it."

In another experiment, researchers were presented with two groups of rats. They were told that one group was bred for increased intelligence and that the other group was rather stupid. The researchers were asked to test each group of rats to see how much faster the intelligent rats learned to run through a labyrinth. As expected, the intelligent rats did indeed learn significantly faster to run through the maze. Then came the surprise: All the rats from both groups were genetically from the same stock. The only difference was the expectations of the researchers. In a similar experiment, school teachers were told that certain students were especially intelligent. And although the students were of only average intelligence, they did excel in their courses when their teachers expected them to excel. These surprising results, which are in perfect agreement with quantum theory, cast doubt upon the accuracy of much of the scientific research performed throughout history. These examples imply that in this universe of ours, there is a tendency to find what you are looking for!

Another basic premise of quantum theory is the "superposition principle," which states that everything is related to and connected with everything else. In a universe such as this implies, it is impossible to make any definite statement about cause and effect. In order to make some sense of observed phenomena, it is necessary to isolate and abstract them from the all-encompassing quantum world into the special, classical world of time and space. Then the system researched has individuality, measurements can be taken, and statements about its nature can be made. But any such measurements and statements about the "reality" of the system researched are dependent upon the point of reference, the context of the investigations and the expectations of the researchers themselves.

Although quantum theory has been accepted by most branches of science, many in the world of medicine cling to the cause-effect mentality defined by Newtonian mechanics. Classical medicine still bases its diagnostic and treatment techniques upon the concept of the lock and key, in which the lock is a disease and the key is a medicine or medical technique (chemical medicines, surgery, etc.). This linear thinking model implies that each part of the body and indeed each cell is an independent entity that may be treated for its independent disturbances. However, in a multi-cellular being such as the human body, cells do not exist individually. Historically, the abstract concept of the separate cell and its pathologies (Virchow, 1858) led to the linear idea of "for one disease, one specific cure." Within this thinking, the individual phenomena one experiences when ill are ignored in favor of defined models of illness. Symptoms are quantified and used as indicators of specific syndromes. If the values of a certain test are above a defined level, you have the syndrome. After effective treatment, the values must again fall below the defined level. An effective treatment within this perspective means "normalizing" the values—bringing them back into the accepted range of tolerance. At its worst, this scientific dogma leads to treating the model of the disease instead of the patient.

For example, a patient had breast cancer that had spread to many other areas of her body. In May, after surgery to the breast and chemotherapy, she was told to prepare for death before September. Her T-lymphocyte cell count was 18/µl. The normal level is defined as being between 1000 and 3500/µl. She enjoyed running and continued to run 17 kilometers each day. In February, she was still alive and her T-cell count had increased to 76/µl. The doctors said that this increase was too small to have any significance whatsoever. The idea that her regular exercise might be keeping her alive and improving her health was not even considered. She was told that the increase in the number of T cells had no meaning and

not to allow it to produce unrealistic hopes, because she would soon be dead.

This type of medical viewpoint automatically places limits upon which possible therapeutic efforts may even be considered. By only considering lab test values, doctors may diagnose and prescribe swiftly and thereby see more patients per day. The problem is that in this simplistic model, there is no place for individual variation. There is no room in this thinking for the fact that the same symptoms may be produced by different causes. And there is no place for the fact that the same medicine may produce different effects in two individual patients, even though they have the same presenting symptoms. More attention is given to the numerical results of medical tests than to how the patient is feeling or the causes of her symptoms viewed within her personal biology/constitution, or considered with reference to the quality of her lifestyle.

In acute illnesses where physical damage to tissues or infection by a micro-organism is the main cause, traditional medical diagnosis and treatment are extremely effective. In most acute illnesses, one specific cause outweighs all the others. In such cases, the "one disease-one treatment" mentality is usually successful. Doctors using this method have developed effective treatments for most acute medical problems. Because of these great successes, the world is largely free from many of the complaints that were often a cause of death in the past. Today the situation has changed. The most common medical complaints are no longer acute "diseases," but are instead tumors and other chronic degenerative illnesses. And traditional medical thinking is at a loss in dealing with these problems.

Because people today seldom die young from injuries, infections, and infectious diseases, the average age of death has risen significantly. Bodily functions and the ability to recover and regenerate decrease with increasing years. Old people typically die from degenerative diseases. That there are more older people is one reason degenerative diseases are more prevalent today. But the fact that many more young people suffer from degenerative diseases today than in years past indicates that there are other causes besides increasing age.

Thinking along the lines of the lock-and-key model, the doctor prescribes a chemical medicine to kill bacteria, or in the case of a viral infection, a chemical that inhibits viral reproduction. But medical research has revealed that many of the disease-producing bacteria and viruses live upon and within our bodies constantly. Often, the question is not asked as to why the body was susceptible at this particular time to infection. To even be aware that such a question exists, the doctor needs to expand his or her thinking from the classical Newtonian mechanics style of thinking that typically dominates the field of medicine to the more expansive, multi-dimensional concepts of modern quantum theory and chaos theory.

Anyone who has had a garden has observed that insects prefer to infest plants that are already weak. Similarly, anyone who has observed their own changing state of health knows that they are more likely to succumb to the ever-present cold viruses when they are exhausted, chilled, hungry, emotionally upset or otherwise excessively stressed. When the body is under stress, the bacteria that normally live on the skin can more easily infect a cut.

Seen in this light, it seems likely that taking medicines to combat an infecting agent, although temporarily successful against the acute disease, may be ignoring the multiple other causes of why the person got ill in the first place. And evidence indicates that, if not corrected, these multiple stresses may cause a repeat attack or eventually even result in a degenerative disease.

Furthermore, it is well known that those who are prone to infections and get sick a few times each year have less probability of developing our most prevalent disease, cancer. However, this benefit is lost if they take medicines that prevent their immune system from building strength by performing its natural fight against the infecting agents. Research strongly indicates that the immune system needs to battle diseases from time to time to keep in shape. When infectious diseases are severe, medicines may save lives. But their use for every little infectious disease that occurs may actually be one of the causes of severe diseases such as cancer!

Newtonian mechanics defines physical systems as functioning in a linear manner. An example of a linear system is a single pendulum. Its oscillating behavior is independent of the influence of any separate objects in its environment and is relatively independent of the effect of the observer. This is similar to the medical model of the single, isolated cell discussed above.

However, the concepts of cybernetics (Wiener, 1963), chaos theory and thermodynamic open systems of energy (Prigogine, 1979) have demonstrated that biological systems are non-linear. A simple example of a non-linear system is many different pendula linked together with springs. When one is moved, the energy dissipates first into the nearby and then into the more distant pendula and then back again until all are moving together in harmonic resonance. Like these coupled pendula, most structures within non-linear systems are self-repetitive. The same patterns of structure and motion are seen on many levels. This principle is observed throughout nature.

In the eighteenth century, Ernst Chaldni placed sand upon a thin plate of glass and made the plate resonate by stroking it with the bow of a violin. The sand vibrated into beautiful repetitive geometric figures across the surface (Chaldnian figures). Chaldni publicized his discoveries in his book, *Entdeckungen über die Theorie des Klanges,* (Leipzig, 1787). The Swiss scientist, Hans Jenny, spent ten years investigating the power of sound to form geometric patterns in various inorganic substances. The patterns produced by sound vibration in his experiments look like starfish, bacteria, organs and other patterns seen in forms of life. In *Cymatics* (1974), he concluded that where organization is concerned, the harmonic figures of physics are essentially similar to the harmonic patterns of organic nature.

These patterns of physics are seen in all living systems. Their principal characteristic is redundance, i.e., the same patterns repeat again and again on many levels until the available space is filled. For example, in the circulatory system each artery branches again and again into smaller and smaller, but in form essentially identical, arterioles and capillaries. The lung provides a similar example. The lung is basically a bag of air that is subdivided into smaller and smaller bags of air. This redundancy principle may be seen also in the form of most organs, which are segmented with each segment also segmented and so on until each sub-segment is completely filled with nearly identical cells.

Fractal Geometry

Mathematics recognizes such redundant systems of organization in which the same patterns appear repeatedly on various levels of complexity until the available space is filled. In mathematics, these geometric structures are called "broken dimensions" or "fractals." Fractal geometry was developed by the Polish-born French mathematician Benoit Mandelbrot. He coined the word "fractal" from the Latin verb *frangere*, "to break," and the related adjective

fractus, "irregular and fragmented." Fractal geometry deals with structures that repeat on finer and finer scales (Mandelbrot, 1991). Fractal geometric figures are self-similar. This means that when enlarged, their parts are identical with the whole. Fractals are not smooth figures like the curves and circles that exist in Euclidean geometry. They instead have a step-wise, jagged quality.

Mathematical fractals are perfectly symmetrical and remain geometrically identical on any level of magnification. They exist between strict order and chaos in the realm of "determined chaos." If the definition of fractals is expanded a bit to include some non-linear qualities (some deviation from mathematical perfection), such geometric forms can be found in nearly every natural phenomenon. Outside certain defining limits, forms may be very rough (but not self-similar) or very smooth—thus defining them as not fractal but rather Euclidean. As already described, life can only exist in an area between chaos and structure. Too rough is too chaotic. Too smooth is too structured. Within these limits, virtually everything is fractal. For example, almost any-sized piece

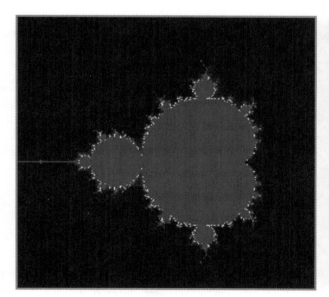

DIAGRAM OF A BASIC MANDELBROT SET

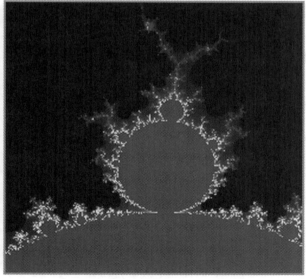

MAGNIFIED TOP SECTION OF THE FIRST DIAGRAM

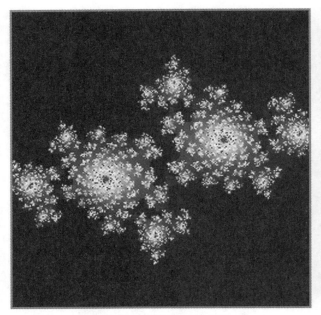

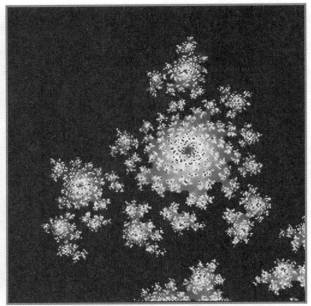

DIAGRAM OF A JULIA SET   MAGNIFICATION OF THE TOP PORTION

of cauliflower looks much like a whole head of cauliflower. The pattern "cauliflower" is clearly present on all these levels of observation. Thus the design of cauliflower is fractal. Fractals are an essential part of the mathematics of all natural phenomena, including life.

Fractal geometry has been used to understand disorder (chaos) in natural systems. In 1961, Mandelbrot applied his fractal theories successfully to turbulence in moving fluids, the distribution of galaxies, and even to predicting fluctuations of the stock market. In 1967, he showed that the irregular shorelines of the English coast are fractal.

Two American mathematicians, John Hubbard and Adrien Douady, developed the most known and useful set of non-linear fractals and named it after Mandelbrot. The more the bud-like geometrical figures derived from this set are magnified, the more the unpredictability increases. The Mandelbrot set is central to the science of dynamic systems.

Note that whereas the first figure of a Mandelbrot Set has one single line extending from it, in the magnified figure the line divides into two lines of unequal length. In further magnifications, the amount of such unpredictable changes continues to increase.

The French mathematician, Gaston Julia, used the Mandelbrot set to develop a mathematics of non-linear transformations in a complex plane. The "Julia sets" he devised are used to produce computer graphic images that often strikingly resemble natural forms.

Note that when the top portion of the first figure is magnified, nearly identical geometrical figures are revealed. This is the nature of fractals, within which the same figures can be found on many levels of complexity.

The chaos theory of mathematical physics uses fractals to describe the routes a dynamic system takes from order to chaos. A chaotic system is sensitive to initial conditions. A slight uncertainty in the beginning develops into greater and greater unpredictability (chaos) over time. In all chaotic systems, a tiny change in the beginning produces great effects later. Chaotic systems include all living forms, ecosystems, social systems and the universe as a whole including the atomic, geological and astronomic levels.

On the atomic level, fractals and chaos theory have contributed to the understanding of chemical reactions, wave motion and electrical currents in semiconductors. Geological fractals exist both in the external structures of the earth and also in internal structures such as faults. Earthquakes occur in a fractal pattern across the surface of the earth. Earthquakes under a magnitude of 6 occur in self-similar (fractal) clusters over time. Rain falls in a fractal pattern over time. In biology, the temperature-related shape of proteins is fractal. In astrophysics, fractal patterns have been observed in the pulsations of variable stars (stars whose observed intensity of light vary over time). The pattern of atoms on the surface of a protein molecule is fractally distributed. And since proteins are the basic chemical building blocks of all biological systems, the patterns of living structures are fractal.

Biological systems are many-sided, complex and highly interconnected. They can take in energy (food, light) and use it to more highly organize themselves. They are interconnected in a complex manner and have feedback systems that allow them flexibility to react to the situation of the moment in spontaneous ways. They can optimize their behavior. Biological systems, like all non-linear systems, exist within natural laws but tend toward a chaotic state ("determined chaos"). They exist in a dynamic balance between utter chaos and rigid order in both structure and function. Too much order (as in a crystal) or too much chaos means death, i.e., destruction of the system. In the determined chaos of biological systems, small changes in the current state of the system can produce large future changes. This fact provides a possible explanation for the effectiveness of such healing treatments as acupuncture or homeopathy in which tiny stimuli may produce system-wide changes that cannot be explained within traditional medical models.

In a complex interconnected system with great redundance such as within a specific organ with millions of essentially identical cells, many parts can be destroyed without reducing the quality of the function of the organ. The quantity of the chemicals produced or the other functions of the organ will be reduced but it will essentially function as before. This redundant quality of non-linear systems is an important factor for survival.

HOLOGRAMS

It is interesting to note that a hologram demonstrates characteristics similar to those of life. In a hologram as in a living being, "the whole information is present and repeated in all parts" and "portions of parts may be removed without disturbing the function qualitatively." These attributes of a hologram are in harmony with the superposition principle that states that everything exists in relation to and has an effect upon everything else.

A visual hologram is produced on photographic film by utilizing one laser beam of light divided into two. One of these beams goes directly to the photo film. The other one bounces off the object to be photographed and then onto the film. The two light beams interact and form interference patterns over the surface of the film. When that film image is viewed by ordinary light, there is no recognizable image. But when a laser beam is directed toward the film, a three-dimensional image of the item photographed appears in the air above the film.

In such a visual hologram, a complete three-dimensional picture is present in all parts of the film. Cut a small corner of the film and the whole picture is still present, though in reduced clarity. This may be compared to an organ in which many cells may be destroyed but the organ still performs the same activity with no change in quality, only a reduction in the quantity of activity. A hologram is clearly a quantum mechanical phenomenon in which all parts are interconnected and the whole is present in the parts.

There is much evidence to suggest that the brain stores information holographically, that is, that each specific bit of information is replicated over wide areas of the brain. Rats that have learned to run a maze still remember how to do so when up to 50% of their brain cortex has been removed. And it doesn't matter which 50%! This implies that the learning is stored all over the brain like visual information in a hologram.

Holograms can be produced with almost any source of energy, not only light. In producing a holograph, there are always two reference sources of energy. The bilateral structure of the human body may provide similar energy pairs for the formation of holographs within the nervous system. Evidence indicates that the nervous system functions holographically with respect to sensory and motor systems. Perhaps this is why there are two hemispheres of the brain that each receive signals from two eyes and two ears. These separate pairs of images likely are the two references necessary to form holographic sensory images in the brain.

If the nervous and organ systems function holographically, then it is logical that one may act upon one part and produce effects on any other part. This is the concept underlying the many systems of reflex therapy.

When two similar but not identical holograms are placed one upon the other in laser light, interference patterns appear. These are called "Newton rings." Goodheart believes that something similar occurs in the human body. Goodheart proposed that the brain has a perfect holographic image of all the parts of the body. When the local hologram in one part of the body (for example, an injured knee) does not correspond accurately with the perfect hologram of the knee in the brain, the brain is alerted that something is wrong. Symptoms then occur, and the healing process is initiated (Goodheart, 1986; Walther 1988, p. 26).

The many similarities between human functioning and the properties of the hologram suggest that many of the structures and functions of the human body have holographic qualities and may be accurately described and analyzed within the models of quantum theory.

One advantage of a non-linear system is that when it is disturbed and moved out of its normal position or activity, it quickly returns to its basic position or rhythm. In chaos theory, this quality of a non-linear system is called an attractor. Biological systems have attractor activities that repeat on a constant time cycle. Under normal conditions, they can react and adapt to small disturbances and swiftly return to their basic rhythm. Examples of such rhythms are heartbeat, respiration, temperature, permeability and metabolic rate. In chronic illnesses and especially in tumor tissues, such activities no longer occur rhythmically. If these rhythms cannot be reestablished, the prognosis for cure is poor. For example, the temperature of the surface of the skin changes regularly with a 24–hour cycle. However, changes in the temperature of the skin over a tumor have no regularity. Thus chronic illnesses are marked by a loss of natural rhythmic periodicity in the affected tissues. Therapeutic efforts that return normal periodicity to diseased tissues are especially important and effective in restoring health.

Under normal physiological circumstances, the homeostasis of an organism is extremely stable. Outer and inner stressful influences are quickly adapted to and the system returns to balance. For example, if adequate food is not available, the system will adapt to the situation in a reversible way. Minerals may be removed from the bones to replace those not currently in the diet. If this process goes far enough, there will be noticeable symptoms. Later, when the missing food elements are provided, the system can return to its prior state of balance. This exemplifies the interconnectedness and redundancy of non-linear systems. However, when a biological system is sufficiently stressed, it may not spontaneously return to balance. Once such an imbalance becomes established, small further disturbances of various types are not automatically corrected but rather may resonate with and thereby add their weight to the existing imbalances. When the combination of imbalances stresses the system enough, illness is the result. Seen in this light, illnesses are recognized to be system-wide disturbances that are often the result of many different causes.

The inferences of quantum mechanics concerning

the state of determined chaos of living organisms allow us to understand nature more deeply and accurately than the classical models of cause and effect. The possibly multiple causes of a patient's disease may each be considered within their own individual contexts. Internal and external factors (bio-chemical individuality, diet, posture, exercise, weather, social situation, the effect of prior experiences, expectation, occupational stress, etc.) may be analyzed for their contributing part in health and disease. The attention of the patient is focused upon his personal responsibility in promoting or combating disease. The patient is helped to help himself. Both the patient and his physician are operating from a far more complicated multi-dimensional picture of the processes of health and disease. Because this picture more accurately represents reality, it provides a better basis for both an evaluation of the totality of the health situation and for the application of the wider spectrum of therapeutic efforts needed to solve health problems, particularly those of chronic and degenerative diseases. These "new worldview" ideas are being pursued today by medical doctors and other scientists in the emerging field of "biological medicine."

Biological Medicine and the Systems of Regulation

This section is for the advanced student who desires to better understand the biochemical and electrical aspects of health and disease. Although an attempt has been made throughout this book to define every new term used, in this chapter I won't even try. The complete definitions would more than double its size. Obviously only a most superficial view is possible given the small amount of space that can be devoted here to this huge field. By giving an overview of this fascinating world of knowledge I hope to inspire my readers to inquire further on their own. Because so much of the new knowledge has been recently gathered, I urge you to read only the newest standard textbooks of anatomy, physiology, neurology and functional histology. For the advanced student with

a good understanding of the German language, I can highly recommend the best single textbook I have found on this topic: Hartmut Heine's, *Lehrbuch der biologischen Medizin*.

In the new medical discipline of "biological medicine," attention is given in both diagnosis and treatment to almost every factor that may make an individual ill.

Modern medicine conceives the gene to be one of the controllers, or the direct controller of biological functioning. The contrary view of biological medicine is that:

1. the gene is the repository of blueprints of instructions on how cells and higher systems should operate, not a direct activator, and

2. the actual *regulation* of biological activities in cells and all higher levels of organization lies in a so-called "system of ground regulation."

The tissues of higher life forms are built of three basic structures; the capillary, the ground substance or matrix, and the cell. The basic structure of the system of ground regulation is the ground substance. The ground substance is a complex connective tissue that lies between all the cells of the body. It consists of two groups of components, the amorphous ground substance and the structural ground substance. The amorphous ground substance is a transparent, half-fluid gel produced and sustained by the fibroblast cells of the connective tissues. It consists of highly polymerized sugar-protein complexes. One of its main families of components is the glycosaminoglycanes. Glycosaminoglycanes are bound to proteins in the tissues, forming huge chains (polymers) with a molecular weight of several million. They do not bend around into a circle like most other proteins but rather lie flat and take up lots more room than other molecules of the same molecular weight. On their flat sides they bind large amounts of water and positively charged ions (especially sodium), which assists the amorphous ground substance to become viscous and gives the structural ground substance turgor (fluid pressure) or even hardness. They twist together and partially form the permeability barrier around cells.

The structural strength of the ground substance is also provided by various kinds of fibers. The structural ground substance consists mainly of bendable reticulin fibers that can mature into inelastic collagen, stretchable elastin fibers, and the recently discovered structural glycoproteins fibronectin and laminin that are a part of cell surface membranes. The components of the structural ground substance form other types of connective tissues such as those of fascia, tendons, ligaments and cartilage as well as fat tissues, veins, arteries, lymphatic vessels, bones and teeth. These other types of connective tissues are durable, strong and long-lasting. They represent a kind of "long-term memory" of the ground substance.

The smallest structural element of the ground substance is the matrisome, which has a polygon network structure formed of various glycoproteins and transitorily bound proteins. The matrisome structure is arranged in many self-repetitive layers. Each layer is slightly rotated the same amount with respect to the next layer. We will return to the matrisome again later in this section.

The ground substance surrounds and interconnects the cells. It acts as a molecular sieve, determining what chemicals enter and exit the cells. The maintenance of homeostasis in the cells requires that the ground substance reacts swiftly and precisely to complex changes. This is made possible by the diversity of molecular structures of the sugar polymers of the ground substance, the ability to swiftly generate new such substances, and their high interconnectedness. This creates a redundancy that makes possible the controlled oscillation of values above and below the dynamic homeostasis present in all living creatures. This is a kind of fast-responding, "short-term memory" of the ground substance. Without this capacity, the system would quickly move to an energetic equilibrium, which would bring inactivity and death.

The ground substance contains a network of fibrous and non-fibrous connective tissue paths through which interactive information can flow. Such information flows into the ground substance as chemical, electrical and electromagnetic signals from blood, lymph, nerves, glands, etc., plus formatted information on proper "how to's" from the genes into the ground substance; then from the ground substance to the cells defining "what" to do. This interchange of information over the interactive network of the ground substance determines the reactions to internal and environmental influences. These stereotyped responses form the ever-repeating and yet ever-individual patterns of metabolism, development, growth, repair and behavior, etc.

Only about 2% of all illnesses are produced by the functioning or malfunctioning of a single genetic element. Biological medicine contends that most of the other diseases are produced by a combination of factors that interfere with the processes of the system of ground regulation. The system of ground regulation controls the relationship between cells and their environment—how energy and matter are exchanged in the thermodynamics of open energy systems of the human body. A knowledge of this system allows doctors to recognize malfunctions in tissues early so that corrective measures may be taken before disease develops. Thus the biological medicine approach provides for true preventative health care.

The function and composition of the ground substance can change swiftly under the various influences of the nervous and immune systems plus a wide variety of chemical influences including hormones, neuropeptides, enzymes, growth factors and cytokines.

The end of the motor nerves of the vegetative nervous system project out from their insulating myelin sheaths into the ground substance. They do not form synapses or enter the cells that they influence but rather end naked in the ground substance. Their signals are carried up to 2000 nm through the ground substance along fine collagen fibers to the basal membrane of the connective tissue or organ cells. Thus the nervous control of cells does not occur through synapses but through the chemical medium of the ground substance. Not only electric signals emerge from the end of nerves. Chemicals (neurotransmitters, neuropeptides and cytokines) are also released.

These bind to receptors on the connective tissue and organ cells and cause the cells to release short-lived chemicals (cytokines) that have a reciprocal influence upon the cells themselves, upon nearby cells, and upon distant cells via the circulatory system. Fine hollow tubes within the cells carry the chemical signals into and out of the cells, providing for fast communication and reciprocal reaction. The chemicals that are released by nerve endings are also involved in the process of inflammation.

Inflammation is a basic reaction of the tissues of the body against various damaging stimuli. These may be mechanical (friction, pressure, foreign bodies), chemical (acids, bases, toxins), physical (temperature, radiation), damaging internal processes (uremia, tissues destroyed by tumors, or microorganisms (bacteria, virus, yeast, parasites). Thus inflammation is the basic reaction of the body in all diseases. Inflammation of a tissue indicates that the body is fighting against a disturbing factor, substance, stimulus, process, or infecting agent.

Mast cells control the process of inflammation. Mast cells can move like amoebae and many of them gather near the end of nerves of the autonomic nervous system. These nerves are concentrated on the basal membranes of capillaries so the mast cells are concentrated here as well. Within mast cells is a great variety of preformed biologically active chemicals. Sometimes mast cells selectively release chemicals. Under the influence of progesterone they release serotonin. Under the influence of estrogen they release histamines. When the mast cells degranulate their various chemicals are released. These react with other chemicals such as prostaglandins and leukotrienes and become extremely biologically active in the ground substance. It is mainly through degranulation, releasing their stored chemicals, that the mast cells direct the complete process of inflammation. They are rightly called one-celled endocrine glands and "the guards of the ground substance."

There is much reciprocal effect between nervous signals coming into the ground substance and structural constitution of the ground substance itself. This plays an important role in development, growth, the healing of injuries, and also in pathological processes such as inflammation and the formation of tumors. The autonomic terminal axons (nerve endings) and the mast cells of the ground substance influence each other directly. Any sort of shock causes the nerve endings to release catecholamines (adrenaline or epinephrine, noradrenaline, dopamine). These chemicals are needed to produce the central effect of inflammation—the degranulation of the mast cells. In the case of an allergic reaction or a septic condition in the tissues, the mast cells degranulate directly, which then causes the nerve endings to release catecholamines.

The capacity of the ground substance to become inflamed is dependent upon the intactness of the sensory innervation of the tissues. The signals from nerve endings travel toward the central nervous system. Along other branches of the same nerve some of these signals return to the cell from which they originated (the axon reflex). When the signals return, they cause the ends of these sensory nerves to release active chemicals including pain neuropeptides such as substance P (SP) and calcitonin gene-related peptide (CGRP). These cause the mast cells to degranulate and cause the macrophages, monocytes and neutrophils to go into attack mode and digest the infecting agents, substances, or tissue remnants. In the process enzymes, oxygen radicals and many mediating chemicals are released that promote the transformation of the composition and structure of the ground substance. SP also promotes the proliferation of T lymphocytes, the differentiation of the B lymphocytes and an increased production of immunoglobulins. Thus inflammation is partially controlled on a local scale in and near the affected tissues.

Sensory signals from the ground substance also have the task of signaling the central nervous system to stimulate the release of adrenaline, noradrenaline, acetylcholine, cytokines, neuropeptides, etc.

Furthermore, sensory nerves also act as receptors of immune-related chemicals. These toxins, antigens and antibodies are transported along the sensory axons to the central nervous system, evidently for processing there. This has an effect upon the central nervous system and the peripheral release of neurotransmitters and neuropeptides.

While struggling with this extremely complicated information, my partner suggested that the axon reflex and the transmission of immune-related substances, through sensory nerves to the nervous system for processing there, may be one of the reasons that people feel better and get well faster when lovingly stroked. Sometimes all this complex scientific nomenclature and information needs to be so translated into more human terms!

The system of ground regulation has four main systems of communication. One is chemical, as in the many processes described above. The others are electrical impulses through the nerves, electrochemical synapses (found between fibroblasts and between functional organ cells helping them to act together), and electromagnetic vibrations. Thus the wide variety and vast quantity of internal and external information is coded and exchanged in only these four ways. This simplification is necessary for the creation and maintenance of living systems. However, this also presents the danger of false transmission of information through genetic or environmental influences. And poor nutrition or environmental pollution can change the chemistry of the ground substance so that incoming signals are incorrectly processed. All this indicates that the genetic and environmental factors cannot be considered separately or simply additively. They are inseparably networked together in the ground substance.

No other system unites the huge amount of genetic, biochemical and environmental information like biological medicine with its basic foundation in the system of ground regulation. In this system, the individual is not only seen to be a product of his genetic composition, but rather is considered in the rich network of functional relationships of his DNA and the complete environment around it, including the mechanisms of the cell, the ground substance, the circulatory system, and the totality of the mental, emotional, and physical environment in which he lives.

For its biochemical survival, every organism requires the ability to rapidly construct, destroy and reconstruct the constituents of the ground substance. The ground substance itself has a polygonal net structure. The smallest unit of the ground substance is called the matrisome. The matrisome structure is oriented in a self-repetitive (redundant) manner through many anatomical layers of organization throughout the ground substance. No matrisome is identical to another but all have the same pattern of organization. A dividing plane through any matrisome yields a polygon. The matrisome may be imagined as a series of identical line drawings placed one over the other, with each one a bit more rotated and further away than the last (see the diagram). This creates the appearance of hyperboloid spiraling tunnels through the many layers (Heine, 1997, p. 52).

Between the molecules that make up the ground substance there are minimal surfaces. The formation of soap bubbles provides a well-known example of

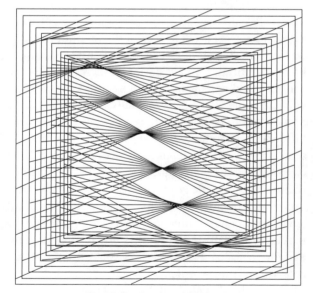

DIAGRAM OF A MATRISOME

the formation of minimal surfaces. Their spherical shape arises because it is the smallest possible surface that contains the volume of air that the soap bubble encompasses. When one dips a bent clothes hanger or other metal wire into a solution of soap, the so-formed soap membrane has a surface that describes the minimal surface connecting every point on the ring.

Between the molecules of the ground substance there are not only minimal physical surfaces like in a soap bubble but also minimal electrical surfaces. These surfaces are not minimal in size but rather in potential energy. Minimal electrical surfaces have a negative gaussian curvature like a saddle or folds in a skirt (Schnering, 1991).

The electrical charging and discharging of the materials of the ground substance cause electromagnetic field oscillations (photon fields). The interference of these fields creates short-lived (from $10-9$ to up to $10-5$ seconds) tunnels through the ground substance (Popp, 1987). Through these tunnels, shaped like the hole through a donut, large chemicals may traverse from capillaries through the ground substance and into the functional cells of organs and back again. All metabolic processes depend upon this transport mechanism.

The self-repetitive structure of the ground substance identifies it as a system of determined chaos. The cyclic appearance and disappearance of the tunnels through the matrisomes identifies them as attractors (Heine, 1997, p. 27). The spontaneous appearance of order in chaos and chaos in order is well known in chaos theory. The mathematics of minimal surfaces shows that tiny changes in one area can cause large changes in distant areas of the same (ground) substance. Coupling and resonance are qualities that always appear in the non-linear systems of determined chaos. Under the conditions of minimal surfaces as found in the ground substance, the energy of one single photon can cause extensive effects throughout the ground substance (Heine, 1997, p. 55). This is the likely explanation of the phenomena of homeopathy, acupuncture and bioresonance, in which the application of tiny stimuli may produce system-wide changes.

In order for a nerve to fire, a stimulus of about 60 millivolts must be applied. Pressure upon nerve receptors can create adequate voltage to fire the nerve cells. However, holding a homeopathic remedy or a gemstone near the body cannot logically cause the nerves to directly fire. And yet, AK muscle testing reveals that the body does selectively respond to such remedies, even through glass bottles. How is this possible? The ground substance requires only a shift of one electron to set up a process that can cause a nerve to fire. Apparently, holding some "energized" remedy near the body can be somehow registered in the extremely sensitive ground substance, which then evokes far-reaching responses throughout the body.

Many authors contend that remedies, gemstones, etc., have an electromagnetic field that affects the human body. Fritz A. Popp, a world authority on subtle biological energies, has another idea. In private conversations with the author, he agreed that there is no measurable electromagnetic field around such substances that could have an effect upon the body. He suggested that the effect might be due to some kind of "echo" phenomenon similar to sonar (for example, how a bat sends out auditory signals and maneuvers his flight according to the sound waves bouncing back). The human body produces various electromagnetic fields. Perhaps these pass through the remedy held in the hand and return to the body changed. This returning electromagnetic field may carry information specific to the remedy. This may cause changes in the ground substance that resonate through the body and brings about the changes revealed by muscle testing. But this theory can only be true if humans can be shown to have magnetic field receptors as yet unknown to science.

Many animals are capable of detecting the magnetic field of the earth and use it for orienting themselves. Birds migrate accurately using the magnetic field of the earth, even when cloudy weather prevents them from visually orienting themselves. In one experiment, humans were blindfolded, rotated so as to lose orientation, driven many miles from their original location, and then asked to point in the direction of the location where they were blindfolded. In the countryside, most people were able to do this fairly accurately. But when this experiment was repeated in a city, where trains, trams, electric wires, radios, etc., often produce fields far stronger than that of the earth, people were unable to orient themselves toward the point of origin. The ambient electromagnetic fields present in modern industrial life appear to disorient our electromagnetic receptors.

The eyes are electromagnetic receptors that respond to a small spectrum of wavelengths of electromagnetic radiation. With the exception of the eyes, scientists haven't yet discovered human electromagnetic field receptors and their neurophysiology. However, the above-described experiment indicates that we likely do have them. If so, then the following hypothesis could describe the modus operandi of many hitherto unexplained phenomena observed and applied by therapists who use AK:

1. The human hand has a small magnetic field.

2. All magnetic fields are circular, returning toward their source.

3. When a substance is held in the hand, the hand's own magnetic field passes through the substance.

4. The hand's magnetic field is altered by passing through the substance.

5. The altered field returns to the hand and is detected by the postulated electromagnetic field nerve sensors.

6. These nerve sensors fire in response to the received field.

7. The ground substance is affected by the received signal, either directly or through the secondary firing of nerves.

8. The whole body is affected by nervous system signaling and by the transmission of information through the system of ground regulation.

9. Thus the tiny stimulus of a substance held in the hand may have system-wide effects.

All the systems of the body are interconnected into a functional network. Like many pendula linked by springs, the various systems of the body have an energy coherence; they vibrate together. This creates and is an expression of order or health in the system. All chemical reactions create small electromagnetic energies. But major ordering energy structures in the body are created by the ground substance. One of these is collagen. The chains of collagen in the ground substance are not only able to conduct energy, they also generate energy themselves. Collagen has piezoelectric properties. Like quartz crystal, collagen in the ground substance and the more stable connective tissues (fascia, tendons, bones etc.) transforms mechanical energy (pressure, torsion, stretch) into electromagnetic energy, which then resonates through the ground substance (Athenstaedt, 1974). However, if the ground substance is chemically imbalanced, the energy resonating through the body loses coherence. For example, repeatedly feeding the body highly oxidative white flour or white sugar can cause such loss of coherence of energies with disastrous consequences for the body.

Any stressor (disease to a specific organ, trauma, focus) causes changes in the system of ground regulation in the local area. If this stress continues, other systems are affected until the system of ground regulation for the whole body becomes involved. This is what occurs in the adaptation response described by Hans Selye. In this condition, the body is then liable to break down under any new stress. For example, the extra stress caused by a chill may result in an attack of rheumatism. When the system of ground regulation is stressed and out of balance, the probability of the occurrence of chronic illness also increases.

Pischinger originated the concept of the system of ground regulation. He found that one main block to the function of the system of ground regulation is infection. The popular medical terminology is "focus of infection." The typical areas of focal infection include the tonsils, teeth, appendix and gall bladder. Further experimentation by Pischinger revealed that foci that block the function of the system of ground regulation include areas that have no infection such as scars and dead teeth. Such a tooth can be rotted out but upon examination is found to no longer contain any active infection. For this reason, already in the 1960s, Pischinger gave up the term "focus of infection" and replaced it with the term "focus." The treatment of scars with laser, neural therapy or various creams (Bach Rescue Cream®, APM Creme®, Ionen Salbe Forte®, etc.) may remove the disturbances that scars may produce. Dead teeth may be "provoked" with an osteitis nosode. If a long-term or extreme inflammation around the tooth results, it is advisable to have the tooth pulled. If the reaction heals quickly, the body can clear up the focus and the tooth may be able to stay without negatively influencing the health.

Since foci interfere with the system of ground regulation and thus with the health of an organism, removing foci is of utmost importance in the healing process. This may involve surgically removing dead teeth or an organ, or removing pathogenic agents and fetid matter from an organ such as the large intestine in order to restore it to normal function.

Organisms are energetically open, highly networked systems. Open systems are generally capable of rhythmic oscillation. Biorhythms are an example of such rhythms (Heine, 1997, pp. 18–20). Open systems require a regular input of energy in a form that they can utilize and which can dissipate throughout the system (food). They are feedback-coupled, which defines them as non-linear. Because of this they are capable of self-organization. That means that although they seem to be without fixed rules and no accurate long-term prognosis can be made, they do have an ordered structure (determined chaos). This order is characterized by coherence, meaning that they, like a laser, contain phase and frequency-identical bundles of energy.

The order within an organism is maintained by a coherence of electromagnetic field oscillations. These arise from reactions within the body and from electromagnetic fields in the environment. The most important fields within the body are created by the piezoelectric and pyroelectric qualities of collagen located in the ground substance and in all connective tissues. There are many levels of electromagnetic fields within the body. Atoms at body temperature vibrate at more than 10–15 Hz. Molecules (groups of atoms) vibrate at about 10–9 Hz. Cells (groups of molecules) vibrate near 10–3 Hz. The human organism as a whole vibrates with a frequency between 7 and 10 Hz. Thus the community of cells and ground substance also vibrates at 7–10 Hz.

These frequencies are found in nature as well. The atmosphere between the surface of the earth and the ionosphere forms a resonant body with a resonant frequency from 8–10 Hz (Schumann, 1954). This means that all electrical discharges around the earth are damped except for those of 8–10 Hz (the main Schumann frequency), which can resonate freely and extend around the earth (Bergsman, 1994). We live within this constant, vibrating field. This rate of vibration can be detected upon the surface of the brain and especially in the hippocampus, an ancient brain structure in vertebrate animals that uses smell and visual input to direct behavior. In the hippocampus the decision is made as to whether a situation is of emotional importance or not. In mammals and especially in humans, the hippocampus is connected to the limbic system (including the hypothalamus) that controls the emotional reactions and the function of memory. As the hypothalamus is the main director of the autonomic nervous system and directs the functions of the master gland, the pituitary, anything that affects its function has far-reaching effects upon health and behavior.

It is highly possible that the human body as a whole, and the hippocampus specifically, vibrate at this rate because of having evolved within the Schumann waves upon the surface of the earth. In this way at least, we are in resonant harmony with our environment. However, in industrial countries, humans are subjected to powerful electromagnetic fields of similar frequency. For example, the alternating-current electricity that powers trains in Europe has a frequency of 15 Hz. It is likely that these external electromagnetic fields have a negative effect upon brain and other bodily functions. We are the first few generations to be subjected to such human-generated fields. It may take a number of generations before we become aware of the consequences that such fields produce upon human structure and functioning.

The hypothalamus directly and indirectly controls the release of neurotransmitters and related chemicals called neuropeptides. The hypothalamus is the area of the brain where emotions are generated. Via the hypothalamus, emotional states cause the release of a great variety of neuropeptides including adrenaline, serotonin, dopamine, endorphin, insulin and glutamine. These directly affect the ground substance and thereby the health of the whole body. Specific neuropeptides are generated in the brain and travel through the nerves to target organs. Some of these are disease-preventing. Others promote disease in the target organ. It seems likely that this is one of the ways that emotional states affect health.

Research by Heine indicates that unresolved emotional traumas cause the release of the neurotransmitter substance P from nerve endings in the junction of muscles and tendons. This causes the collagen to take on a hexagonal structure, which he has observed under the electron microscope. This hexagonal form of collagen is far more ordered than the forms collagen normally has in the body. And as we have discussed, too much (or too little) structure means death. This form of collagen is present in the exact areas of the pain produced by fibromyalgia. Heine refers to this overly-structured collagen as an "emotional scar." (Heine, 1990, pp. 127–159). His breakthrough research provides an important scientific verification that diseases can have psychological causes.

Many electromagnetic fields originate within the body. All chemical reactions generate electromagnetic fields. Some of the most important electromagnetic fields are generated in the ground substance and in the related connective tissues. Collagen fibers are piezoelectric and pyroelectric. This means that stretched or warmed, they produce an electrical potential. The collagen fibers and the sugar-protein complexes that are attached to them bind water and electrically charged metal ions in the ground substance. Together they function as bio-sensors that signal electrically the smallest changes that occur within the organism. Collagen fibers are diodes; they allow electrons to pass through them in only one direction. Collagen fibers in the ground substance are arranged so that some of them allow energy to move toward the cells (afferent) and others provide an electrical path away from the cells (efferent). So defined, the afferent paths of collagen fibers bring the coherent electromagnetic energy from the neuronal net of the ground substance into the cells. The efferent paths send energy out of the cells into the ground substance.

The bio-sensor network in the ground substance is quite different from other typical electric circuits characterized by a classical cause-effect and yes-no logic. A normal network will fail when any of its components fails. Until measured values reach a defined critical level, no correction occurs. The biosensor network functions in quite a different manner, one that can be best described by a concept from quantum physics termed "fuzzy logic" (Heine, 1997, p. 143). Fuzzy logic is used in modern video cameras to produce a stable picture. This is effectively a kind of "camera homeostasis" that maintains a steady picture even when the camera is held unsteadily. Working on a "when-then" rule, fuzzy logic networks are very robust. Many parts can fail but the function itself, though reduced in intensity, does not suddenly fail. Such systems only step-wise lose their capacity to function. Thus, even under duress, the bio-sensor network allows the ground substance to continually make small "when-then" type adjustments to maintain bodily homeostasis. When such a system has suffered partial debilitation, internal repair mechanisms or external therapy can usually return it to full function.

The biosensors are set to recognize patterns, not absolute values. This provides a good example for comparing the parallel differences between Newtonian and quantum mechanics on one hand and between classical and biological medicine on the other hand. Classical medicine looks for absolute values. If you complain of discomfort, one of mainstream or "school" medicine's major tools is laboratory analysis of the current condition of your blood. If your blood sugar, for example, is found to be above a specific level, that constitutes a specific problem. School medicine characteristically then prescribes a specific chemical to offset this rise. Thus it tends to treat the symptom, often without seriously looking for an underlying cause and only very rarely looking for possible multiple causes.

By contrast, biological medicine looks for connections among the patterns in behavior, structure and functioning. Health is considered to depend upon the continual monitoring and correcting of the intake of nutrients and water, exercise, electromagnetic fields, the social situation and all the various inner and outer factors that have an effect upon the ground substance. By testing for all likely causative factors, often with the techniques of Applied Kinesiology, the biological medicine practitioner develops a much broader picture of what is amiss throughout the patient's entire system. He or she is then in a position to treat causes rather than symptoms. The practitioner is able not only to effect immediate corrective measures, but also to instruct a patient that with the concepts of biological medicine, every day one has the chance to make choices that improve the quality of the ground substance and thereby one's overall health.

The combination of collagen fibers and sugar-protein complexes produces its highest piezoelectric energy values at 37° C, the temperature of the human body. And the liquid crystal molecular structure of water is highly ordered with minimum energy also at 37°. This combination allows signaling to traverse the watery medium of the ground substance of the human body easily and with practically no energy loss and no consequent warming (Heine, 1997, p. 142). Thus a disturbance anywhere in the body is registered almost immediately everywhere within the body.

This transfer of energy through the ground substance allows information transfer throughout the body. Without it life would cease! In addition, for life to be possible, there needs to be a difference of temperature between the cell and the intercellular spaces occupied by the ground substance. In fact, the cells must be warmer than the ground substance. When the difference is small, metabolic processes take longer to occur. When the difference is zero, metabolic processes don't occur at all, which means death. Since all life processes occur through the ground substance, it is important that the energy- and heat-producing chemical processes of the ground substance require less energy than those of the cell.

The functions of the ground substance form a system of regulation for the whole body. This system of ground regulation contains various levels of subsystems that, while relatively independent, have an effect upon and are affected by the whole system and all of its parts. This fractal repetition of patterns of function on many levels is typical of all non-linear systems of determined chaos, as discussed earlier in this chapter.

Acupuncture points have a functional connection with the system of ground regulation. The concept of the acupuncture "point" once hindered research greatly. G. Kellner, under the direction of Pischinger at the University of Vienna, searched for special nerve endings in the skin that might be the physical aspects of acupuncture points. He came to the conclusion that there is no definite physical structure corresponding to acupuncture points (Kellner, 1979).

However, in the Mandarin Chinese language, the word translated as "point" (Xue-Wei) actually means "hole." Applying this literal translation has proved to be more fruitful in defining acupuncture points. Indeed, 82% of the 361 classical acupuncture points have been found to be located over perforations of the superficial body fascia. The smallest (e.g. Lung 8) are about 2 mm in diameter. The largest (e.g. Bladder 52) are about 8 mm. Most the remaining 18% are over other kinds of perforations through bones and dura mater or in other well-marked anatomical areas. In all cases, the acupuncture points consist of a small bundle of nerves and blood vessels wrapped in a loose coating of connective tissue that penetrates other tissues to reach near the surface of the skin (Heine, 1997, pp. 179–186; Zerlauth, 1992).

Both the water and chemical contents of this bundle of blood vessels and nerves are electrically conductive. In comparison, fascia tissues are electrically resistant. For this reason, acupuncture points have a greater conductivity than other points on the skin. Small devices for measuring electric conductivity are popular for locating the exact position of acupuncture points. As we shall see, groups of acupuncture points (meridians) are associated with the function of particular organs and operations in the body and therefore may be meaningfully assigned to particular systems of regulation. When the system of regulation associated with the particular acupuncture point is out of balance, the electrical conductivity of the point will change measurably and the point may become painful to the touch ("trigger points"). Proper stimulation of such "active" points may have profound therapeutic effects upon the system of regulation. Thus the acupuncture points are a window for detecting and affecting the functioning of the systems of regulation (Bergsman, 1990).

In traditional Chinese medicine, the acupuncture points are connected by lines that we in the West refer to as *meridians*. The acupuncture points of a meridian lie along muscles and tendons that are connected with each other. These muscle groups work together in producing specific bodily movements. Therefore the muscles and related connective tissues (fascia and tendons) upon which the meridians are located are referred to functionally as kinetic chains. This has been demonstrated by Bergsmann and Bergsmann (1988) and further developed by Stecco (1996) in electro-myographic studies. These authors showed that during simple motions such as straightening the arm, the frequency of muscle contraction potentials along the complete chain of fascia-muscle-tendon increased, even in muscles not involved in the motion. Furthermore, stimulation of "active" acupuncture points may cause pain to appear at areas remote from the points but always along the related chain of muscles and connective tissue.

In neural therapy, painful trigger points are injected with a local anesthetic. This causes a temporary equilibration of energy potential between the nerves and the ground substance in the area, which temporarily inhibits the pain. This can also promote a lasting regeneration of the local ground regulation that eliminates the disturbing symptoms. Simply placing a needle (without injecting any substance) into the point creates a short-circuit between the nerves and the ground substance with similar results. Moreover, the process of healing the tiny wound produced by the needle involves an inflammation; a prolonged, complex, bio-chemical process which produces a continuing therapeutic stimulation in the area where the needle was placed.

The chains of muscles and connective tissue upon which the acupuncture points are located are the physical carriers of the meridians of oriental medicine. Goodheart's research has correlated the various muscles, glands and other organs of the body and their function into fourteen groups associated with the fourteen major meridians of oriental acupuncture. All AK treatments are aimed at affecting one or more of these fourteen systems.

Based upon the work of Pischinger, it is indicated to define any area of the body that is connected to a specific meridian-organ system as belonging to one (sub-)system of regulation. So defined, it is the work of AK to determine and correct whatever is interfering with the function of these fourteen systems of regulation. By specifically correcting imbalances, the ground substance in these systems is improved in quality and function.

Hauss (1994) determined that there is an "unspecified reaction of the mesenchyme" in the most common diseases of the industrially developed countries. Mesenchyme is the mother of all the connective tissues including the ground substance. Which disease and which organ is affected depend upon genetic factors, the type of stress or injury, and the individual stress factors such as foci, nutrition and disturbing fields of energy.

All the techniques of biological medicine have the same goal: to improve the function of the ground substance. In the multi-dimensional approach of biological medicine, all the various factors that influence the ground substance are considered in the diagnosing and prescribing of corrective measures for any illness. These methods promote the health and optimal functioning of the ground substance through personal attention to the individual and all aspects or his or her life situation.

AK provides an ideal diagnostic method for biological medicine. Individual stresses may cause weakness or hypertonicity in the muscles associated with the affected system of regulation. Sufficient stress of any kind will eventually cause the body to go into an adaptation reaction. This is usually accompanied by general hypertonicity and blocks many functions of the ground substance throughout the body. Much of the primary work in modern AK (at least in the ICAK-D) has the goal of removing the blocks to the function of the system of ground regulation as revealed by muscle testing.

The various causes of disturbance to any of the systems of regulation can be determined by testing the items that make a normotonic or a hypertonic muscle related to that system test weak. For example, if the rectus femoris (which correlates with the small intestine) tests hypertonic, a tiny quantity of candida antigen may be placed upon the tongue. If the hypertonic muscle now tests weak, there is very likely an overgrowth of candida in the small intestine

that needs attention. If muscles test hypertonic because of histamine-related allergies, holding a bottle of histidine will likely make the hypertonic muscle test weak. And holding a bottle of histamine in homeopathic dilution D 12 will likely make the hypertonic muscle test normotonic. The various methods of improving the health of a system of regulation can be similarly determined by using a weak-testing muscle from that system and testing what makes it normotonic.

In the example above, the rectus femoris was made weak by placing candida antigen upon the tongue. If the candida antigen remains upon the tongue, the rectus femoris will continue to test weak, making it an excellent indicator for possible anti-candida treatments. The anti-candida substance (lapacho, grapefruit seed oil, Nystatin®, Ampho-Moronal®, etc.) that makes the rectus femoris normotonic is the one that will work best for this particular patient (Gerz, 1996, p. 291). If no weak-testing muscle from that system can be located, therapy localization to the affected organ or bodily area itself may be used to provide a weak-testing indicator muscle related to the chosen system of regulation. These genial and simple techniques are rapidly making AK the tool of choice for diagnosis and for determining the proper individual treatment in biological medicine today.

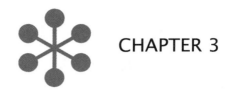 **CHAPTER 3**

The Muscle Test

Theory, Procedure, and Interpretation of Muscle Testing

Muscle testing is the central tool of Applied Kinesiology. Muscle testing, when performed with the necessary sensory awareness and experience, accurately tests the physiological reaction of the muscle, its nerve receptors, and the nerves involved with its contraction. It is a strong muscle test, requiring activation of the full strength of the muscle tested. It is a patient-initiated muscle test, which gives the examiner the full responsibility of reacting correctly by applying equal counterpressure to the patient's continually increasing pressure. Since the patient initiates the test and the examiner responds, the patient does not have to be specially trained before being tested.

For those who muscle test and have so far tested in ways that differ from the AK muscle test technique, a study of AK techniques and a comparison of the results may bring an enlightening surprise and enrichment. In the sort of muscle testing that one learns in a Touch for Health course, the examiner initiates the test pressure. The responsibility is placed upon the client to react correctly to the examiner's slowly increasing, gentle pressure. (Touch for Health practitioners have "clients" not "patients"). For this procedure, the client must first be taught how to react correctly. Since (hopefully) the examiner has more experience than the client/patient, the chances of

something going wrong and creating false results in muscle testing are smaller with Applied Kinesiology muscle testing.

Perhaps both types of muscle testing have their own particular merits and areas of application. Be that as it may, it behooves any serious student of kinesiology to study and learn the original concepts and techniques of Applied Kinesiology. In any field of endeavor, it is wise to go to the source first, before exploring the value of subsequent diversions.

To perform an Applied Kinesiology muscle test, the bones attached to each end of the muscle are positioned to place the muscle into a partial or a complete contraction. The test position is chosen to make the tested muscle the prime mover with as little synergistic help from other muscles as possible. The test position and the point of contact are also chosen to give the examiner a clear mechanical advantage. This ensures that the examiner can almost always be able to more than match the strength of the pressure applied by the patient. Exceptions occur when a lightly built examiner tests a powerful and heavily muscled patient.

The examiner makes a broad soft contact with his hand upon an area of the body appropriate for exerting pressure against the contraction of the desired muscle. This is usually upon the distal (away from the trunk) end of the bone upon which the insertion of the muscle is attached. When possible, direct pressure upon joints or bones lying near the skin is avoided. Care is taken that pain is not produced in the area where the test pressure is applied. The examiner must continually increase the counter-pressure, but only fast enough to exactly match the steadily increasing pressure exerted by the patient. Any muscle will test weak, even with a small amount of pressure, if the counter-pressure is applied by the examiner too rapidly.

In Applied Kinesiology muscle testing, the patient receiving the muscle test contracts the muscle tested with increasing force until maximum force is achieved. The examiner provides resistance, in a direction exactly opposite that produced by the patient's contraction of the muscle, to maintain the limb or other body part in its original test position. The critical part of an Applied Kinesiology muscle test is a subsequent attempt by the examiner to move the insertion away from the origin and thus extend the contracted muscle. When the examiner senses that the patient has "locked" the joint against his test pressure, i.e., has reached a maximal or near maximal strength of contraction in the muscle tested, the examiner presses a bit (only 2–5%) more firmly. Either the patient can match this extra pressure and the body part remains in position (the muscle tests strong), or she can't resist this extra pressure and the body part tested moves away from the initial test position (the muscle tests weak.)

In the first stage of the muscle test, the examiner and patient exert identical counter-pressures and the muscle contracts without movement (isometric contraction). In the second part of the muscle test, the examiner pushes past the patient's maximal isometric contraction and begins to lengthen the patient's muscle (eccentric contraction). To maintain the initial test position, the patient must exert more than her maximal strength. How could this be possible to accomplish?

The maximal strength one can willingly exert is less than the amount available in a stress situation. When a child or pet is under a car, people can and have lifted cars. This strength goes far beyond what they are capable of doing in normal circumstances. We have a reserve of energy (estimated to be at least 30%) above what is willfully available. The second part of the muscle test requires that the patient muscularly resist more than she normally can, which puts her into stress. Thus, the muscle test examines if she can involuntarily access some of this extra reserve of energy available for stress situations.

For AK muscle testing to function, the one receiving the muscle test (the patient) must mentally agree to being tested and decide to resist the pressures applied. The pressure upon her limb will then be monitored by various nerve receptors in her muscle (tendons, ligaments, joints, and skin) and transmitted through the sensory nerves to the central nervous system. The central nervous system processes this incoming nerve signal and generates the needed signal to resist the test pressure. This signal is then transmitted through the motor nerves to the muscle being tested. The muscle reacts by contracting. Ordinarily, a muscle will be unable to resist the test pressure if any link of its nervous and muscular circuit is malfunctioning. In this case, it is said to test weak.

It is easy for an experienced examiner to differentiate between weak-testing muscles and normotonic muscles. A normotonic muscle being tested feels like pushing upon a wall. The muscles lock the bones in place without a great sense of effort, and can resist the extra pressure applied after the muscles reach maximal conscious contraction. On the other hand, a weak-testing muscle soon gives way and feels mushy or melting.

A "weak-testing" muscle is not necessarily the same as a muscle that is muscularly weak. Physically strengthening a truly weak muscle requires weeks of fitness training. Correcting a weak-testing muscle so that it tests strong usually requires only moments. This is the unusual and valuable basis for the muscle testing and strengthening techniques. And fitness training proceeds more rapidly and with less chance of injury when the muscles test strong in muscle testing.

Applied Kinesiology muscle testing does test if the muscle can exert a reasonable degree of brute muscular strength. The patient is given every possible advantage. She starts the test and increases the pressure at her own rate. During the first part of the test, she need not adapt to the examiner. On the contrary, it is the examiner's responsibility to exert an equal and opposite steadily increasing isometric pressure. The examiner must then be able to estimate when the strength of contraction in the muscle tested approaches maximum. Although brute strength is a factor measured here, it is not the most important factor being tested. Brute strength is a measure of how much weight or force the muscle can support. Sequentially lifting objects of increasing weight until the patient reaches the maximum that can be lifted into the test position would be one way to measure the brute weight-bearing strength of the muscle. Placing a weight upon the patient that he must support upon his outstretched arm would be another way to measure brute strength. In both these examples, the weight is taken by the patient all at once. Therefore the force upon the patient, after taking the weight, remains constant. During muscle testing, the force is constantly increasing.

In the second part of the test, muscle testing measures the capacity of patient's nervous system plus the "system of ground regulation" (Pischinger, 1975) to automatically call upon reserve energy to match the extra test pressure applied after the normal maximal contraction has been reached. At this stage, muscle testing measures how well the nervous system is monitoring and responding to the test. It is at this point that the muscle tests strong (holds) or weak (gives way). However, some patients will be unable to attain the beginning position of the test or apply pressure at all. A muscle in this condition is also considered to have tested weak, though more extremely so.

All people have, at least under certain conditions, "weak-testing" muscles. Making these muscles test normotonic again is one of the main goals of Applied Kinesiology. The so-called strengthening of a weak-testing muscle

is actually a fine-tuning of the nervous system's awareness and control of the body. This conditioning process produces a higher level of personal functioning. For a discussion of muscles that test "too strong," see the section "General Hypertonicity" page 93.

Examiner Prejudice or Impartiality

The responsible examiner will try to keep an open mind at all times concerning the new discoveries and developments in AK. This openness should also extend to his or her muscle testing of patients. As soon as the examiner expects the muscle should test strong or weak, this thought is likely to influence the results of muscle testing.

Even well-known professional therapists can become prejudiced about the outcome of their muscle testing and thereby arrive at misleading results. In an example of this, John Diamond, who made Applied Kinesiology popular through his books and who works exclusively with the "delta" muscle (the middle deltoids), was convinced that everyone would test weak with white sugar in their mouths. The one exception, he contended, occurs if the patient is "switched" (see Neurologic Disorganization, page 84). When other examiners tested this hypothesis, not

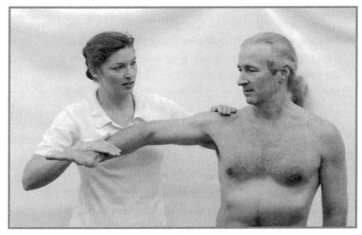

THE ARM PULL-DOWN OR "DELTA" TEST

knowing whether the test patient had the sugar in his mouth or not, the same results were not obtained. Indeed, in cases of low blood sugar, white sugar was found to sometimes even strengthen weak-testing muscles. If one desires dependable results in muscle testing, if one desires to determine the true reaction to the stimulus, it is best to avoid having opinions as to the expected outcome.

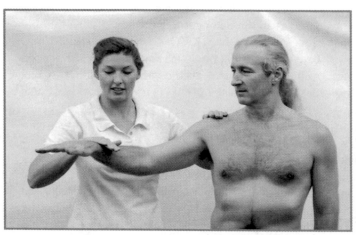

THE DELTA MUSCLE TEST WITH SHOULDER ROTATION

Beyond the problem of prejudice in the examiner, many therapists who use AK contend that the delta muscle test itself, which John Diamond uses exclusively, is one of the least reliable muscle tests. Since the patient may rotate the shoulder (consciously or unconsciously) without changing the position of the hand, this change of the parameters of the test may go unnoticed. Since such a change brings other muscle fibers into play in the muscle test, the results may vary from test to test.

When the examiner wants or fears a specific result in muscle testing, his mental-emotional state will change how he tests. He may press in a slightly different direction or with a different pressure or velocity. Mental intention may also influence the results of muscle testing. The examiner should be pleased when the results are not always as he expects. This likely indicates that the results of his muscle testing are not being controlled by his prejudices. An excellent examiner has only neutral curiosity, not preconceptions. He is interested only in finding out what is true, not in proving his own preconceptions to be correct.

Applications of Muscle Testing

There are two applications of muscle testing. In the first as described above, one tests various muscles without permitting any other stimulus to be involved *(muscle testing in the clear)*. In this type of muscle testing, one is simply investigating the functional integrity of the complete circuit of that portion of the nervous system involved with that muscle, the "system of ground regulation" (Pischinger), plus the function of the muscle itself. This type of muscle testing is taught in standard medical school curricula. For example, after an injury to the spine, a doctor will test the muscles connected to nerves that emerge from the spine near the area of the injury. If these muscles test weak, this is considered evidence that the injury has pinched or damaged the nerve activating the weak-testing muscle.

In the second type of muscle testing, one uses a muscle that tests normotonic in the clear as an *indicator muscle* to assess various possible problems and functions. For example, the examiner can apply a "challenge" by presenting the patient with some kind of stimulus (nutrition, medicine, allergen, emotion, assuming poor posture, stressful memory, etc.). and check the effect of this challenge upon the results of muscle testing. Also, if a patient touches a bodily area where a problem exists, a previously normotonic indicator muscle will usually test weak. This phenomenon, wherein the muscle's test strength may be affected by the patient touching himself or herself, is known as "therapy localization." Therapy localization is actually a "touch challenge." Much of the magic of AK lies in the fact that most factors that influence health may be tested using an indicator muscle with challenge or therapy localization.

Challenge

Challenge, in Applied Kinesiology, is a diagnostic tool used to test the body's reaction to stimuli as measured by manual muscle testing. The stimuli may be either positive or negative and affect the structure of the body, the chemistry of the body, or the functions of the mind. Challenge reveals the interplay of the three sides of the triad of health (structural, chemical, mental). By applying a challenge to one side of the triad, factors of another side may be significantly altered. Some kinds of challenge will affect the test strength of any muscle in the body. Other kinds of challenge will selectively affect specific muscles only.

In conjunction with muscle testing, challenge helps the examiner to discover the underlying factors and corrective measures for any disturbance. In general, any challenge that can correct a problem will strengthen and make normotonic a muscle that tests weak because of the problem, when the correction implied by that challenge is appropriately implemented.

That which will make a problem worse will weaken most normotonic muscles. When a muscle tests weak due to any kind of problem, challenge may be employed to locate the needed corrective measure. Any challenge that causes the weak-testing muscle associated with a problem to become normotonic will help to correct the problem. With challenge, Applied Kinesiology provides a unique method of diagnosis that enables the therapist to determine both the type of disturbance to the organism and the precise type of treatment best suited to the particular patient. And after the application of therapeutic measures, one may similarly challenge the correction to see if it had the desired effect.

Originally, Goodheart used the word "challenge" only to refer to the effect (upon simultaneous or subsequent muscle testing) caused by pushing upon bones. Today, the meaning of the word challenge has been extended to include anything that occurs to the patient between two muscle tests.

For their training of medical doctors in AK, the German-speaking AK association has created the following definition of "challenge."

Definition of Challenge (IMAK)

In AK, challenge refers to the testing of one or more muscles during or immediately after a chosen provocation or other application of a stimulus. With challenge the patient is stimulated with a chosen structural, chemical or mental test stimulus.

Types of Challenge:

1. Structural/Mechanical

    a) Vertebrae and pelvis
    b) Cranial bones and the stomatognathic system of head, neck and jaw.
    c) Musculature
    d) Joints of the extremities
    e) Inner organs (visceral osteopathy)
    f) Skin

2. Considered in the largest sense possible, with challenge, we can examine how a patient reacts to any kind of stimulus. The stimulus can be any kind of disturbing factor but can also be a medicine or supporting factor. In this case we needn't necessarily use the known correspondences of muscles, organs and meridians, but rather work with an "indicator muscle" according to the following principle:

Possible Reactions of an Indicator Muscle to Challenge

A weak-testing muscle can
– Stay weak-testing, become hypertonic, or become normotonic

A normotonic muscle can
– Become weak-testing, stay normotonic, or become hypertonic

A hypertonic muscle can
– Become weak-testing, become normotonic, or stay hypertonic

The following areas can be investigated:

• Medicines and all other kinds of healing remedies

• Disturbing fields or foci

• Allergens and other substances that the body has difficulty digesting or otherwise processing

• Toxins

• Psychological problems

• All other stress-causing factors (environmental, geopathic, etc.)

The results of examination with challenge should be compared with the clinical experience, the physiology and with good common sense. Above all, with difficult decisions or examinations, this is urgently recommended. In no case should AK-examination be used alone as the single diagnostic method. (Gerz, 1996, page 66).

In order to perform challenge correctly, the examiner needs to know what to look for. As Goodheart often said, "You can only find what you know." The success of applying challenge lies in knowing what to challenge for and how to perform the challenge precisely and adequately. Anything that causes too much stress to the organism should, when tested correctly, produce a positive challenge.

There are four major forms of challenge:

• Structural or mechanical

• Emotional

• Functional-neurological

• Chemical-physical/Energetic-electromagnetic

1. STRUCTURAL OR MECHANICAL CHALLENGE

In this kind of challenge, the examiner can test the structures named in the definition above (a–f). There are three sub-divisions of this category:

The sustained (or static) challenge,

The dynamic (rebound and non-rebound) challenge, and

The respiratory challenge.

The Sustained (or Static) Challenge

Definition: "A sustained or static challenge is a form of mechanical challenge in which one or more structures of the body are moved and remain in the new position until the following AK muscle tests are completed." (Gerz, 1996, page 69.)

In the "sustained" challenge, the effect of a change of position or the application of a static pressure upon the body is tested. It is often observed in AK examination that muscles that were strengthened while the patient was lying become weak-testing again when the patient stands. Thus in this example, standing is a sustained mechanical challenge. Mechanical challenge may also be used to determine if various kinds of physiotherapy would be useful to the patient. Statically pressing and holding a subluxated (out of position) bone in the direction it needs to go will strengthen a muscle that tests weak due to the subluxation.

The Dynamic (Rebound and Non-Rebound) Challenge

Definition: "A dynamic challenge is a mechanical challenge in which one or more structures of the body are actively or passively moved and then released before or during an AK muscle test." (Gerz, 1996, page 68.)

An example of a positive dynamic challenge that is often encountered in AK examination is the return of weak-testing muscles after walking, climbing stairs, or some other physical activity is performed.

Classical osteopathy calls all problems between bones "lesions." German manual therapists call these "Blockierung". Certain schools of American chiropractors further divide these lesions into "subluxations" and "fixations." Goodheart studied in one of these chiropractic schools. For these reasons, AK also divides lesions between bones into the subgroups of subluxations and fixations.

a) Subluxations

When the two bones that meet in a joint (articulation) of the extremities are not in proper alignment (a subluxation), stress is produced by movements of the articulation. In such a case, a structural challenge (movement of the two bones by the examiner) can reveal both the existence of the subluxation and the direction of the corrective thrust needed to realign the bones. In practice, most examiners test articulations of the extremities by pushing the two bones in opposite directions, releasing them and then subsequently testing if this challenge weakens an indicator muscle. Unless they have an assistant, they don't have enough hands to hold this new position static while they test an indicator muscle. So, as performed, this is a type of dynamic challenge. But unlike challenges of the vertebrae, pelvic and cranial sutures, the rebound effect is not being tested. Gerz calls this type of challenge a "non-rebound challenge."

If a specific muscle tests weak because of the subluxation, the non-rebound challenge direction that most strengthens the muscle is the correct adjustment direction. This is the preferred technique. If such a muscle cannot be located, or cannot be tested, almost any muscle of the body that tests normotonic in the clear may be chosen as an indicator muscle. In this case, the joint is challenged to determine the direction that most weakens the indicator muscle. This is the direction in which the joint is subluxated. The adjustment is then performed in the opposite direction. In both cases, the adjustment is performed in a direction toward the natural position of the bones involved. For this reason, it is called a "direct" correction. Classical chiropractic technique is to perform one or more single strong thrusts in the correction direction. Some examiners prefer to press gently and wait until the body releases and goes back to its natural position. When successful, such an adjusting thrust or more gentle mobilization brings the bones back into proper orientation, and further challenge of the joint will no longer weaken the indicator muscle.

b) Fixations

Definition: In AK, a fixation refers to a dysfunction between two or more bones without being out of normal alignment. Sometimes vertebrae become locked together (fixated), preventing motion between them. Unlike to subluxations, fixations cannot be

Challenge of a Subluxation of an Extremity

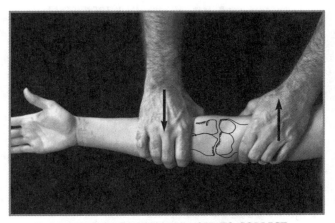

THE DIRECTION OF PRESSURE USED TO CORRECT
A SUBLUXATION WILL STRENGTHEN A MUSCLE
THAT TESTS WEAK BECAUSE OF THE SUBLUXATION

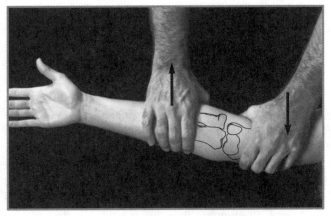

THE DIRECTION OF PRESSURE THAT INCREASES
A SUBLUXATION WILL WEAKEN MOST
STRONG-TESTING INDICATOR MUSCLES

detected by TL to the area alone (Gerz 1996, p. 203). Sometimes adjacent vertebrae are immobile because of muscular and proprioceptor disturbances in the area. They are then said to be in fixation. Movement between them is reduced or absent altogether. Such fixations cannot be identified by TL alone. To check for such fixations, the examiner may palpate the vertebrae for freedom of movement, or dynamically challenge the suspect vertebrae by pushing them simultaneously in opposite directions. This may be accomplished in a general way by applying TL to the area while the patient flexes and extends that part of the spine. To do so more specifically, the tip (spinous process) of one vertebrae may be pushed to the left and the tip of the next one to the right with a twisting pressure applied by the examiner's thumb and first finger. Neither the patient flexion (or extension) nor the twisting pressure applied by the examiner need to be held during the subsequent testing. In both cases, the TL to the suspect area must be applied during the motion and be continued while muscle-testing an indicator muscle. If the motion of the spine causes the indicator muscle to weaken, a fixation may exist between the vertebrae in the area moved. To correct a fixation, one of the involved vertebrae must be stabilized while the next one is moved. An audible release (crack) may be heard when the fixed vertebrae move apart from one another. However, the correction may occur without a sound being produced.

The Rebound Challenge
The Respiratory Challenge

The term "rebound challenge" is in itself illogical. In reality, rebound is not a form of challenge, but rather a possible reaction to a dynamic challenge applied to a specific part of the body. Be that as it may, the term "rebound challenge" is utilized in AK to refer to a dynamic challenge used to determine the direction for correction of misaligned vertebrae, cranial or pelvic bones. The bone in question is pushed with 0.5–3 kg pressure and then released. Then a normotonic indicator muscle is tested for weakening. The direction of

pressure that most weakens the indicator muscle is the direction for the corrective thrusts or gentle manipulations. Then the patient holds various phases of respiration while the direction of most positive challenge is repeated. The test may look like this:

1. The patient breathes halfway in and holds his breath. The examiner presses the bone in the previously weakening direction and tests the indicator muscle.

2. This process is repeated while the patient breathes fully in and then holds his breath.

3. This process is repeated while the patient breathes half out and then holds his breath.

4. This process is repeated while the patient breathes fully out and then holds his breath.

In one of these phases of respiration, the muscle will not weaken. In AK, the corrective thrusts are provided gently and repeatedly in the direction that previously weakened the indicator muscle while the phase of respiration that abolished the indicator muscle weakening is held by the patient.

Notice that in this example, the phase of respiration is a "respiratory challenge." Since the breath is held, it is also a kind of sustained challenge. When holding a phase of respiration alone causes an indicator muscle to weaken, cranial faults (or problems with the diaphragm or other muscles involved in breathing) are indicated. The specific phase of breath that makes an indicator muscle test weak or a weak-testing muscle test strong indicates the specific kind of cranial fault. For the exact correspondences, challenges and corrections, the reader is directed to the literature (Walther, 1983, Vol. II; Gerz, 1996, pp. 195–219). After respiratory challenge has revealed the presence of a cranial fault, it is then confirmed by challenging the fault. Note that simple cranial suture faults will therapy-localize, but most cranial faults will not. Therefore, the presence of cranial faults must be confirmed by challenge.

Originally in AK, the phenomena of rebound challenge were explained as follows: Pushing the bone toward its normal position further stretches the overly tight muscles that are holding it out of position. It was believed that when the bone is released, these muscles respond by temporarily tightening even further, which pulls the already subluxated bone further out of position, causing enough stress that indicator muscles subsequently test weak. This is the "rebound" aspect of this kind of challenge. This belief still appears to be correct with respect to vertebral and sacral subluxations and simple sutural faults of the cranium, but not with other cranial faults or faults of the extremities.

Formerly in AK, it was believed that the direction of positive rebound challenge to a cranial bone indicated the direction the bone needed to move to return to its natural position. However, osteopaths correct such cranial faults in exactly the opposite direction! This discrepancy was solved by AK changing its wording to "we are moving the bone into further lesion and accompanying it back into its correct position." By taking the phase of respiration that abolishes the positive challenge, this AK technique does work. But the description of the technique and how it functions needed to be changed to be in agreement with osteopathy and with the actual physiology involved. For this reason, the term "rebound challenge" is also being questioned and redefined. What examiners using AK do with cranial faults may be more accurately described as a kind of "rebound correction!" The cranial bone is not pushed toward its natural position but rather pushed toward further lesion on the phase of breath that neutralizes the positive TL. For this reason, this method is called an "indirect" correction. It appears in this case that the therapist is pushing the cranial bone into greater lesion while the held phase of breath is providing a pressure out of lesion toward correction. When he does so, the elastic tissues connecting the cranial bones are stretched. When they are released, they tend to pull the bones back toward their natural position. One could also correctly say that the phase of breath held during the correction is a motive force in the correction, moving the cranial bones toward their actual position

when the gentle corrective pressures are released.

However one describes the challenges and corrections, the AK technique for detection and correction of cranial faults is relatively fast and easy to perform. Unlike osteopathic methods, it does not require fine palpatory ability. The precise vector for the corrections can be tested in advance. A tested phase of breath assists the correction. And both the examiner and the patient are involved in the process of diagnosis and correction.

As the well-intentioned but untrained practitioner can easily and unintentionally inflict injury, all bone manipulations should be left to the trained chiropractor or osteopath.

2. EMOTIONAL CHALLENGE

"In an emotional challenge, the patient is muscle-tested during or immediately after being exposed to a potentially positive or negative emotion or imagination." (Gerz, 1996, page 69)

Mental-emotional factors may be challenged by having the patient look at, visualize, or think of any possible factor while the examiner tests an indicator muscle. For example, thinking of a stressful emotional experience will weaken an indicator muscle. The pectoralis major clavicular muscle associated with the stomach and with Chapman's emotional reflex will more consistently weaken with emotional stress than other indicator muscles.

Sensory impressions from any of the five senses may become mental factors that function as emotional challenges. Such challenges may include looking at someone or at oneself in the mirror, listening to someone or to one's own voice, thinking of being heard, smelling one's own body odor, etc. Psychologists may use this technique to quickly identify unresolved emotional stresses requiring attention.

In general, an "emotional challenge" involves the patient experiencing any emotion or imagination of a situation and testing the effect upon an indicator muscle. If a normotonic muscle becomes weak-testing or hypertonic, the tested emotion had a negative effect. If a weak-testing or hypertonic muscle becomes normotonic, the tested emotion had a positive therapeutic effect.

If the patient has emotional difficulties with being touched, such mental factors may be inadvertently tested when the examiner touches the patient to perform a challenge. To eliminate such possibilities, the examiner is wise to first assess the effect (upon an indicator muscle) of touching a new patient in some bodily area known to be distant from reflex points or possible disturbances.

3. FUNCTIONAL-NEUROLOGICAL CHALLENGE

The test for "ocular lock" (see page 85) is an example of a challenge of neurological function. In such challenges, complex movements that require integrated function of various proprioceptors, the right and left sides of the brain and the related centers in the brain are tested. These types of challenges form an important part of the advanced AK diagnostic techniques.

4. CHEMICAL-PHYSICAL/ ENERGETIC-ELECTROMAGNETIC CHALLENGE

"This is the AK testing during or immediately after the patient is exposed to a chemical or physical test stimulus." (Gerz, 1996, p. 69.)

Chemical-physical challenges include

- Healing remedies of all sorts
- All foods and drinks
- All other non-toxic substances taken into the mouth (dental repair materials, mouthwash, mild drugs . . .)
- Room air tests
- Air tests of carpets, mattresses, pillows, closets, etc.
- Material tests for toxic or allergic vapors (carpets, wood, etc.)
- All kinds of cosmetics
- All kinds of perfumes, essential oils, and other substances with fragrance

Energetic-Electromagnetic Challenges

- Homeopathy, Bach Flower Remedies, etc.
- Temperature

- Physical therapy treatments
- "Geopathic energies"
- Light, color
- Sounds, Music (Gerz, 1996, pages 69–70)

Chemical-physical challenges include oral, nasal, and skin contact challenges that test the influence of substances such as foods, allergens and medicines. Also included in this group are the electromagnetic and "subtle" energies and energetic medicines such as homeopathic remedies and flower essences. Such challenges may test the effect of temperature, any kind of physical therapeutic technique, geopathic energies, sounds and music, light and colors.

A positive challenge may be given to the chemical side of the triad of health by placing a nutritional substance (food, vitamin, mineral, gland extract, or other nutritive factor) or a medicine in the mouth and instructing the patient to chew and taste it. This is an "oral challenge." If the chewed substance makes a weak-testing muscle normotonic, it is an appropriate corrective measure. Conversely, a substance that has a negative effect upon a specific organ will, when in the mouth, cause the associated muscle and possibly many or all other muscles to temporarily weaken or become hypertonic. For the testing of individual nutrients, the use of extremely pure samples not mixed with other chemicals, binders, coloring agents, etc., is highly recommended.

The standard AK method to test non-toxic materials is to put them in the mouth or, if they have an odor, they may be tested by smelling them—a "nasal challenge." Walther (in Synopsis, p. 135) recommends testing and applying herbs, homeopathic preparations and Bach Flower Remedies by inhalation using a vaporizer. Inhaling the odor of an herb and testing if this can make a weak-testing muscle normotonic is an excellent application of nasal challenge. Air samples may be gathered in a clean bottle and sniffed for testing. Similar tests can be made of the gases exuded by carpets, furniture, etc. To do so, the bottle should be left open against the item to be tested for 30 minutes and then closed. Better still is to test the item directly, but this is not always convenient. The aroma of essential oils can be therapeutic. Aromas of all kinds can be tested by smelling them and assessing their effect with muscle testing.

While acceptable with herbs, Walther's recommendation to use nasal testing of a vaporized Bach Flower Remedy or homeopathic remedies is not a good idea. Such testing causes the patient to absorb small quantities of these substances, which are effective even in extreme dilutions. Testing many different remedies in this manner would definitely not be a good idea! This standard ICAK technique is, in the ICAK-D, considered obsolete.

Subtle energy medicines such as Bach Flower Remedies and homeopathic preparations appear to have an extra energy component that can be tested accurately by skin contact, even through a glass bottle. Various well-established European diagnostic methods utilize this phenomenon (e.g. Voll Electro-Acupuncture). The mechanism is not fully understood and will likely be found in the extremely sensitive ground substance and in the energy fields of the human body.

Babies and children often respond accurately to skin testing of any substance. There is no clear dividing line as to when this questionable technique will work or not. For this reason, it is highly recommended to test all normal, non-toxic substances by oral or nasal application.

In order to avoid errors, the various forms of substances must be tested in particular ways. A vial of a homeopathic remedy like Traumeel® may test perfectly to negate a weakness caused by a injury, etc. A tablet of Traumeel will test just the same when held in the hand. The energy component of such homeopathic remedies is easily tested when the remedy is held in the hand. However, homeopathic tablets are made with a base of lactose. With hand-held testing, the body doesn't seem to recognize the nutritional substance lactose but does recognize the energetic remedies in Traumeel. If a patient is intolerant to lactose, hand-held testing will not detect this problem. Gerz reports causing major neurodermatitis reactions by

missing the lactose intolerance with hand-held testing. These problems are immediately revealed by putting the test substance on the tongue. If the examiner puts such a tablet upon the tongue of someone with a lactose intolerance, most normotonic muscles will weaken or become hypertonic. To differentiate such problems, pure lactose tablets may also be tested.

Hans Selye considers extremes of temperature to be maximally stressful to the body. This can easily be tested by applying hot or cold to the body as a challenge.

Heat, cold, microwaves, electrical stimulation and other techniques of physical therapy can be applied as a challenge and the effect muscle-tested for appropriateness. A helpful therapy form will, when applied to the area to be treated, strengthen a muscle that tests weak due to the problem. Alternately, TL to the problem area may be used for such testing.

The effect of geopathic energies can be determined by muscle testing. To do so, the examiner accompanies the patient and tests her in various areas of her home and place of work.

Various systems of music and color therapy are popular today. With muscle testing and challenge, the effects of sound, music, light and colors can be tested for their usefulness as therapeutic measures.

For a step-by-step description of the use of challenge, see the section entitled "Testing Substances and Other Stimuli" (page 119).

Therapy Localization

If a patient touches a bodily area where a problem exists, a previously normotonic indicator muscle will test weak. Goodheart named this phenomenon therapy localization. It is not a form of therapy but rather a diagnostic technique. It could be more accurately called "diagnostic localization."

Goodheart discovered therapy localization quite accidentally. With a female patient, the results of muscle testing kept changing for no observed reason. Various muscles would test strong, then weak, then strong again without Goodheart doing anything. He called a colleague in to perform the muscle tests upon this patient while he watched what was going on. He observed that the woman crossed her arms and held one wrist with the other hand. Then she would switch hands and grasp the other wrist. He experimented and found points upon the area of the wrist where the pulse is taken that, when touched, will weaken or strengthen the various muscle tests. He later learned that these points are well known in Chinese medical diagnosis. As so often occurred in the history of AK, Goodheart utilized this anecdotal observation to create a very useful AK technique.

Therapy localization is actually a "localization challenge." In contrast to other kinds of challenge, where the examiner applies some stimulus to the patient, therapy localization involves the patient touching herself (or the examiner touching her). In most cases, it makes no difference whether the patient or the examiner touches the point. However, in some cases, the results are different when the examiner touches the point. To avoid such errors, it is recommended, whenever possible and convenient, to instruct the patient to touch herself for all tests of therapy localization.

A positive therapy localization (one that changes the response of the muscle test) indicates that something is wrong at, or related to, the point touched. The indicator muscle may at first test weak, normotonic or hypertonic. Any change of tonus in subsequent muscle testing that is produced by touching the body is a positive TL. Areas that will therapy-localize include damaged tissue, infection, muscle dysfunction, subluxation, diseased tissue, malfunctioning or damaged proprioceptors, active reflex points and active acupuncture points. However, *therapy localization alone does not, in itself, indicate what is wrong at the point touched*. Other diagnostic techniques must be used to find out what is causing the positive therapy localization.

To simplify the search for areas of active TL, large areas may be touched using the whole surface of the hand. If this produces a positive TL, the precise area may be determined by touching with an individual finger. This is standard AK practice. However, due to minute differences in polarity, TL with one finger may produce a different response than with another finger. To avoid this problem, Gerz recommends performing TL with two or three fingertips together.

Therapy localization can be used to determine, in advance, which treatment(s) will be effective for a specific problem. If a reflex point is involved with the muscle weakness, the weak-testing muscle will test strong when that reflex point is touched by the patient. For example, if a muscle tests weak, rubbing its associated neurolymphatic points will often make it test strong. To see if this will work in a specific case (before any correction is performed), the patient touches a neurolymphatic point for this muscle. While touching this point, the muscle is retested. If this touch alone causes the muscle to temporarily test strong, applying the correct stimulus (firm massage for neurolymphatic points) will cause the muscle to subsequently test strong and remain so. Other reflex points or correction techniques that could strengthen a weak-testing muscle may similarly be tested for their potential strengthening effect.

Therapy localization can be used to test how long to treat a point. When a muscle tests weak, touching its neurolymphatic point may cause it to temporarily test strong. If so, after massaging the neurolymphatic point, the muscle will most likely test strong and continue to do so. Even though this is the case, the muscle may still need more such neurolymphatic massage. To determine if this is the case, therapy-localize the neurolymphatic point while retesting the muscle. If this causes the muscle to again weaken, the neurolymphatic point massage was incomplete. When massage is sufficient, touching the point will no longer weaken the muscle.

The main use of therapy localization is as a technique for discerning the causes of known problems. For example, a successful treatment to a subluxated ankle may be lost when the patient stands or walks. Having the patient touch the ankle with one hand will weaken an indicator muscle. If another point can be found by searching, i.e., by having the patient touch with her hand, in succession, a series of likely points, one point may be found, which (when touched by the patient's other hand at the same time as the ankle) causes the muscle to restrengthen. It is then reasonable to infer that something associated with that strengthening point is a probable cause of the ankle problem. Correcting the problem associated with that other point will usually prevent the recurrence of the ankle subluxation. Note that since both of the patient's hands are used in this process, a leg muscle must be used as an indicator. This *two-handed therapy localization* (double TL) is an accepted Applied Kinesiology technique used to search for the underlying causes of a problem.

As mentioned, touching a problem area with one hand will usually cause the indicator muscle to test weak. If simultaneously holding the forehead with the other hand (two-handed or double TL) causes the weakened indicator to test strong, a main cause of the problem is emotional in nature.

In some cases, a muscle tests normotonic even though the associated organ/gland is known to be malfunctioning. However, having the patient therapy-localize (touch) over the organ (or over a reflex point to the organ) usually causes the associated muscle to weaken and may cause any normotonic indicator muscle to weaken. Any challenge (medicine, nutritional substance, or other therapeutic intervention) that restrengthens the muscle while the point is again touched should help the gland or organ to regain proper function. Note that in this example, the patient provides a therapy localization by touching herself, which makes the indicator test weak. At the same time, the challenge provided by the correct medicine, nutritional substance or therapeutic intervention makes the muscle test strong again.

Sometimes a reflex point for a condition needing treatment will not therapy-localize unless another factor is tested simultaneously. For example, swollen tissue may indicate the need for better lymph drainage to the area. Touching the tissue itself may therapy-localize, but touching the related neurolymphatic point (which should improve the lymph drainage to the area) may not therapy-localize by itself. If simultaneously touching the tissue (which weakens the indicator muscle) and touching its related neurolymphatic point causes the indicator muscle to regain its

strength, neurolymphatic massage of the point is indicated. It is not fully understood why particular points that need treatment may not therapy-localize when tested alone but do when TL is applied to another factor simultaneously. This appears to be due to some mechanism of compensation in the body.

Touching an active point for too long (more than 10 seconds may be too long in some cases) may cause the point to no longer therapy-localize. As the active "positive" therapy localization soon returns, this seems not to be therapeutic. For this reason, do not let the patient touch any point too long or the positive therapy localization may be temporarily lost. It is also important to have the patient hold her hands away from her body during muscle testing to avoid the possibility of inadvertently touching active points and thereby changing the results of the tests.

When skin sensation is absent, therapy localization will normally not function. However, Goodheart found that by activating the half of the brain opposite the side of the body which lacks sensation, therapy localization could sometimes be brought to function in areas lacking skin sensation. The left hemisphere can be activated by doing mental mathematics such as reciting aloud the multiples of 7. The right hemisphere can be activated by humming an improvised melody—a melody spontaneously composed on the spot. Though not always effective, this technique is worth attempting with clients who have points to be tested that are located upon body areas lacking skin sensation.

Walther reports that a "high-gain" therapy localization can be obtained by holding the thumb and little finger tips together and touching the body with the other three fingers. When the results of therapy localization are unclear and more sensitivity is desired, this technique may be useful. It is postulated that by activating the opposing thumb (which is unique to humans and has made our precise use of tools possible), higher brain centers are activated, resulting in the therapy localization being more sensitive.

Some evidence suggests that therapy localization is an energy phenomenon with electromagnetic characteristics. Therapy localization energy appears to flow through a metal wire connecting an active point to the patient's hand because touching with a wire held in the hand has the same effect as touching directly with that hand. Cutting the wire in half and inserting a diode between the two lengths limits electrical energy to flowing in one direction only. Using such a test circuit, it can be demonstrated that therapy localization energy flows from the patient's hand to an active point before treatment. After incomplete treatment of a point, it can be shown that therapy localization energy flows from the active point to the hand. Why the direction of energy flow reverses is unknown. However, this experiment does at least suggest that therapy localization is a phenomenon similar in some respects to electricity.

Dehydration will weaken the effect of therapy localization. Drinking water or wetting the fingertips will increase the effect of therapy localization upon muscle strength. As electricity flows more easily through a wet junction, this provides a bit more evidence that therapy localization has certain characteristics in common with electricity.

Like electricity, therapy localization energy is blocked by ceramic pottery and synthetic materials such as nylon and plastic. However, therapy localization energy will flow through substances known to block electricity such as wool, cotton, paper, and wood. Furthermore, it will not travel through lead, although lead will conduct electricity. There are likely many other types of energy than just those with which we are currently familiar. Nonetheless, it is puzzling that such evidence clearly demonstrates that therapy localization is not exactly comparable to electricity. In any case, therapy localization does indicate the presence of a complex system of signaling in the body about which there is still much to be learned.

Perhaps the ancient Chinese concept of the meridian system is nearer to the truth about energies, such as those involved in therapy localization, than any Western concepts yet developed. Even though we lack a complete understanding or explanation of the mechanisms involved in therapy localization, it would certainly be foolish not to employ such techniques simply because we can't explain exactly how they function. Extensive clinical application has repeatedly demonstrated the value of TL in

1. locating hidden problems,

2. locating treatment modes for known problems, and

3. determining when treatment has been adequate.

Surrogate Testing

In some cases, muscle testing is not possible. The patient who is unconscious, in a coma, or physically injured cannot be muscle tested. Patients who are extremely weak may not have enough muscle strength to be easily muscle tested. Children may be too young to understand and perform the muscle test procedure. For all people who cannot be directly muscle tested, surrogate testing may be used.

Goodheart inadvertently discovered surrogate testing even before he learned of therapy localization. The teres minor muscle of a woman tested strong. He was interrupted by a phone call. When he returned, he tested the teres minor again and it tested weak. She was holding her child, so he had her put her child down and retested the teres minor. It was again strong. He suspected that the weakness had to do with how she was holding her child. To test this hypothesis, he had her simply reach out and touch the child with one hand. Teres minor again tested weak. Goodheart reports, "I thought I was taking leave of my senses." (*You'll Be Better*, chapter 3, page 2.) Further experiments revealed this to be a demonstrable and repeatable phenomenon. He reasoned that some kind of energy transference was taking place.

The chances of error with surrogate testing are greater than when testing a patient directly. Care must be taken that the surrogate does not have a reaction to the TL or challenge, or this may be interpreted as the patient's reaction. A change in posture or other parameter may also change the results of muscle testing.

Surrogate Testing a Baby

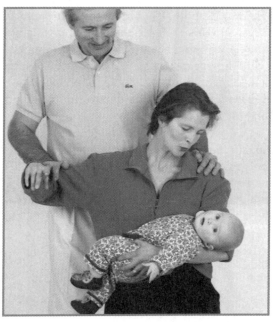

MOTHER HOLDING HER BABY
WITHOUT SKIN CONTACT

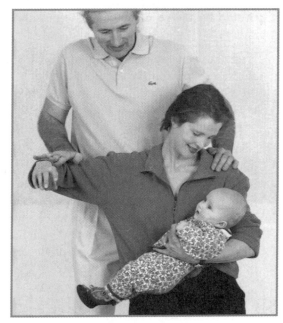

MOTHER HOLDING HER BABY
WITH SKIN CONTACT

TECHNIQUE FOR SURROGATE TESTING

1. Find an easily testable normotonic muscle in the surrogate person. Test in the same posture as will be used for surrogate testing. If a mother will be holding her child, she should first be tested while holding her child but having no skin contact. The surrogate may need correction techniques to make the chosen indicator muscle normotonic before proceeding.

2. Surrogate and patient make skin contact. Sensitive areas where energy is easily exchanged such as the navel, palms of the hands or soles of the feet are recommended. Neither TL nor challenge is applied yet.

3. If the indicator muscle remains normotonic, it can be used with TL or challenge to test what is bad for the patient. TL or challenge should be applied (by the surrogate or by the patient herself) directly

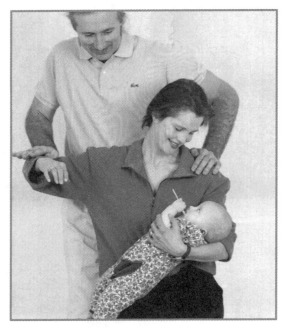

MOTHER PRESENTING STIMULUS TO BABY

to the body of the patient. Medicines or foods should be tested directly in the mouth of the patient.

4. If the muscle tests weak, it can be used with TL or challenge to identify the medication, food, or other therapy that will have a positive effect upon the patient. These will make the muscle test normotonic.

5. If the simple contact of the surrogate and the patient makes the surrogate's indicator muscle test hypertonic, either change the surrogate or try to find out what will make the muscle normotonic. This can be difficult as the cause can lie with the patient, the surrogate, or the interaction between the two. If the surrogate cannot be changed because, for example, a child only wants to be touched by its mother, a third person can serve as surrogate. In this example, the examiner tests the surrogate who touches the mother who touches the child. Surrogate testing will work through such a chain of people, but the chance of errors arising increases with each extra person in the chain (Gerz, 1996, p. 85).

Goodheart recommends using the surrogate technique only in difficult situations where the patient is not directly testable (Goodheart, *You'll Be Better,* chapter 3, page 2). For an example of using a surrogate to test a baby's foods, see Appendix VIII, "Case Histories."

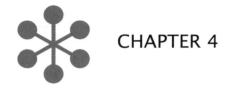

CHAPTER 4

Pretests

How to Prepare an Indicator Muscle for Accurate Testing

Before one can use a muscle as an indicator for other functions (by using challenge or therapy localization) its own function "in the clear" must be established. A scale requires a "pre-test" calibration in which it is set to zero before it can be counted upon to measure weight accurately. Similarly, until certain pre-checks and necessary corrections are completed, one may receive unreliable results when using a muscle as an indicator. This explains why many novices to muscle testing receive, at best, mixed results. For an indicator muscle to give accurate results, it must be in a normotonic state: It must test strong yet be able to be weakened. Furthermore, the nervous system as a whole and especially those portions of the nervous system associated with that muscle must be functioning in an organized manner as described below.

A. Is Dehydration Present?

There is no single direct test in Applied Kinesiology for dehydration. However, it is to be suspected when the patient has:

- dry, scaly skin
- dry mouth
- edema
- many muscles that test weak but become normotonic after drinking water

- neurolymphatic reflex points that are consistently active
- congestion of the lymphatic system and/or
- therapy localization does not function well until the patient wets her fingers first.

Many of these items may only become evident later in an examination. Dehydration is very common. Almost no one drinks too much water. Other drinks do not have the same positive effect as pure water. Unless there is some suspicion of kidney failure or congestive heart disease, recommending that the patient drink more water is always a good idea.

Furthermore, when the body of the patient lacks adequate water, therapy localization may not function well. If the examiner touches the patient for TL tests, he too must be adequately hydrated. It appears that therapy localization is an electrical-type phenomenon, which requires adequate water in the tissues for the exchange of energies. For the following pretests, therapy localization must function correctly. Therefore, it is a good practice for both the examiner and the patient to drink a glass of water before beginning to perform these pretests.

B. Does the Muscle Test Strong in the Clear?

To muscle-test, the examiner first asks permission. If the patient is new to muscle testing, the examiner explains what it is, and what is actually being tested.

Then he guides the patient into the correct position for participating in the test. He explains any postural requirements, such as keeping the elbow fully extended for testing latissimus dorsi. The range of motion of every muscle test describes the arc of the actual movement of the body parts, not a straight line. The examiner demonstrates the range and direction of the test with precisely this arc of motion.

The examiner then informs the patient that she will initiate the muscle test by contracting her muscle in an attempt to move her arm (or other body part tested) against the examiner's stabilizing hand. She should take about two seconds to build up her tension to the maximum contraction of which she is capable. She is to press only once with a continuous increase of pressure (no bouncing!). After she has reached maximum contraction the examiner presses a little bit harder. The patient is to maintain maximum contraction against the examiner's pressure.

Next, the examiner places his hand where it needs to be for testing. If necessary for the specific test, he stabilizes the patient with his other hand. Then he says, "Press as hard as you can" or some such verbal signal to indicate that she is to begin contracting the muscle. It is the examiner's responsibility to provide the exact counter-pressure needed to stabilize the arm (or other area tested) and prevent it from moving. Then, after maximum contraction has been attained, the examiner goes beyond simply resisting and gives an extra pressure of about 2–5% more.

When the examiner gives the extra pressure, either the muscle "locks" the joint in place (tests strong) or the muscle strength characteristically "breaks" and gives way (tests weak).

If a muscle tests weak, it may be strengthened by several different techniques which are applied as needed. These include:

• Massage of the origin and insertion of the muscle,

• Neurolymphatic point massage,

• Holding plus tugging upon neurovascular points, and

• Manipulation of the muscle proprioceptors.

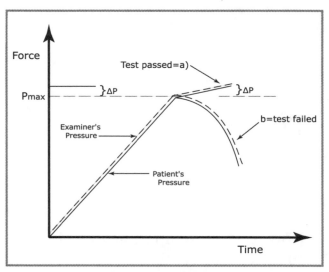

THE RELATIONSHIP OF PRESSURE APPLIED
IN MUSCLE TESTING VERSUS TIME

After the application of each strengthening technique, the muscle is retested to evaluate the success of the treatment. If the muscle now tests strong, the correction is challenged by retesting the muscle with the patient's hand over the last area of treatment. If the muscle still tests strong, the muscle has been adequately treated. If it again weakens, further treatment is required. This is an example of one of the finest aspects of Applied Kinesiology: It is possible to determine whether one has adequately corrected a problem or if further correction is needed.

Any muscle that can be properly isolated and directly tested may be used as an indicator muscle. If the muscle chosen to serve as an indicator tests weak, and the examiner has difficulty in strengthening that weak-testing muscle, he should find another muscle that does test normotonic in the clear to use as an indicator muscle.

Various muscles are typically used as indicator muscles in AK. The best ones are those that require no stabilization. This leaves the examiner's (and the patient's) other hand free for TL. Latissimus dorsi is often used. However, care must be taken that the patient does not bend the elbow during the test, which would make a weak-testing latissimus dorsi appear to test strong. Leg muscles are the best choice because they leave both of the patient's hands free for double TL. Rectus femoris is an excellent choice. It is one of the strongest muscles in the body and can withstand repeated testing without tiring. However, the rectus femoris of a strong client may be extremely strong. If so, a lightly built examiner may not be able to repeatedly resist the complete contraction of the muscle as is required for AK muscle testing. In such cases, an excellent alternative indicator muscle is the piriformis. To use the piriformis as an indicator muscle, the knee of the patient can be stabilized against the therapist's chest (see page 189).

The rectus femoris connects the pelvis just superior to the hip socket (acetabulum) with the kneecap

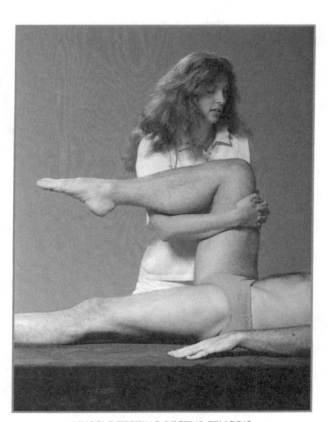

MUSCLE-TESTING RECTUS FEMORIS
USING BOTH HANDS

(patella). A ligament connects the kneecap to the shin bone (tibia). The rectus femoris flexes the thigh over the hip socket and extends the leg around the knee. In the muscle test of the rectus femoris described below, only the action of flexing the thigh is tested.

Muscle-Testing Rectus Femoris

1. First the examiner demonstrates the test. The initial position is with the patient supine, the knee and hip bent 90°. This brings the rectus femoris into a position of partial contraction. It is tested by pushing or pulling upon the thigh just superior to the knee in a direction away from the head (inferior). This moves the leg straight down toward the table and toward a resting position parallel with the other leg. No rotation of the thigh is allowed during the test.

2. While explaining the test to the patient, the examiner guides her through the range of motion (the arc) of the test without the patient resisting. This alerts the involved portion of the nervous system to anticipate similar moves during the upcoming test. Then he brings her leg back to the beginning position.

3. The examiner makes contact with his open hand proximal to the patient's knee on the upper thigh.

4. The examiner says, "Press as hard as you can," and responds with the necessary counter-pressure to stabilize her leg in place.

5. When she has reached maximum contraction, the examiner goes beyond just stabilizing and actively presses with about 2–5% more pressure. The examiner then carefully senses whether the patient's leg held firmly in place (the muscle tested strong) or fell away when the final pressure was applied (the muscle tested weak.)

6. If the examiner is not certain if the muscle tested weak or not, he asks the patient to attempt to contract her rectus femoris even more strongly. Then he repeats the test. Normally a normotonic

muscle will continue to test strong even after being tested a few times. However, a weak-testing muscle will test weaker when tested more than once. If the muscle does test weak, he may use it in its weak state to determine by TL or challenge, what is needed to make it test strong. Or if he desires to begin with a normotonic indicator muscle, he may either strengthen it or choose another muscle and begin again.

C. CAN THE MUSCLE BE WEAKENED?

In AK, four techniques are typically used to check that a normotonic muscle can be weakened (i.e., is normotonic and not hypertonic). These are neuromuscular spindle cell manipulation, meridian sedation points, application of a magnet and stroking the associated meridian against its natural direction. In tests performed by AK diplomats in the European meeting in Monte Carlo in 1994, it was determined that TL to the meridian sedation points is statistically the most effective technique for checking if a muscle can be made to test weak. Spindle cell manipulation was next best, but finding the exact location of the spindle cells in a large muscle may be difficult. In that meeting the European AK diplomats decided upon a working definition of "normotonic" and "hypertonic" muscles:

Definition of Normotonic Muscles

When a muscle has been identified as strong, a further differentiation must be used to determine if this muscle is hypertonic or normotonic. In AK, a normotonic muscle is defined as one which is strong, but is perceived as weakening when one of the following procedures is used:

a) TL to the sedation point of the meridian associated with that muscle, on the side of the body where the muscle being tested is located.

b) "Running the meridian in reverse."

The associated meridian can be contacted and stroked lightly, but quickly, with the palmar aspect of the hand, in the direction from the highest point to the lowest point on the meridian. This should inhibit (weaken) the related muscle for approximately 10 seconds.

c) Spindle cell manipulation.

Contact is made in the center of the muscle belly so that the fingertips of each hand are oriented toward each other at a distance of about 5–10 cm apart. The two hands are then pushed together five times with short bursts of relatively intense pressure, which approximates (shortens) the muscle belly and its fibers. This should inhibit (weaken) a muscle for up to 10 seconds.

d) Either of the two poles of a strong, axially polarized magnet (minimum 2000 Gauss), centrally placed upon the belly of the muscle, should temporarily inhibit (weaken) the muscle. Regarding the effects of the N and S pole of magnets on the strength of muscles, seemingly contradictory responses have been observed. Therefore, at this time, it is suggested that both poles be tested.

If none of the above methods causes weakening of the muscle, it is defined as hypertonic. It is recommended that at least two of the above procedures be used when evaluating the status of a muscle (Gerz, 1996, p. 27).

Muscle-testing rectus femoris as an indicator muscle, continued:

7. After applying one of the four weakening stimuli described above, the examiner retests the rectus femoris. If it tests weak, it passed the second test for preparing an indicator muscle. When it tests weak, the new patient receives his or her first clear experience of a weak-testing muscle.

8. When the examiner removes the magnet or the TL from the sedation point, the muscle should again test strong. If spindle cell manipulation or "running the meridian" was used, the muscle should test strong again after about 10 seconds. The examiner should retest the rectus femoris to confirm that it again tests strong before proceeding. If the rectus femoris now tests strong

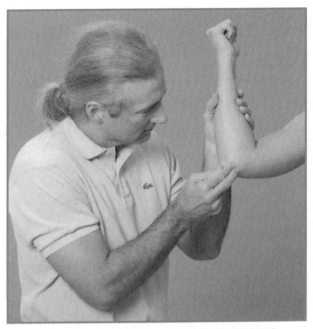

WEAKENING THE RECTUS FEMORIS BY TAPPING
UPON ITS SEDATION POINT, SMALL INTESTINE 8

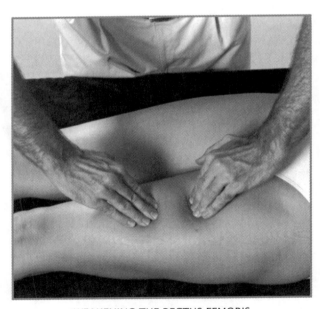

WEAKENING THE RECTUS FEMORIS
BY NEUROLOGICAL SPINDLE CELL MANIPULATION

and can be weakened, it is ready to use as an indicator muscle.

Techniques for the correction of hypertonic muscles are included in the next section. If the rectus femoris (or other indicator muscle) cannot be made normotonic with methods known to the examiner, he should choose another indicator muscle and begin again.

D. Is the Individual Muscle in a Hypertonic State?

Sometimes the above techniques fail to make the muscle test weak. When a muscle tests strong but cannot be weakened, it is said to be hypertonic. Various names have been applied to this state of muscle tone in AK. This state was first described by Sheldon Deal as a "frozen muscle." Joe Schaffer uses the term "over-facilitated." Hans Garten calls them "hyper-reactive." The cause of hypertonic muscles is usually stress. When individual muscles test hypertonic, finding and correcting the cause with the following techniques can sometimes make them again testable.

If a patient is *mentally* preoccupied with something besides the test (mentally stressed), she is not mentally present and some or all of her muscles may test hypertonic. In such a case, the patient may be called back into the present and made testable by saying, "Be here with me now. Relax. Breathe while I am testing and be testable." This is not a standard AK technique.

The stress may be *chemical*. A muscle may be hypertonic because the body is lacking some nutrient, or in need of some remedy (medicine, herb, vitamin, mineral, etc.). When the patient puts the needed nutrient or remedy in her mouth, the hypertonic muscle may become testable. Nutrients for specific muscles are given in the section on muscle tests (pages 153–231).

The stress may be *structural*. Hypotonicity in muscles can be caused by malfunctioning muscle proprioceptors. In such cases, proprioceptor work (spindle cell pinching or Golgi tendon organ stretching) will often relax a hypertonic muscle and make it normotonic.

Hypotonicity in an antagonist muscle can cause the muscle tension of the agonist to increase and become palpatory hypertonic. Such muscles also typically test hypertonic. In these cases, Goodheart strengthens the hypotonic muscle, which has the effect of lowering the tension in the hypertonic agonist and making it test normotonic. This is an example of the structural cause and correction of hypertonic muscles.

Another possible structural cause of hypertonic muscles is dehydration. The upper trapezius is particularly prone to this problem. During a kinesiology training course, I had very tight and painful upper trapezius muscles. As a massage therapist was present in the course, she was asked to massage the tight muscles. She walked away, returned with two large glasses of water and commanded, "Drink them!," which I did. About twenty minutes later she asked, "How are your tight muscles now?" Amazingly, all pain and most of the excess tension was gone!

Richard Utt, founder of Applied Physiology, is the discoverer of the seven states of contraction of a muscle. This concept was introduced into AK by his therapist and teacher, Sheldon Deal. Richard Utt created the following technique that can sometimes make individual hypertonic muscles testable: The patient extends the muscle to the maximum. The examiner supports the limb in this position and then has the patient contract the muscle (isometrically) against the examiner's supporting pressure. Next the muscle is put into a position of complete contraction, the limb is supported in this position, and the patient attempts to extend the muscle (contract its antagonists.) This activates all the nerve receptors in the muscle itself, in its antagonists, and in its tendons and joints at both extremes of the muscle's activity.

A tennis player awaiting the serve jumps about to activate the proprioceptors in his muscles. This sends a flood of sensory information to his central nervous system about the exact position and weight of his body parts. With all this kinesthetic information, the central nervous system can direct more accurate responses. Like the tennis player's jumping about,

this technique of stretching and then tensing the muscle and its antagonists sends to the central nervous system a flood of sensory information about the two extremes of contraction and extension of the muscle. The neuromuscular spindle cells and other proprioceptors then respond more accurately. Now when these "freshly activated" neuromuscular spindle cells are pinched, they should cause the muscle to test weak.

Individual hypertonic muscles are a nuisance but may be corrected by one or more of the above techniques. A much greater problem is caused when most or all muscles test hypertonic. This will be discussed in detail in the section, "General Hypertonicity" page 93.

Is Neurologic Disorganization (Switching) Present?

Neurologic disorganization indicates a lack of proper integration, that is, a state of confusion in the nervous system and body. Neurologic disorganization is popularly referred to as "switching" because diagnostic results may be reversed. Switching can change the results of muscle testing, giving false information. When switching is present, indicator muscle-testing may locate a problem on the left side of the body, which is actually on the right side. For example, a patient may be carrying his right shoulder high. This could logically indicate that either the upper trapezius (which lifts the shoulder) is hypertonic on the right side or that the latissimus dorsi (which pulls the shoulder down) is hypotonic on the right side. Yet muscle testing may reveal that the latissimus dorsi is weak not on the right as expected but rather on the left side! In this case, the visual body language and the results of muscle testing do not concur. The results are switched from side to side. When such a lack of integration exists, as indicated by diagnostic results that are contradictory, it is necessary to correct it (with the techniques explained below) before proceeding with other tests. Otherwise, the results of some tests, and the application of therapy based upon such results, will be inaccurate. Pretests E through H that follow are all tests and corrections for neurological disorganization.

E. OCULAR LOCK

One popular test for neurologic disorganization (switching) is ocular lock, a disturbance of the coordination of the two eyes.

Until the two brain hemispheres begin to synchronize their activity, normally at an age of 2–5 months, a child cannot synchronize the movements of the two eyes. In some cases, the desired synchronization does not become stable and may easily be lost, even decades later in life. Under enough stress, we all may lose certain aspects of proper synchronization and go into a state of switching.

Patients with neurologic disorganization (switching) often have difficulty coordinating the two eyes. When patients have this "ocular lock" condition, looking in one specific direction will cause an indicator muscle to test weak. The original test for ocular lock involved the patient looking as far as possible in one direction, and then testing an indicator muscle. The directions typically tested are up, down, right, and left. Some examiners also test the four diagonal directions. However, in some patients with ocular lock, the precise angle for the eyes must be obtained very specifically or the indicator muscle will not weaken. The above eight eye positions may all test strong because the exact problem angle lies between two of them.

People who cannot stay awake when attempting to read in bed often suffer from ocular lock. The activity of moving the eyes back and forth in reading disturbs their neurologic functions enough that they become uncontrollably sleepy. As driving a car also requires back-and-forth motions of the eyes to observe the road conditions, driving may make such people sleepy, which could be very dangerous.

Leaf (1995) tests ocular lock by having the patient turn her head to one shoulder and look in the opposite direction. This is repeated with the patient turning the head toward the other shoulder. Another popular test for ocular lock is to have the patient read aloud normally (from left to right) and reversed (reading the words from right to left). After each of the above procedures, an indicator muscle is tested. Weakening of the indicator muscle indicates ocular lock.

A more modern test has been devised to easily check all positions of the eyes. The patient visually follows the examiner's finger as he traces a circle clockwise in front of and around her face. Then he tests an indicator muscle. The circle is then traced counterclockwise and the indicator muscle is tested again. The circles should be made large enough that the patient must look about as far as she can in all directions. The circles should be far enough away from the patient that she has no difficulty focusing on the examiner's finger. Otherwise, the effort to focus may make the indicator muscle weak even when ocular lock is not present.

The patient's eyes will usually make erratic, jerky motions when passing over the problematic direction. If they do, the direction of difficulty has been located. Looking specifically in this direction will make the indicator muscle test weak. Some patients experience disturbing emotional states and develop excessive muscular tension in the back of the neck or other muscle groups when the eyes are maintained in the weak-testing direction.

Permanent correction of ocular lock usually requires chiropractic correction of cranial and pelvic faults. Until this is performed, certain physical activities such as walking will cause the condition of ocular lock to return. Ocular lock can be temporarily corrected by massaging the navel and the end points of the kidney meridian (the K 27s). This is the same correction that is performed to correct switching as described below. Most effective is to have the patient look in the weakening direction while the K 27s and navel are massaged.

Although the above simple correction for ocular lock is most often only temporary in its effect, it can be very helpful for the patient to use on her own before reading or other activities that require coordinated eye movement. As with all types of switching corrections, this will improve the accuracy of further kinesiologic testing. Therefore it is recommended that the examiner check and correct ocular lock as part of the pretest procedure.

F.   KIDNEY 27 AND OCULAR LOCK CORRECTION

To test for switching, the patient touches (therapy-localizes) specific points while the examiner muscle-tests an indicator muscle. The points most often used to test for switching are:

- the navel;

- the K 27s—the end points of the kidney meridians located just below where the clavicle meets the sternum, at the junction of the sternum, clavicle and first rib;

- CV 24—the end point of the central meridian (also called the conception vessel) located just below the center of the lower lip;

- GV 27—the next-to-the-last point of the governing meridian (governing vessel) located just above the center of the upper lip;

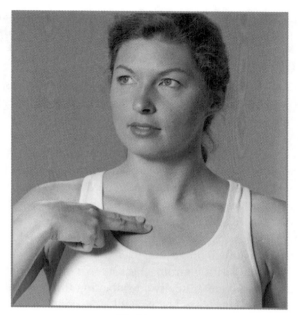

TL TO K 27

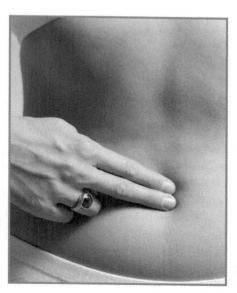

TL TO THE NAVEL

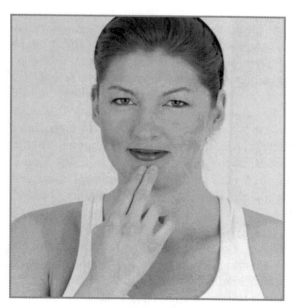

TL TO CV 24

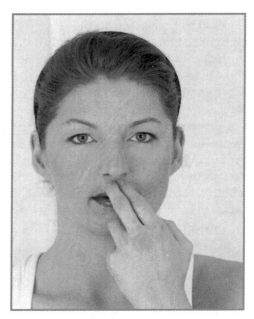

TL TO GV 27

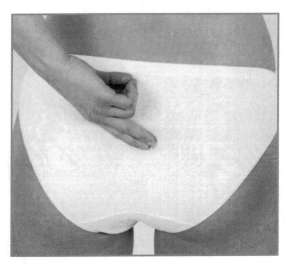

TL TO GV 1

• GV 1—the beginning point of the governing meridian (which is also referred to as the governing vessel) at the tip of the coccyx (tailbone).

If touching any of the above points (with the exception of the navel) causes a previously normotonic indicator muscle to test weak, switching is present. Attention must be given to having the patient touch the exact area of the K 27s. Massage of the points that tested weak will temporarily correct the switching. The exact procedures are as follows:

Since the navel is used in the first two switching tests, a TL to the navel must test strong before proceeding with other tests. If touch to the navel alone weakens the indicator muscle, the disturbance caused by the scar of the navel needs to be cleared. To do so, rub into the navel some Bach Rescue Remedy® cream, APM Creme®, Ionen Salbe Forte® or shine a laser upon the scarred tissue in the navel. Then recheck that the TL to the navel no longer weakens the indicator muscle before proceeding.

The main diagnostic tests for switching are:

• TL to the navel and the left K 27.

• TL to the navel and the right K 27.

• TL to both K 27s.

• Cross TL to both K 27s. To perform this, the patient touches her left K 27 with her right hand and her right K 27 with her left hand. There is a tendency for the patient to not touch the K 27s accurately, so extra care must be taken. Also, the two hands must not touch each other.

To temporarily correct imbalances detected in any of these four tests, massage for 20 seconds both points that tested weak (navel + left K 27, navel + right K 27, both K 27s or crossover K 27s). If cross TL to the K 27s tested weak, be sure to also cross the hands while massaging the points. The correction is checked for success by again performing the TL to the points that were active, and testing the indicator muscle. It should now test strong. If ocular lock was present before massaging the K 27s, it should now be absent.

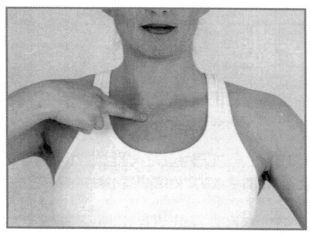

TL TO THE NAVEL + ONE K 27

This is checked by having the patient look in the direction that weakened the indicator muscle. If the indicator muscle no longer weakens, ocular lock has been corrected. Some authorities state that when correcting ocular lock, the patient should look in the weakening direction while massaging the K 27s.

If ocular lock is still present, Walther suggests that the patient look in the weakening direction and take two deep sniffs in through the nose. If the indicator muscle tests weak after these two sniffs, the examiner taps on both sides of the patient's nose for about one minute. This will almost always eliminate, at least temporarily, the ocular lock condition.

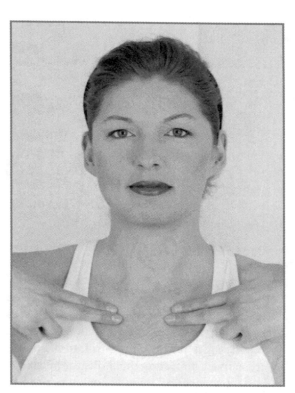

TL TO BOTH K 27S

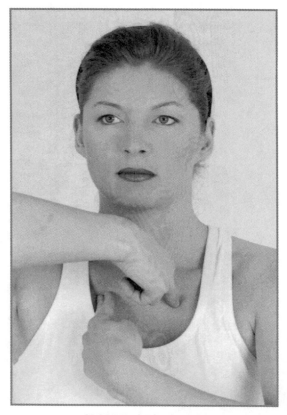

CROSS TL OF THE K 27S

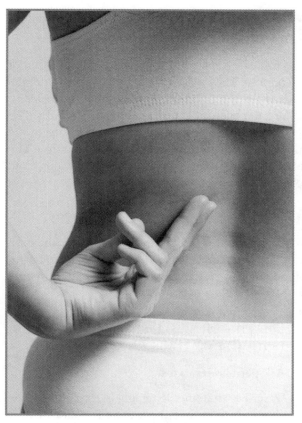

TL OF THE AUXILIARY K 27

G. Auxiliary K 27

If signs of switching are still present after massaging the K 27s and the navel, the patient therapy-localizes each of the "auxiliary K 27" points located next to the transverse processes of the thoracic vertebra 11. If TL to either of these points weakens the indicator muscle, the auxiliary K 27 that tested weak and the navel are massaged. Then TL to the auxiliary K 27 that tested weak should no longer weaken the indicator muscle. These points are described in this way by Walther (1988, p. 149). Gerz (1996, p. 88) locates these points a bit lower in the areas to the sides of L1–L2, directly behind the navel.

H. Central (Conception) Vessel and Governing Vessel (CV 24, GV 27, GV 1)

If therapy localization to CV 24, GV 27 or GV 1 weakens the indicator muscle, the examiner presses firmly upon CV 24 and CV 2 (at the top of the pubic bone) for 20–30 seconds. Then he gently touches GV 1, located at the tip of the coccyx, and CV 2 simultaneously for 20–30 seconds. Another way to correct these points is simply to massage the CV 24, GV 27 or GV 1 that tested weak. The correction is checked by therapy-localizing CV 24 and then GV 27 while testing an indicator muscle as before. The indicator muscle should now test strong. If not, the space between thoracic ribs 6 and 7 near to where they meet the vertebral column should be therapy-localized. If this weakens the indicator muscle, the patient may need a chiropractic adjustment in that area before correction of CV 24, GV 27 or GV 1 will succeed.

Switching, even when corrected, may return in any single moment of an AK diagnostic session. To avoid the false responses that switching produces, it is wise to learn to detect (from the body language) when switching is present. Body language that may indicate switching includes poor coordination, bumping into things, mixing up numbers, words or syllables, stuttering, the voice suddenly taking on a higher pitch, a change of skin coloration, asymmetrical posture and doing the opposite of what was requested. When a patient exhibits any of these behaviors, the examiner ought to check (again) for switching and correct it as necessary.

There are many advanced Applied Kinesiology procedures to determine and correct the underlying causes of switching. When these causes are found, the source of the patient's health problems will also be found. Until these causes are located and corrected, switching will recur again and again. Several of these advanced techniques, not described in detail in this book, are listed below to incite further study. However, until these advanced techniques have been mastered, it is recommended that the examiner at least eliminate switching temporarily through the use of the simple techniques in this section before performing any further AK tests.

To discover the causes and more lasting corrections of switching (neurologic disorganization), do not massage the navel and the K 27s or stimulate the GV and CV points. Instead, TL the active switching points and simultaneously TL (double TL) or challenge suspect causes of the switching. Any TL or challenge that eliminates the active TL to the switching points is a cause of the switching. Correctly treating this cause should provide a more lasting correction for switching. Typical causes can be on any of the three sides of the triad of health—structural, chemical and mental.

Structural causes include dental occlusion, jaw function, cranial faults and subluxated bones. When ocular lock is present, the cause of switching is almost always structural. The most common areas of subluxation that cause switching are in the cervical spine, the pelvis and the feet but may be anywhere in the body. Other structural causes of switching include cloacal synchronization, "pitch, roll and yaw," the gaits, and dural tension.

Chemical causes of switching may relate to nutritional substances that influence the neurotransmitters. Typical substances to test are adrenal substance, choline, and RNA.

When double TL to the active switching points plus the forehead (frontal bone eminences) eliminates the positive TL, the cause of switching is mental/emotional. Emotional switching is also indicated when the cross K 27 TL is active. In this state, same-sided arm and leg movements will test strong, and opposite-sided (contralateral) movements will test weak. Normally the results are just the opposite. Also, when cross K 27 is active, sensory disturbances including hypersensitivity will occur. Cross K 27 is often present in cases of schizophrenia. However, active TL to the cross K 27s in itself does not indicate schizophrenia.

Again, it is highly recommended that all the above pretests and at least the temporary corrections be performed before attempting other Applied Kinesiology procedures.

Muscle Testing Pretests
A Summarized Overview

The following is a brief summarized description of the pretests. They serve as a kind of calibration of the muscle test and should be conducted in order to ensure the accuracy of muscle testing results. The reader should review any pertinent portions of the previous text for more complete information. The labels A-H are the same in this and the previous, more extensive, description of the pretests.

A. Is Dehydration Present? (Page 79)

When a patient is dehydrated, therapy localization may not function well. For this reason, before beginning to muscle-test, the examiner and patient should both drink a glass of water.

B. Does the Muscle Test Strong in the Clear? (Page 79)

1. Ask permission to test.

2. Describe what muscle testing is. Explain that the patient is to initiate the muscle test and steadily increase the force of contraction to attain maximal contraction within 2 seconds. Provide resistance to prevent any movement during the contraction. Then apply a bit more pressure. The patient is to resist so that the arm or other body part tested does not move.

3. Gently guide the patient into the correct position for the test.

4. Demonstrate the range and direction of the test without resistance. Explain any patient postural requirements such as holding the elbow completely extended during the test.

5. Place your hand where it needs to be for applying the resistance.

6. Stabilize the patient with your other hand as needed.

7. Say "Press as hard as you can" to indicate that the patient is to begin the test.

8. Resist until you feel the muscle lock the joint and the force of contraction reach a maximum. (At maximum, the force of contraction will stop increasing.)

9. Then add about 2–5% more pressure.

10. If the muscle continues to hold the test position, it tested strong. If it "breaks" and the tested body part gives way and moves, the muscle tested weak.

If the muscle remained strong, it passed the first test. If not, either strengthen it before continuing or find another muscle that tests strong.

C. CAN THE MUSCLE BE WEAKENED?
(PAGE 82)

1. Firmly pinch the spindle cells in the belly of the muscle together, parallel to the length of the muscle. Avoid the extreme ends of the muscle.

Other options include:

a) TL or tap the acupuncture sedation point for the meridian associated with this muscle.

b) Place the north pole of a magnet upon the belly of the muscle. "North pole" means the one that has the same polarity as the north pole of the earth. A compass needle will point toward this end of the magnet or,

c) Stroke along the meridian against its natural direction.

2. Retest the muscle. If it now tests weak, it passed the second test. After the weakening stimulus has been removed, the muscle should self-correct within 10 seconds. Test it to confirm that it again tests strong.

3. If it did not weaken, either clear the hypertonicity so that it can be weakened, or find another muscle that passes both tests (tests strong and can be weakened).

D. IS THE INDIVIDUAL MUSCLE HYPERTONIC?
(PAGE 83)

If the muscle cannot easily be weakened with the above techniques, try to correct the muscle with the following techniques:

1. Ask your patient to "Relax. Be here with me now. Tense only the muscle we are testing. Breathe during the test and be testable."

2. Move the limb to put the muscle into extreme contraction. Stabilize it there and have the patient attempt to move the limb toward extension of the muscle. Then move the limb to put the muscle into extreme extension. Stabilize it there and have the patient attempt to move the limb toward contraction of the muscle. Pinch the neuromuscular spindle cells together as in step C (1) above and retest the muscle.

3. Have the patient drink a large glass of water. Then retest the muscle.

4. Try any other technique you know that may make hypertonic muscles normotonic.

5. Apply one of the four weakening techniques listed above and retest the muscle. Try with at least two of the weakening techniques. If the muscle still cannot be weakened, choose another muscle and begin again.

For the treatment of bilateral hypertonic muscles or general hypertonicity of many or all muscles, see the section on "General Hypertonicity," page 93.

IS NEUROLOGIC DISORGANIZATION (SWITCHING) PRESENT?

E. OCULAR LOCK (PAGE 85)

1. Guide the patient to look at your hand as you move it around in a clockwise circle in front of her face. Make the circle large enough that the patient has to look about as far as possible in all directions without moving her head. Watch the patient's eyes for any erratic movements.

2. Test an indicator muscle.

3. The patient looks at your hand as you move it around in a counterclockwise circle. Watch the patient's eyes for any erratic movement.

4. Test an indicator muscle.

5. If looking around in either direction causes the indicator muscle to test weak, ocular lock is present.

6. Have the patient look in the direction where the patient's eyes jumped or made jerky movements and retest the indicator muscle.

7. If the indicator muscle tests strong, have the patient look in a slightly different direction and retest.

8. The direction in which the eyes look that weakens the indicator muscle is the direction of ocular lock. This will be corrected and retested in the next step below.

F. Kidney 27 and Ocular Lock Correction (Page 86)

1. TL the navel. If this weakens the indicator muscle, apply Bach Rescue Remedy® cream, APM Creme®, Ion Salbe Forte®, or the light of a laser to clear the influence of the navel scar.

2. Muscle-test an indicator muscle while the patient touches the navel and the left kidney 27 located just below where the clavicle meets the sternum. Repeat the test with TL to the navel and the right K 27. Test TL to both K 27s. Test crossover TL to both K 27s.

3. If the indicator muscle weakens on any of these four tests, massage the two points that tested weak for 20 seconds.

4. Test the indicator muscle while touching the two points that tested weak. This should no longer weaken the indicator muscle.

5. If ocular lock was present before massaging the K 27s, it should now be absent. Have the patient look in the previously weakening direction and retest the indicator muscle. If the indicator muscle now tests strong, ocular lock is no longer present.

6. If ocular lock is still present, have the patient look in the weakening direction while massaging the K 27s.

7. If ocular lock is still present, have the patient look in the weakening direction and take two deep sniffing inhalations.

8. Test the indicator muscle while the patient continues to look in the weakening direction. If the indicator muscle tests weak, tap on both sides of the bridge of the patient's nose for about one minute.

9. Have the patient look in the previously weakening direction and take two sniffs.

10. Retest the indicator muscle. It should now test strong, indicating that ocular lock is no longer present.

G. Auxiliary K 27 (Page 89)

1. If signs of neurologic disorganization are still present (conflicting diagnostic information still exists), therapy-localize each of the auxiliary K 27 points located lateral to the transverse processes of thoracic vertebra 11 (T11/L2).

2. Test the indicator muscle.

3. If the indicator muscle tests weak, massage the active auxiliary K 27 point (lateral to T11/L2) and the navel simultaneously.

4. Again therapy-localize lateral to T11/L2 and retest the indicator. If the indicator muscle now tests strong, this problem has been corrected.

H. Central (Conception) Vessel and Governing Vessel (CV 24, GV 27, GV 1) (Page 89)

1. Therapy-localize CV 24 (below the lower lip) and test an indicator muscle.

2. Therapy-localize GV 27 (above the upper lip) and test an indicator muscle.

3. Therapy-localize GV 1 (tip of coccyx) and test an indicator muscle.

4. If touching either CV 24, GV 27 or GV 1 weakens the indicator muscle, press firmly CV 24 and CV 2 (on the top center edge of the pubic bone) for 20–30 seconds.

5. Then gently hold GV 1 (at the tip of the coccyx) and the navel for 20–30 seconds.

6. Therapy-localize CV 24 and test the indicator muscle. Therapy-localize GV 27 and test the indicator muscle. Both tests should now test strong.

7. An alternate correction is simply to massage the CV 24, GV 27 or GV 1 that tested weak. Again TL the previously weak-testing point and test the indicator muscle to confirm the correction.

General Hypertonicity

"General hypertonicity" refers to the state in which most or all muscles are hypertonic (test strong but cannot be weakened by the usual techniques). The causes of general hypertonicity in muscles are also the causes of the major health disturbances in the patient. Finding and correcting these causes will often eliminate many secondary problems, including neurologic disorganization. For this reason, many examiners experienced with this aspect of AK techniques no longer make it a standard practice to test for switching at the start of an examination.

The theme of hypertonic muscles is receiving more attention lately by those who use AK. Until recently, most examiners analyzed the results of muscle testing with the simple categories of "strong=normal" and "weak=too little—not ok."

For anyone with some knowledge of the scientific process, AK muscle testing is easy to understand. It is just an experiment. The muscle tests strong or weak. If it tests strong, it is OK. If it tests weak, there is a problem. When it tests strong, other factors can be added to the equation (the test situation) to see what will cause the muscle to test weak. The factors that weaken a strong-testing muscle are considered to have a negative effect upon the body. When the muscle tests weak, other factors can be added to the test to see what will make the muscle test strong. The factors that strengthen a weak-testing muscle are considered to have a positive effect upon the body and especially upon the organs and glands associated with the weak-testing muscle. This simple "strong or weak" model is still used by many in AK and by most in the Touch for Health-based kinesiologies today.

However, in the field of medicine, the results of diagnostic measurements are judged as being too low, the right amount, or too high. The right amount is usually a range of values within which the body is considered to be functioning normally. Blood pressure, heart rate, amount of nutrients, constituents of the blood, level of hunger, temperature, reactions of the skin, reflexes and most other parameters tested in medicine are rated as being too low, in a normal range, or too high.

As discussed above, AK historically defined the results of muscle tests as too low (weak) or strong (normal). Where is the "too high" result? The hypertonic muscle is logically this missing "too high" result. If AK is to be recognized as the effective medical diagnostic method it is claimed to be, a reliable technique to test this third category of "too high" needs to become part of the standard AK diagnostics. This has been provided recently by Wolfgang Gerz and is now accepted by the ICAK-D as standard practice. ICAK in America moves much more slowly. Typically, any new AK technique requires ten or more years of consideration before being officially accepted by the ICAK in America. But medicine moves more swiftly than the ICAK. The many medical doctors who use AK in German-speaking lands cannot wait ten years or more for new knowledge to become official. They want theoretical models and therapeutic techniques that can be integrated with their medical work to increase their ability to help their patients now.

German medical doctor and ICAK diplomat Wolfgang Gerz acquired the extra diploma to practice complementary medicine *(Naturheilverfahren)*. His work has done much to integrate the various diagnostic and therapeutic techniques of AK with allopathic and complementary medicine. His medical background provided him with the needed knowledge to recognize and tackle the missing "too high" result in AK muscle testing.

In his practice, Dr. Gerz noted that in more and more of his patients, all muscles tested strong and almost nothing provided a positive challenge or therapy localization. Many of these patients had obvious health problems, but the muscles associated with the diseased organs all tested strong. However, further testing revealed that many or all such muscles could not be weakened by normal means: They were in a hypertonic state. But Gerz did not know what to do. He read the available literature and found general information indicating the existence of the problem, but few ideas concerning how to correct it.

The basic problem was stated in a general way by the founder of chiropractic, D. D. Palmer, "I wish that all chiropractors could take in this basic principle of our science - that too much or not enough energy is disease."

Early in AK, in *You'll Be Better,* (Chapter 6, page 7) Goodheart said, "If the liver has a disturbed energy pattern, this disturbance 'overflows' into a muscle associated with that energy pattern, and the muscle will *test either too strong or too weak*." Walther (1981, p. 167) discusses an example of individual palpatory hypertonic muscles under the topic of reactive muscles. The treatment to lower the tension of a palpatory hypertonic muscle in the case of a reactive muscle is through manipulation of the nerve receptors. But the case of AK hypertonic muscles (that test strong and cannot be weakened) appears to have been mostly ignored. Goodheart only mentions that such a state may exist but does not explain how to correct it. And no mention is given in the early literature of cases in which many or all muscles test hypertonic. One reason for this is that twenty years ago, there were few such cases. The phenomenon has emerged only recently as a widespread problem. The pollution of food, water and air plus the stress of modern lifestyles are suspected to be the major causes of this increase in the prevalence of general hypertonicity of muscles.

Walther in *Synopsis* writes about a lack of correlation between other diagnostic factors and the muscle test: "Persistence in investigating an apparent lack of correlation finds that there is muscle association; however, it may be a hypertonic muscle or a subclinical involvement." (1988, p. 15.) By "subclinical" he means that there is a problem but the body has compensated for it. Thus the problem is not directly observable. For example, the body may tighten muscles and alter the posture to avoid putting painful stress upon an injured knee. As long as the body remains in this compensated posture, the pain in the knee may well be absent. However, the problem still exists and may be provoked by removing the compensation, i.e., by having the patient stand and walk upright with correct posture. Walther goes on to describe how to search for subclinical involvements (by muscle stretch reaction, etc.), but fails to define, discuss or give any directions whatsoever concerning hypertonic muscles.

In Brussels in 1992, W. Gerz asked Goodheart about hypertonic muscles. Goodheart said that he was aware of hypertonic muscles and that in his experience they were usually caused by meridian imbalances, especially of the triple heater meridian. It is noteworthy that the triple heater meridian is associated with the thymus and thyroid glands, which are always involved in stress reactions.

With so little offered in the literature and training, many examiners using AK techniques as well as those in other branches of kinesiology simply ignore the phenomenon of "hypertonic muscles." If a muscle tests strong, they consider it to function correctly and devote no further attention to it. Other examiners, upon finding a muscle that tests strong but cannot be weakened, simply ignore it and find another muscle that can be weakened to use as an indicator muscle. But when all muscles test strong and cannot be weakened, some kind of solution must be found.

A sentence by Michael Lebowitz, D.C., finally gave Gerz a clue: "Sometimes, in the all-muscle-strong-patient with a multitude of problems, copper helps." (Lebowitz/Steele, 1989.) From his complementary medicine training, Gerz recognized that copper is given as a homeopathic remedy for cases of muscle spasticity and cramping. Spasticity and cramping are examples of extreme hypertonicity. Experiments revealed that giving orthomolecular (pure substance) amounts of copper or copper in homeopathic dilutions sometimes caused the hypertonic muscles to become normotonic. In such cases, the expected muscle weaknesses characteristic of the patients' problems appeared. However, the oral application of copper only produced these desired results in a small proportion of the patients in whom all muscles test hypertonic.

With one patient who had all muscles hypertonic, suddenly and unexpectedly many muscles tested weak. Gerz noted that the patient was holding one hand in the other. Experimenting, he found one specific point that, when therapy-localized, often makes blocked muscles test weak. The spot was triple heater 3, located proximal to the space between the hand knuckles of the little and ring fingers. This confirmed Goodheart's observation that blocked muscles relate to imbalances in the triple heater meridian. Gerz reasoned that this was a new kind of challenge. He named any challenge that could make one or more hypertonic muscles test weak a *superchallenge (SC)*.

Further experiments revealed that various challenges could "break" the hypertonic muscle. Some challenges had the effect of making the hypertonic muscle test normotonic—strong but able to be weak-

ened. Gerz named any challenge that makes a hypertonic muscle normotonic a *normotonic challenge (NC)*. The superchallenge was found to indicate the cause of the hypertonic muscles. The normotonic challenge is often precisely what the patient needs to correct the cause of the hypertonic muscles.

Furthermore, a challenge can make either a weak-testing or a normotonic muscle hypertonic. Such a challenge is a *hypertonic challenge (HC)*. The body is extremely stressed and immediately put into a strong adaptation reaction by such a challenge.

Gerz determined that all patients with general hypertonicity were extremely stressed. And, as expected, he found that these patients had stress-related disturbances of the immune system such as allergies, low resistance, rheumatic problems, clinical ecology illnesses, disturbances of the intestine including overgrowths of candida, psychosomatic complaints, weakness of the adrenal and/or thymus glands, and "vegetative stress syndrome." Often such patients are taking antirheumatic medicine, cortisone or "mood-altering" medication. (Gerz, 1996, p. 312.)

Gerz found that when he therapy-localized or challenged the causes of the stress/hypertonic muscles, some or all of the hypertonic muscles tested weak (a superchallenge). Thus this provides a useful method to locate the cause of the patient's stress and dis-ease. Besides TL to triple heater 3, the superchallenges that are most often effective include histidine, pcck, "eyes up," the antigen substance of candida, emotional challenge, the challenges that reveal neurologic disorganization (switching), and TL to the thymus, adrenals, pectoralis minor NL, neurovascular stress points on the frontal eminences of the forehead, and to functionally disturbed focal points such as the tonsils, teeth, sinuses or scars. (Gerz, 1996, p. 312.) For example, if TL of a dead tooth makes the hypertonic muscle test weak (a superchallenge), the tooth is likely a focus and may need to be removed. If the candida antigen is a superchallenge, the patient likely has an overgrowth of candida in the intestine and needs a candida cure. The examiner ought to test many different possible superchallenges. He or she should determine and perform the indicated therapeutic steps (or direct the patient to the needed therapy) for each positive superchallenge.

The substances Gerz found that make hypertonic muscles normotonic (a normotonic challenge) are the substances that are effective in correcting the above conditions: zinc, magnesium, copper, histamine D12, homeopathic remedies (mostly single substances in mid to high potencies), neural therapy to the focal points that one found as active superchallenges, Bach Flower Remedies and Iliocaecal valve treatment, etc. (Gerz, 1996, p. 312.)

Finding the cause and determining how to correct general hypertonicity as described above is certainly more difficult than just finding and massaging the switching points with an active TL. But the results not only produce a more long-lasting correction for switching they also reveal the most important steps needed for improving health.

A full explanation of all the above causes of stress, superchallenges and normotonic challenges will not be attempted here. For further information, the interested reader is advised to peruse the literature; especially Gerz's book quoted above. Sources for the superchallenge and normotonic challenge substances listed above are given in the appendix, "Contact Addresses and Sources."

How to Detect Hypertonic Muscles

1. Test a muscle.

2. If weak, strengthen it with the techniques you know. It should test strong before you continue.

3. Pinch its spindle cells together, touch or tap upon the associated meridian's sedation point, place the north pole of a magnet upon the belly of the muscle, or stroke the meridian against its natural direction and retest the muscle.

4. If the muscle fails to weaken after application of at least two of the above weakening techniques, it is hypertonic.

5. If many or all the muscles test hypertonic, this problem of general hypertonicity needs to be addressed.

How to Correct Hypertonicity in Individual Muscles

This technique will often work for both palpatory hypertonic muscles and AK hypertonic muscles (test strong but cannot be weakened).

1. Locate a normotonic indicator muscle.

2. TL various points in the contractile part of the hypertonic muscle. Points that TL are malfunctioning neuromuscular spindle cells. If an active TL point is found, continue with the following step:

3. Place a finger on each side of the malfunctioning neuromuscular spindle cell. Press into the muscle and then press the fingers toward each other. In other words, pinch the spindle cell together in a direction parallel to the fibers of the muscle. Repeat this process, pressing firmly several times.

4. Check that the area no longer has an active TL. If more than one area had an active TL, repeat this technique with the other active TL areas.

5. TL the junction of each end of the muscle with its tendons. Points that TL here are malfunctioning Golgi tendon organs. If a active TL point is found, continue with the steps below.

6. Press the fingers into the muscle on the muscle belly side of the malfunctioning Golgi tendon organ and pull it toward the tendon/bone end of the muscle.

7. Check that the Golgi tendon organ no longer has an active TL.

8. The muscle should now feel softer (palpatory normotonic) and should weaken when normal weakening techniques are applied.

How to Correct Hypertonicity in Bilateral Muscle Pairs

Bilateral hypertonicity logically indicates an adaptation reaction in the system of regulation (organ, gland, etc.) associated with the muscle. To correct such a problem, use the same technique as for General Hypertonicity. The normotonic challenge will likely be a remedy or corrective technique known to improve the function of the associated organ of the system of regulation.

How to Correct General Hypertonicity

1. Test many muscles, attempt to weaken them, and note their reaction. Though most test hypertonic, a few may test weak or normotonic.

2. Choose a hypertonic muscle that is convenient to test.

3. Find the superchallenge(s) that weaken it. This gives information about the nature of the stressors against which the body is currently fighting.

4. Continue one of the superchallenges and find the normotonic challenge(s) that make the weakened muscle again test strong.

5. Repeat the process (steps 4 and 5) with each of the superchallenges found in step 3 above.

6. If possible during the session, apply the therapeutic corrective measures corresponding to each of the normotonic challenges.

7. Check the chosen muscle and the other muscles tested in step 1. If the chosen muscle or other muscles are still hypertonic, locate other superchallenges and repeat the process. Note also that the tested therapeutic procedures may need to be implemented for a period of time before the hypertonic muscles return to being normotonic.

8. Instruct the patient concerning further processes for a more complete correction of the state of general hypertonicity. The patient may need to have dead teeth removed, clear foci and waste from the sinuses, the intestines, the tonsils, etc., avoid allergic substances, get more exercise in the fresh air, improve posture, replace missing nutrients, and reduce all kinds of stress.

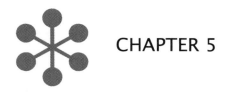

Diagnosis and Correction Techniques

The Origin-Insertion Technique

As mentioned in the section on the history of Applied Kinesiology, in 1964 Goodheart first strengthened a weak-testing muscle quite inadvertently. He was trying to detect a reason why one of his patients had one shoulder blade that stuck out from the back of his rib cage. It had been this way for fifteen or twenty years. He recalled reading about " . . . a muscle that pulled the shoulder-blade forward so that it would lie flat on the chest wall." (Goodheart, *You'll Be Better*, Chapter 1, p. 2). He looked in a copy of *Muscles—Testing and Function,* the original reference on this topic by Kendall, Kendall and Wadsworth (1949). There he read that the serratus muscle pulls the shoulder blade against the rib cage. Upon testing, he found that the serratus muscle did test weak, but only on the side where the shoulder blade protruded. While palpating the serratus muscle of his patient, he detected small, sensitive, "BB"-sized lumps at the origin of the serratus muscle on the ribs on the weak-testing side. As he was firmly touching a few of them to try to identify them, they disappeared. He strongly massaged the rest of these lumps, which also disappeared. Subsequently, the shoulder blade lay flat and the serratus muscle tested strong.

This technique was often successful in strengthening other weak-testing muscles. It is likely that some of the time, the effect was due to the stimulation of the Golgi tendon organs (page 29), located in the junction of the muscle with its tendon. The small lumps that indicate the need for the origin-insertion technique are located where the tendon attaches to bone. In many muscles, these two areas are very near each other. Golgi tendon organs require a linear pushing or pulling for optimal stimulation. The origin-insertion technique requires only a heavy massage on the lumps.

Part of the muscle-strengthening effect of the origin-insertion technique is likely due to the vibrating stimulation given to the nerve receptors and nerves in the area massaged. It is an established fact that relatively slow vibratory stimulation, such as the massaging hand produces, facilitates the activity of the alpha motor neurons responsible for raising the tone in a muscle. When the alpha motor neurons are facilitated, they send more nerve impulses per second to the muscle. Thus, the muscle has a greater force of contraction (tests stronger) when tested.

It is theorized that the need for origin-insertion treatment results from a prior trauma that partially tore the tendon away from the periosteum, the skin that surrounds bones. It is believed that the little lumps are micro avulsions—small areas where the tendon is partially torn away from the periosteum. When the little lumps are felt in the tendon-bone junction, the need for this treatment is confirmed. Treatment consists of firmly pushing and rubbing the tendon back down upon the periosteum of the bone to which it is attached.

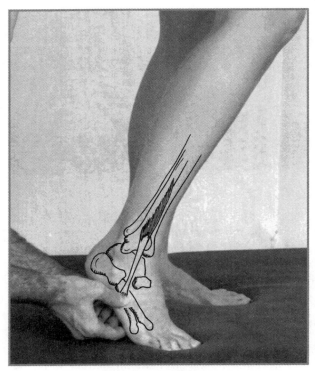

MASSAGE OF THE INSERTION
OF PERONEUS TERTIUS

HOW TO PERFORM
THE ORIGIN-INSERTION TECHNIQUE

Indications:

- A weak-testing muscle with a known history of prior trauma and/or small, palpable lumps where the muscle's tendon attaches to bone.

- The weak-testing muscle tests strong when these lumps are therapy-localized.

- A normotonic muscle weakens when the origin or insertion of the suspect muscle is therapy-localized.

Correction:

Use heavy massage upon the lumps to press and rub the tendon back down onto its attachment to the bone.

Confirm the Correction:

The muscle should no longer test weak. Or the normotonic indicator muscle should no longer weaken when the treated origin or insertion is therapy-localized.

Neurolymphatic Reflexes

Goodheart's first method of strengthening weak-testing muscles was the origin-insertion technique. When this technique worked, the muscle returned to testing strong, and the function of the related organ improved. This was so successful that many other chiropractors began using muscle testing and Goodheart's origin-insertion technique. In many cases, however, the origin-insertion technique failed to strengthen the weak-testing muscle. In such cases, Goodheart and other chiropractors including Walther prescribed exercises to increase the strength of these muscles. Exercises often did slowly increase the mass and weight-bearing ability of these muscles, but they still tested weak. This was the beginning of the realization that a weak-testing muscle is not the same as a physically weak muscle. Other solutions to the problem of weak-testing muscles had to be found.

Most of Goodheart's discoveries occurred in the context of trying to solve the problems his patients brought to him. He had a patient with sciatic nerve pain on one side when lying, sitting or standing. Only walking brought relief. The fascia lata muscle, which covers the outer part of the thigh and moves the leg diagonally forward and away from the body, tested weak on this side. Neither chiropractic efforts nor his origin-insertion could make it test strong. Goodheart reasoned that since walking pumps the lymph out of the muscles, perhaps his patient's problem involved inadequate lymph drainage. He palpated the lymph nodules over the fascia lata but found no difference between the involved and the uninvolved sides of the body. He also palpated the area of the sacroiliac because sometimes there are swollen lymph nodules here when patients have sciatic pain. He found nothing unusual. Then his patient said, "That's the first

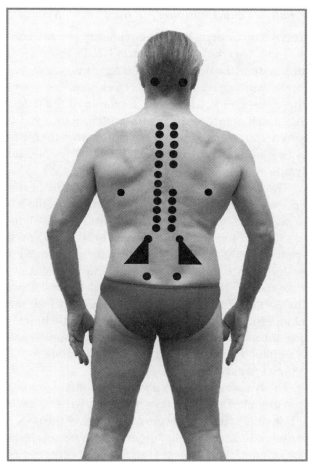

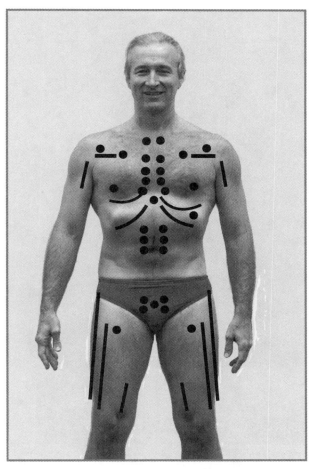

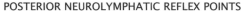

POSTERIOR NEUROLYMPHATIC REFLEX POINTS

ANTERIOR NEUROLYMPHATIC REFLEX POINTS

relief that I've ever gotten." Goodheart remarked, "That's what you came here for." (Goodheart, *You'll Be Better,* Chapter 1, p. 3.) In reality he was quite astonished at his quick success! He continued to palpate and massage these two areas, and the patient's pain completely disappeared and never returned.

He next tried out this technique with a woman's weak-testing neck muscles, but massaging the area of the muscles didn't work at all. He reasoned that his prior success must have been not because he was pressing upon the lymph nodes in the muscle itself, but perhaps because he inadvertently stimulated some kind of reflex points for lymph drainage like the

osteopath Frank Chapman had postulated in the 1930s. Chapman used his reflex points to stimulate the elimination of excess lymph in various areas of the body. Goodheart experimented with Chapman's reflexes and had success using them to strengthen various weak-testing muscles. He also discovered a few more such reflex points that strengthened muscles for which none of Chapman's reflex points were effective. Chapman had correlated these reflex points with specific organs and with various health problems. This added evidence to Goodheart's growing conviction of a connection between specific muscles and organs. In fact, Goodheart found through x-ray,

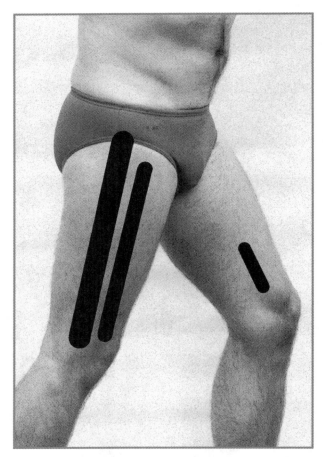

SIDE NEUROLYMPHATIC POINTS

Anatomy and Physiology of the Lymph System

The lymph system, like the circulatory system, consists of a branching net of vessels. Unlike the circulatory system, the lymph system is an open system that begins with tiny vessels at the extremities. The size of these vessels increase in the direction of the trunk. At certain areas (especially the crotch, belly, armpits and neck), many lymph vessels flow together into lymph nodes and from there into the next larger lymph vessels.

The largest lymph vessel, the thoracic duct, gathers the entire lymph from both legs, the trunk, the left arm and the left side of the head into the left lymphatic duct located behind the left clavicle. Lymph from the right arm and the right side of the head is gathered into the right lymphatic duct behind the right clavicle. The left and right lymphatic ducts empty the gathered lymph from the entire body into the bloodstream at the junction of the internal jugular and subclavian veins. The spleen, thymus, tonsils and lymphatic tissue of the intestines also belong to the lymph system.

The lymph system has no heart, no pump to keep it in motion. The lymph flow in smaller lymph vessels is primarily "pumped" by the contraction of the body's muscles. In addition, the largest lymph vessels have smooth muscular walls that rhythmically contract to propel the lymph forward. Even the tiny lymph capillaries, although they don't have a muscular wall, do contain contractile fibers. It is postulated that the effect of massaging the Chapman reflexes (called neurolymphatic reflexes in Applied Kinesiology) is to stimulate the muscular action of the lymph vessels to increase the removal of lymph from the corresponding tissues.

Lymph vessels contain one-way valves that allow the lymph to flow forward but not to reverse. So, when muscles contract, the lymph vessels passing through them are squeezed and the lymph moves forward. This creates a tiny vacuum effect—a negative pressure of about -6 mm of mercury in the interstitial spaces. This effectively sucks the fluids from the interstitial spaces into the lymph capillaries.

biochemistry, or other accepted biological tests that revealed dysfunction and weakness in an organ that such problems were always associated with weakness in specific muscles. His list of muscle-organ correspondences grew larger and more certain with further observation and experimentation by himself and his colleagues.

Chapman's original technique was to observe for edema or other symptoms of excess lymph and then to palpate the reflex points related to the organ or body area requiring lymphatic drainage. He considered tenderness and swelling of the reflex point to confirm the observation of excess lymph and the need for improved drainage.

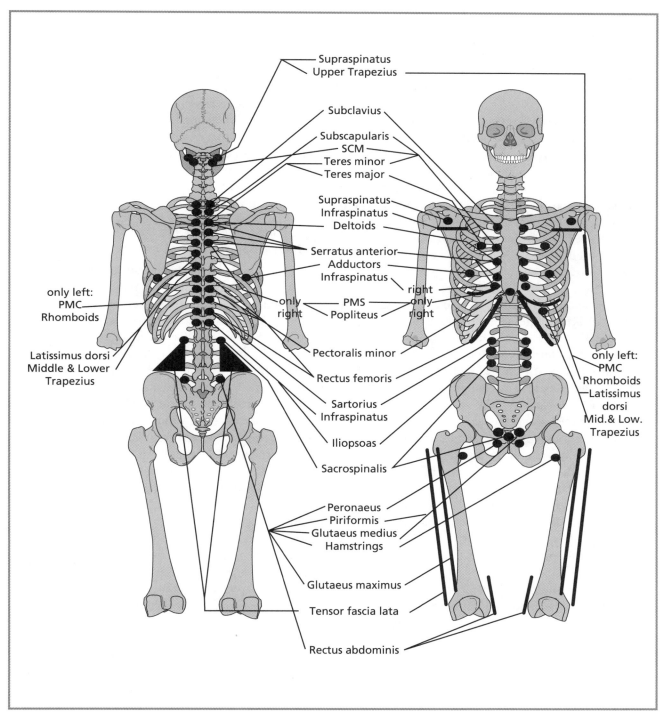

THE NEUROLYMPHATIC REFLEX POINTS

Respiration and all activities that raise the abdominal pressure (coughing, sneezing, lifting, evacuating the bowel) pump the lymph from the legs and abdomen toward the ultimate destination at the base of the neck. There the lymph empties into the venous system.

The human body has twice as much lymph as blood and twice as many lymph vessels as blood vessels. The blood capillaries carry nutrients to the cells. Fats and proteins leave the capillaries and bathe the cells. Some are used by the cells as needed. The unused fats are too large to return to the (blood) capillaries. They are received into the lymph capillaries through tiny one-way valves. If the proteins from the blood capillaries are not used by the cells, they must be absorbed into the lymph capillaries to be eventually returned to the blood. Because the blood contains so much protein already, the protein that leaves the capillaries cannot return directly to them due to osmotic pressure. It is estimated that every 24 hours, 50% of the total amount of protein circulating in the blood exits the capillaries, is mostly unused by the cells, and is then reabsorbed back into the lymph system from which it is delivered back into the venous blood through ducts near the base of the neck.

Besides transporting water, fats and proteins, the lymph system is mainly a waste removal and defense system. In the lymph nodes, bone marrow, thymus and spleen, lymphocytes (white blood cells) are generated. These agents of the body's defense reside mainly in the lymph system. White blood cells there act as "phagocytes," which surround and digest the filtered waste particles and pathogens in the lymph nodes.

The waste products of cell metabolism exit the cells and gather in the interstitial (intercellular) spaces. The waste fluids then flow by osmotic pressure into the lymph vessels. When any tissues are infected, the infectious material and products of cellular destruction (pus) are also gathered into the lymph system. There they are transported to the lymph nodes, which filter out the tissue remnants, foreign bodies and microorganisms to be digested by the white blood cells.

Whenever there is infection in the body, the next lymph nodes in the direction of the circulation of the lymph become swollen and tender. In order to prevent further spread of infection, the purulent material is gathered into the lymph nodes and given over to the white blood cells.

The lymph circulation through the body is slow. It needs to be slow to have enough time to filter out and break down large bits of matter that cannot be safely passed back into the blood. However, if lymphatic drainage of the tissues is inadequate, lymphatic congestion occurs.

Lymphatic Congestion and the Need for Increased Lymphatic Drainage

When the lymph circulation is too slow, the proteins, fats, waste products of cellular metabolism, and infectious material (if present) build up in the interstitial spaces. This buildup of fluids, which inflates of the spaces between the cells, is called *edema*. Edema moves the cells further away from their capillaries, which interferes with their proper nutrition. It is with this disturbance of the lymphatic system that Applied Kinesiology methods appear to have influence.

Edema stretches the tissues and makes them more porous. If this has become chronic, it will be more difficult to achieve a lasting correction, as fluids can easily return through the more porous tissues. For this reason, corrective measures must be applied over a long period of time to reestablish proper lymph system function.

Medical authorities agree that excess lymph in the tissues does not become observable until it has reached a level 30% above normal. This is likely the reason why Applied Kinesiology techniques indicate the need for increased lymphatic activity, although no edema is observed.

Symptoms of lymphatic congestion include edema (especially in the extremities), low resistance, infections, and wounds that do not heal. Lymphatic congestion may often be seen in the eyes as a "string of white pearls" around the outer part of the iris. In some cases there may no apparent symptoms at all.

When a lymphatic problem is acute, the reflex points will be swollen and firm but squishy over the whole area where the reflex can be stimulated. When a problem is more chronic, the center of the reflex point will feel firm but rubbery. When the problem is very chronic (has existed for a long time), there will be small, hard, BB sized lumps (in the fat just under the skin) in the middle of the reflex area.

Chapman's reflex points are located in the intercostal spaces between the ribs anteriorly where they meet the sternum and posteriorly where they meet the vertebrae. There are also some on the lower abdomen, around the scapula, on the low back and on the legs. Most of the reflex points are about 3 cm in diameter. Some, such as those for fascia lata, cover large areas.

Active lymphatic points are massaged with a firm, rotary pressure for at least 15 seconds. In certain cases, such as for the correction of repeated muscle weakness (page 123), the points are massaged for 2–4 minutes or even longer. The points on the anterior side of the body are generally more tender. The more chronic a condition, the greater the amount of tenderness. When the points are very tender, they should be massaged more gently and for a longer time.

As mentioned, Goodheart correlated Chapman's reflex points with specific muscles (and organs). Each muscle was found to have at least one anterior and one posterior reflex point. Goodheart also discovered a method to determine when massage of these reflex points would be useful in strengthening weak-testing muscles. If therapy localization of the reflex point makes a previously weak-testing muscle test strong, massage of the point is indicated. After adequate massage, the muscle should test strong. To confirm the correction, the patient again therapy-localizes (touches) the point and the same muscle is again tested. In Applied Kinesiology, if (after successful strengthening) the muscle again tests weak with therapy localization of the treated reflex point, further stimulation of the *same* point is indicated.

In some patients, every muscle in the body will test weak. A muscle may test strong, then after two or three further tests of the same muscle, it tests weak. In such patients, it is impossible to find an adequate indicator muscle. Typically these people never exercise and are extremely sedentary, spending most of their time sitting (likely in front of the TV). These are often patients with vast quantities of excess lymph in their bodies. A seeming paradox, these patients are often dehydrated. Their excess water is not where it needs to be in the tissues, but rather in the lymph system diluting the concentrated waste products there. These patients respond well to the extended massage of neurolymphatic reflex points as performed in the correction for repeated muscle failure (page 123). When most or all muscles test weak, the patient is in the exhaustion phase of Selye's stress reactions and urgently requires recuperation (see pages 35–39).

Clearing the body of such extreme amounts of lymph requires that the patient assist the process between treatment sessions. One of the best techniques for eliminating excess lymph from the whole body is bouncing on a trampoline. When one bounces up, one is weightless. When one bounces down, one effectively has as much as double the normal weight. Remember bouncing on the family scales as a child, trying to "weigh" as much as possible? These alternate states of "weightless" and "very heavy" act like a pump upon all the tissues of the body. For those whose joints cannot withstand jumping on a trampoline, bouncing while seated on a large gymnastic ball is an excellent and more gentle alternative.

When ill, most people remain in bed nearly motionless. Without muscular activity, the lymph gathers and the tissues swell. During illness, the lymph is full of pus and infectious material. Allowing it to remain and gather in the body is counterproductive to the goal of returning to health. If able, the ill person should be moderately active. Taking walks is recommended. At the very least, bouncing gently on a gymnastic ball is advised as an excellent lymphatic system "pump." Activating the muscles (through muscle testing or other activities) followed by massage of the neurolymphatic reflex points and finished by activating the muscles again will assist the body greatly in eliminating excess lymph from the tissues.

When many different muscles require neurolymphatic stimulation, there is a generalized lymphatic problem. This is usually caused by dehydration. Water is the most common nutritional element needed for general problems with the lymphatic system. The body needs water to cleanse itself via the lymphatic system. Whenever lymphatic problems exist, it is a good practice to advise the patient to drink at least eight, 8 ounce (2.5 dl) glasses of water each day. The same effect is not achieved by tea, coffee, cola or any other kind of drink. For their digestion these other drinks apparently activate specific metabolic processes that interfere with the body getting the maximal positive effects of the water these drinks contain. Imagine taking a shower with cola! Would your body feel clean? Like your skin, your body also needs regular inner "showers"—regular intake of pure water with nothing added.

It is easy to demonstrate the effect of water. Whenever many muscles test weak or hypertonic, have the patient drink a large glass of water and then retest the muscles. Often simply drinking water will make many or all of them test normotonic. This demonstration will assist the therapist in convincing the patient of the need for drinking much more water daily.

It is believed that massage of Chapman's reflex points stimulates nerves that effect better lymphatic drainage in the associated organs and body areas. Following this reasoning, in Applied Kinesiology, Chapman's reflex points are called "neurolymphatic reflexes." The exact anatomy and physiology involved in these reflexes has yet to be demonstrated. However, it has been demonstrated repeatedly that massage of these points does stimulate lymphatic drainage. In this case, the "proof is in the pudding." We don't know exactly what the neurolymphatic points are or how these reflexes function, but the evidence of numerous clinical trials has proven their effectiveness.

NEUROLYMPHATIC REFLEX POINT TECHNIQUE

Testing to determine if NL massage will strengthen a weak-testing muscle:

1. Test muscles.

2. When one tests weak, have the patient therapy-localize (touch) one of the neurolymphatic points associated with the weak-testing muscle. It is often easier for the patient to touch the anterior point than the posterior one.

3. While the patient touches the point, retest the muscle.

4. If the muscle now tests strong, it can be strengthened with neurolymphatic massage.

Correction:

Massage both the anterior and posterior neurolymphatic points for the weak-testing muscle with a firm, rotary pressure. Very tender points should be massaged more gently and for a longer duration. The time for effective massage may vary from 15 seconds to several minutes.

Confirm the correction:

1. Retest the muscle. If still weak, and therapy localization of the neurolymphatic point makes it again strong, the point requires further stimulation. If NL therapy localization no longer strengthens the muscle, it requires some other kind of strengthening technique.

2. If the muscle now tests strong, again therapy-localize the neurolymphatic point and retest the muscle.

3. If the muscle remains strong, the NL massage was adequate and successful.

4. If the strengthened muscle again weakens with therapy localization of the NL, further stimulation of the *same point* is required.

5. When therapy localization of the NL no longer weakens the previously strengthened muscle, the NL correction is complete.

Neurovascular Reflexes

While Goodheart was giving a lecture upon his discoveries, a young boy had an acute asthma attack. When he was placed upon his back, Goodheart noticed that one leg rotated out much further than the other. The sartorius muscle tested weak on this side. Goodheart had already noticed a connection between the sartorius muscle and the adrenal glands. Adrenaline is given in cases of acute asthma, so the connection seemed logical. However, he could not correct the sartorius muscle with any of his techniques. Trying to find something that would help, Goodheart attempted to make an adjustment of the cranial bones. While doing so, he happened to notice a pulsation under his fingers upon the posterior fontanel, one of the "soft spots" on a baby's head. The pulsation was not the same as his own heart rate nor that of his patient's. He continued to hold and feel this pulse, which grew stronger. Then the young patient took a deep breath, continued to breathe easily, and the leg turned back in! (Goodheart, *You'll Be Better,* Chapter 1, p. 78.)

Fascinated by this unexpected success, Goodheart explored these "vascular reflexes" that had already been researched and mapped out by the California chiropractor, Terrence Bennett. Dr. Bennett was a clinician and not a theorist. He never attempted to explain why his reflex points affected vascular circulation. Using an x-ray fluoroscope, he observed that holding specific points caused an increase of blood flow into specific internal organs, which then swelled with the extra blood. Fascinated, he spent hundreds of hours observing the effect of holding his reflex points. As a result, radiation poisoning is said to have been cause of his death.

Goodheart found many (but only a portion) of Bennett's reflex points to be effective in the strengthening of weak-testing muscles. The points that Goodheart found useful lie mostly upon the head. He also found (as with Chapman's reflexes) that when one of Bennett's reflex points strengthened a weak-testing muscle, it also had an apparent positive effect upon the organ and/or gland associated with the muscle in Goodheart's own research. This further confirmed his muscle-organ/gland associations. The Bennett reflexes used in Applied Kinesiology are called "neurovascular reflexes."

The stimulation of the neurovascular reflexes is effected by lightly pressing upon specific points upon the skin and then gently pushing or pulling tangentially to the skin ("tugging") in various directions until a strong pulsation is felt. The examiner experiments carefully until the precise direction which produces maximun pulsation is detected. This precise direction of tugging is then gently and motionlessly held for at least 20 seconds.

The amount of pressure needed to feel the pulse at the wrist is adequate for stimulation of the neurovascular reflex points. The pulsation felt during this procedure is typically between 70 and 74 beats per minute and is independent of the rate of heart contraction. It is speculated that this pulsation is caused by the contraction of the tiny layer of muscles that surrounds each of the blood capillaries in the scalp. This theory has not been conclusively proven, so the exact physiological basis for this observed pulsation remains unknown.

Using sensitive thermometers, Goodheart discovered that properly tugging on the neurovascular reflex points causes warming of tissues in areas of the body far removed from the point. When the stimulation is adequate, the distant area continues to remain warm even after the finger contact upon the neurovascular reflex point is removed. If the examiner changes the direction of tugging and loses the pulsation (which can easily happen if he is not fully attentive to the sensation), the thermal elevation slows and the positive effect of holding and tugging upon the neurovascular point may be reversed and lost. Returning to the correct direction of tugging results in the return of thermal elevation. When adequate attention is given to this detail (tugging the neurovascular reflex point in the direction of maximal pulsation), the results of using neurovascular reflex point holding greatly improve.

Goodheart's research, however, revealed no predictable pattern to this warming. Different reflex points sometimes warmed the same areas. The areas over the corresponding muscles were not specifically warmed. The patterns of warming have not yet been plotted. But this research conclusively demonstrates that holding and correctly tugging the neurovascular reflex points does affect vascular circulation in remote areas of the body.

Vascular Circulation
from the Arteries to the Veins

Arteries (vessels that carry oxygen-rich blood to the tissues) branch into smaller and smaller *arterioles*. Arteries have a heavy muscular coat that gets thinner and thinner until it is only one cell thick surrounding the tiniest arterioles. The smallest arterioles branch into the *capillaries*. Oxygen and nutrients for the cells diffuse through the somewhat porous walls of the capillaries. Some of these traverse the ground substance and enter the cells. Carbon dioxide and small-sized waste products diffuse from the cells through the ground substance and back into the capillaries. Unused molecularly large nutrients (mostly protein and fats), and large waste products from the cells cannot enter the capillaries. These gather in the interstitial spaces, producing enough pressure to push them into the lymphatic vessels where they are processed and eventually delivered back into the venous blood.

The tiny veins that gather the blood from the capillary bed are called *venules*. The venules converge into larger and larger *veins*. Like the arteries, veins also have a muscular cover, but it is much thinner than the heavy muscular coat of the arteries. Venous blood, which carries oxygen-depleted and carbon dioxide-enriched blood and waste products away from the tissues, returns to the heart. The heart pumps the venous blood through the lungs where the carbon dioxide is expelled and oxygen absorbed. This oxygen-rich blood returns to the heart where it is pumped back into the main artery, the aorta, which branches into all of the other arteries of the body.

The amount of blood circulating in the tissues is controlled by the tone of the muscles surrounding the blood vessels. The tone of the muscles surrounding arteries and veins is increased by the hormone vasopressin, which is produced in the hypothalamus and stored in the posterior part of the pituitary, from which it is released into the blood. The tone of the muscles surrounding arteries and veins is neurally controlled by the vasocenter of the brain. This is located in the lower third of the pons and the upper two-thirds of the medulla oblongata. The upper lateral portion of the vasocenter sends continual signals for the contraction of the muscles around all arteries and veins. The medial and lower portions of the vasocenter send inhibiting signals to the upper lateral center, which results in fewer signals with less intensity being sent to the vascular muscles, thereby creating vasodilation. Both the vasodilation and vasoconstriction effects of the vasocenter are influenced by various higher centers of the brain.

At the beginning of a branch of an arteriole into a smaller arteriole (and from the tiniest arteriole into a capillary) is a circular ring of muscle that controls the passage of blood. Surprisingly, the vasocenter has little or no control over these tiny circular muscles. Some believe that when the tiny circular muscles (and the tissues of the surrounding area) require oxygen, the tiny muscles cannot contract effectively. They then open and allow more oxygen-rich blood to flow in. Another theory is that the waste products of cell metabolism act as vasodilators, increasing the blood circulation to remove the waste products from the tissues. Also, the presence in the bloodstream of hormones such as adrenaline definitely affects vasodilation and vasoconstriction, even at the arteriole level.

It is postulated that stimulation of the neurovascular reflex points has its effect by reducing the tension in the tiny arteriole ring muscles and thereby increasing local blood circulation. It is further postulated that the reflex effect upon organs is due to the organ and the particular tissues of the neurovascular reflex point having a common origin in the embryonic tissues. While these theories offer a way to conceive of how the neurovascular reflex points could function, the truth is that we just don't know how they function. But evidence conclusively indicates that when correctly stimulated, they do both increase local circulation and circulation far from the point, do make weak-testing muscles test strong, and do have a positive effect upon the organ or gland related to the muscle so strengthened.

NEUROVASCULAR REFLEX POINT TECHNIQUE

A. To determine if neurovascular (NV) stimulation is indicated for the strengthening of a weak-testing muscle:

  1) Have the patient therapy-localize a NV point associated with the weak-testing muscle.

  2) Repeat the muscle test.

  3) If the muscle now tests strong, NV point-holding is indicated.

In a more complex example, when a muscle first weakens after it has been muscle-tested several times repeatedly, therapy-localize the related NV point and again test the muscle several times. If the muscle tests strong and remains strong while its NV point is therapy-localized, the neurovascular reflex is involved and requires stimulation for the correction of the repeated muscle test weakness (see "Repeated Muscle Testing," page 123).

B. To locate hidden problems in a normotonic muscle:

  1) Have the patient therapy-localize a NV point for the normotonic muscle.

  2) Retest the muscle. If it now tests weak, NV holding is indicated.

Correction:

  1. Touch the NV(s) with the fingertips and gently tug the point(s) in various directions until maximal pulsation is achieved.

  2. Hold this position of maximal pulsation for at least 20 seconds.

Confirming the correction for A & B:

  1. Retest the formerly weak-testing muscle (A) or the formerly normotonic muscle (B).

  2. If it now tests strong, challenge the correction by therapy-localizing the NV point.

  3. If the muscle still tests strong, the application of the NV holding was correct and is complete.

  4. If therapy-localizing the NV point makes the strengthened muscle again test weak, repeat the *same* NV point-holding.

  5. When therapy localization to the treated NV point no longer weakens the strengthened muscle, the correction is complete.

C. When it is suspected that a neurovascular reflex is involved with a problem that therapy-localized, but the related neurovascular points do not therapy-localize (see "Hidden Problems" later in this chapter, page 121):

  1) Therapy-localize both the area of the problem and the NV point simultaneously.

  2) Test an indicator muscle (that tested weak with therapy localization of the problem area alone).

  3) If the indicator muscle now restrengthens, the NV reflex is involved with the problem.

Correction:

  1. Touch the NV(s) with the fingertips and gently tug the point(s) in various directions until maximal pulsation is achieved.

  2. Hold this position of maximal pulsation for at least 20 seconds.

Confirming the correction for C:

  3. Simultaneously therapy-localize the problem area and the NV that previously tested weak with such therapy localization. Test the indicator muscle.

  4. If the indicator muscle tests weak, repeat the correction procedure.

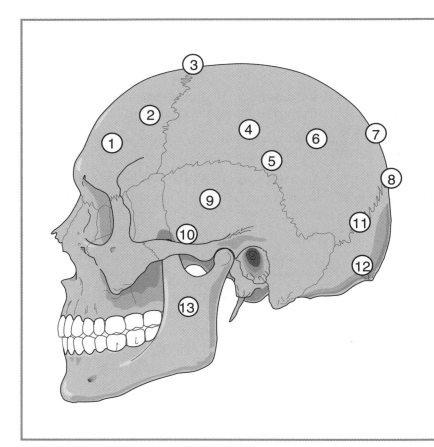

1. Pectoralis major
   clavicular
   Sacrospinalis
   Peroneus (tertius, longus and brevis)
   Rhomboids (Walther)
2. Pectoralis major sternal
   Rhomboids (Leaf)
3. Serratus anticus
   Supraspinatus
   Subscapularis
   Deltoids
4. Rectus abdominis
5. Latissimus dorsi
6. Gluteus medius
   Tensor fascia lata
   Rectus femoris
   Piriformis
7. Hamstrings
   Trapezius, middle and lower
8. Sartorius
9. Teres minor
   Teres major
   Subclavius
10. Trapezius, upper
    Pectoralis minor
11. Gluteus maximus
    Adductors
12. Iliopsoas
13. Sterno-cleido-mastoideus

The Neurovascular Reflex Points

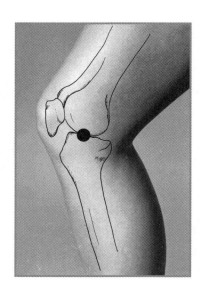
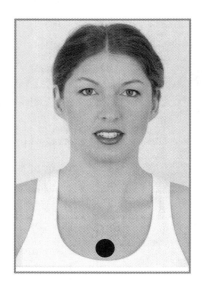
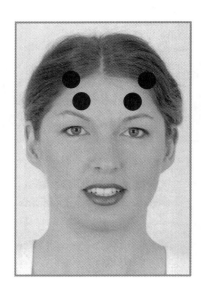

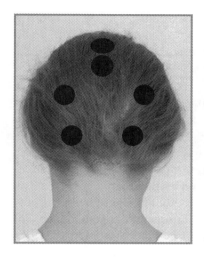 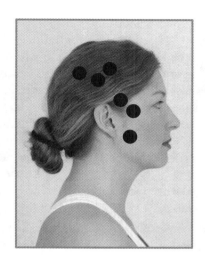 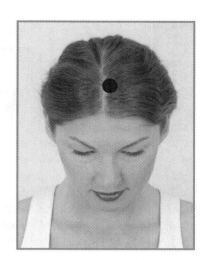

5. If this double therapy localization no longer weakens the indicator muscle, the correction is confirmed.

The Meridian System

The meridian system is one of the most important sources of diagnostic information used in Applied Kinesiology. By comparing and combining the muscle-organ-gland correspondences discovered by George Goodheart with the organ-gland-meridian correspondences of traditional Chinese medicine, muscle-meridian correspondences were discovered. This became the first bridge between Eastern and Western medicine and brought with it many new and very effective muscle-strengthening techniques.

Before the meridian system was included in AK, there were four stages of development of techniques to strengthen weak-testing muscles. First, as already discussed, Goodheart noticed correspondences between specific weak-testing muscles and problems with specific organs and glands. He discovered that massaging the junction of the weak-testing muscle's tendon against the bone where it attached often made a weak-testing muscle test strong and positively affected the related organ. This "origin-insertion" procedure was the first technique for strengthening weak-testing muscles. For the muscles that didn't

respond to this treatment, he prescribed exercises. These often made the muscles able to lift more weight, but they still tested weak. As a result of the failure of this attempt to make the weak-testing muscles test strong, Goodheart realized that although the origin-insertion technique was a valuable breakthrough discovery, it obviously was not enough.

Goodheart's next breakthrough began when he experimented with Frank Chapman's reflexes. Goodheart found that massage of Chapman's reflex points for lymphatic drainage of specific organs and glands not only positively affected those glands and organs, but also strengthened the muscles associated with them. These "neurolymphatic reflex" points became the second technique for strengthening weak-testing muscles. With these he was able to strengthen many of the muscles that his "origin-insertion" technique was unable to strengthen.

The third discovery involved the correction of blocks in the natural motion of the cranial and pelvic bones and the circulation of the cerebrospinal fluid. This forms an important part of AK diagnosis and treatment. A few cranial faults were found to correspond to specific weak-testing muscles. But most could not be correlated with specific muscles. The only example of a cranial fault and muscle correlation that will be discussed in this text is the opening of the sagittal suture as a method to strengthen the rectus abdominis muscles (page 193).

Then Goodheart found that Terrence Bennett's reflex points for increased circulation in organs often strengthened the weak-testing muscles he had already associated with those organs. These "neurovascular reflex" points became the fourth technique for strengthening weak-testing muscles. Goodheart's list of correspondences between weak-testing muscles and organs/glands was rapidly expanding.

The next great breakthrough occurred when Goodheart began to investigate the meridian system. In Chinese medicine, the "meridians" are considered to be invisible energy lines that run along the surface and through the body. Knowledge of the meridian system was brought to the West from China and Japan through the technique of acupuncture. The term "meridian" is a Western term borrowed from sea navigation to describe what in Chinese medicine is seen as a channel for the life energy that the Chinerse call *chi.*

The meridians are not made up of any known kind of tissue. They are anatomically invisible. Despite their vague nature, over thousands of years, uncountable Chinese medical practitioners have agreed upon their location. Meridians have a superficial portion that lies just under the skin and a deeper extension that reaches into the inner part of the body and touches the organ bearing the occidental name of the meridian.

Most of the acupuncture points lie upon the lines of the meridians. And they lie upon the superficial part of the meridian where they are accessible for treatment. Upon charts and anatomical dolls, the acupuncture points are numbered in the direction of the flow of the energy. By stimulating the acupuncture points, one can influence the meridian energy, causing excess energy to flow away from (sedation) or to a point that has a deficit of energy (tonification).

The Chinese define a plethora of differentiations of chi energy. For example, they content that in each meridian both Yin (female) and Yang (male) energies circulate. Although very important and useful in

Chinese medicine, this and their many further differentiations of chi do not as yet have useful application in AK and therefore will not be discussed in any detail in this text.

For some readers, the Chinese explanations of a mysterious life-force circulating through invisible meridians running along the skin are very foreign to our way of thinking. The existence of meridians and how they function may sound mystical and appear to lie beyond experimental proof. Nonetheless, the correspondences between meridians and observed conditions of the body and mind (general health, glands, organs, etc.) have been repeatedly documented for at least three thousand years. Treatments based upon "balancing" the meridian energies have provided undeniable benefits for a like period of time.

In general, modern science only accepts the validity of such healing claims when they are repeatable under identical circumstances. The phenomena connected with the meridian system are definitely repeatable under identical circumstances. However, the explanations from traditional Chinese medicine as to why these phenomena occur may seem very unusual to the Western mind and may require revision at a later date when we have a greater scientific understanding of the processes involved. It is my opinion that the unusual oriental explanations available today in no way affect the worth of our using the meridian system concepts for diagnosis and therapy. This should be held in mind when one begins to consider the philosophy and principles of Chinese medicine.

Applied Kinesiology research has documented that meridian balancing techniques do have a measurable effect upon the results of muscle testing and upon the health of the related organs and glands (Walther, 1988, pp. 203–273).

In Chinese acupuncture theory (more precisely, the theory of the five-elements), the meridians are associated with organs and glands. Proponents of Chinese medicine believe that when the "yin" or "yang" energies in a meridian are deficient (or in excess), the corresponding organs and glands are affected and may become diseased or otherwise dysfunctional.

Even more importantly, practitioners of Chinese medicine believe, and for centuries have demonstrated, that their techniques of meridian energy balancing can positively affect organs and glands; and thereby influence health in general.

With his unique willingness to consider concepts and techniques from other fields of healing, Goodheart initiated new research into this ancient Chinese diagnostic and healing system. For him, the existing correlations between meridians and organs/glands were especially fascinating. He found that by using new-to-him Oriental meridian balancing techniques, he could strengthen weak-testing muscles. By placing a needle, tapping or simply touching the first sedation point, he could make normotonic muscles test weak. Moreover, the organs and glands associated with the meridians proved to be the same organs and glands that his own research associated with specific muscles. In fact, the meridian system proved to fit "like a glove" with his already-established system of correspondences. With this extra piece to the puzzle, his muscle-organ/gland correspondences became associated with the meridians.

There are twelve bilateral meridians (and two that lie on the medial line of the body). Goodheart found that one of the established meridians corresponded with almost every muscle he tested. This provided a simple and useful framework with only fourteen categories for all muscles. According to Chinese medicine, every structure and function of the human body belongs to one or more of these fourteen categories. In this book, these will be referred to as the fourteen *systems of regulation*. Through experiement, Goodheart determined that any technique which improved the balance of energy in a meridian could often strengthen the weak-testing muscle associated with the same organ and gland as the meridian. Conversely, the techniques he had already developed for strengthening a weak-testing muscle often helped to balance the energy of the corresponding meridian.

Until this time, Western science somewhat contemptuously considered meridians to be merely a vague and esoteric concept of oriental medicine.

When acupuncture was introduced into the West, a few open-minded Western doctors were successful in using it to produce anesthesia in their patients. However, no one could explain why it worked. Nonetheless, every true scientist recognized that there had to be some "scientific truth" in any such completely repeatable phenomenon. At that time, there was no way of relating it logically with Western science. The anatomy and physiology of muscles, however, are a researched and accepted area of Western medicine. Goodheart's discovery of the connection of meridians with muscles created the first bridge of understanding between oriental and occidental medicine.

In Oriental medicine, the state of health requires that a normal quantity of energy circulate through all of the meridians. From the AK viewpoint, an "imbalanced" meridian may have an excess of energy or it may have a deficit of energy circulating through it. When a meridian is in a deficient energy state, some or all of its associated muscles will test weak. Therefore, through testing muscles, we can swiftly and easily determine energy imbalances in the meridians. The energy state of the meridian system indicates the imbalances underlying a patient's problems. This provides the examiner with knowledge of areas of possible dysfunction in the muscles, organs, glands and functions associated with the meridian. Such knowledge is the essential first step toward evaluating those dysfunctions. Goodheart's discovery and elucidation of the connection between specific muscles and specific meridians swiftly made the meridian system one of the most important diagnostic factors in Applied Kinesiology.

Goodheart acquired his knowledge of the meridian system from one early book on the topic, *Acupuncture, Ancient Chinese Art of Healing* by the English physician, Felix Mann. Like Felix Mann, Goodheart never attempted to differentiate between the amounts of yin versus yang energy within each meridian. This finer differentiation, which forms an important portion of Chinese meridian diagnosis, still does not exist within Applied Kinesiology.

Within the ICAK-D, the medical doctor Hans

Garten is the current authority for Chinese medicine. In 1991, he and Wolfgang Gerz became the first German medical doctors to receive the status of AK diplomat. Hans Garten went to China several times to study acupuncture. He was in charge of the education program of the German Medical Acupuncture Society (DÄGfA) for several years. He has developed methods of using muscle testing plus Chinese herbal remedies to perform detailed diagnosis of patterns described in traditional Chinese medicine. In private communication, he observed that there is "no AK-way of diagnosing Yin and Yang as they are only acronyms for a myriad of similar qualities." Even without this aspect of Chinese medical diagnosis, AK applications of meridian knowledge are extremely useful.

The most commonly used aspects of meridian theory in AK are the acupuncture sedation points. When the sedation point for a meridian is therapy-localized, all the associated muscles should test weak. Tapping upon this point will usually weaken the associated muscles for about 10 seconds. This is simple to perform and is the most accurate test for hypertonic muscles. Quickly stroking along a meridian in the opposite direction of its natural flow of energy should also weaken the associated muscles for about 10 seconds. If touching or tapping upon the corresponding sedation point or stroking the meridian backward does not weaken a strong-testing muscle, it is in a hypertonic state.

When an organ or gland is dysfunctioning, the corresponding meridian will be found to be in an imbalanced energy state. Is such cases, the corresponding muscles will usually test either weak or hypertonic. However, an imbalance in meridian energy does not necessarily mean that the corresponding organ or gland is already dysfunctioning. The meridian system is highly sensitive. Meridian diagnosis can reveal imbalances long before they could manifest as noticeable dysfunction in the related organs and glands. Thus, it is possible that through diagnosis of the meridian system (by means of AK muscle testing), we can become aware of potential organ and gland dysfunctions before they manifest as illness.

Typically, when meridians become deficient in energy, their associated muscles that normally test strong become unexpectedly weak. This weakening often occurs one to three days before the emergence of the first symptoms of a simple illness such as a cold. If effective corrective measures are taken to bring the meridians back into balance (for example, strengthening the weak-testing muscles) and steps are taken to increase body resistance (vitamins, good food, extra rest and sleep, drinking extra water, immune system stimulators such as echinacea, etc.), the illness may be shorter and milder, or may not appear at all. Illnesses may be thus "nipped in the bud."

Assessment of the meridian system through AK muscle testing not only provides information about the meridians but also indicates both the probable weak-testing muscles and the organs and glands that may be dysfunctioning. Conversely, when a patient has a specific organ or gland that is known to be malfunctioning, the energy in the associated meridian will be out of balance. The testing and strengthening of all the muscles associated with this meridian will do much to correct the functioning of the organ or gland. For specific examples of this process, see case histories #2 and 3 in Appendix VIII.

Oriental meridian-balancing techniques have a positive effect upon both the weak-testing muscles and the associated organs and glands. Oriental diagnostic and correction techniques for the meridian system are not included in this text. For these, the reader is directed to the literature and to personal training in oriental medicine. However, for the examiner who wishes to experiment with the concepts and techniques of oriental medicine, the correspondences between muscles, meridians, organs, and glands (see pages 244) will provide a useful starting point.

For a summary of recent research on acupuncture points and the meridian system, see the discussion in the section on "Biological Medicine and the Systems of Regulation," pages 59–60.

The Meridians

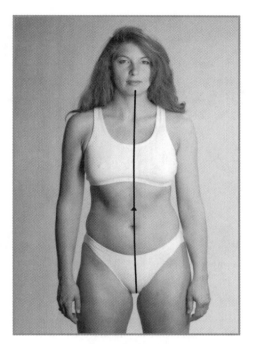

CENTRAL MERIDIAN

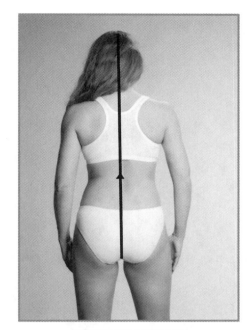

GOVERNING MERIDIAN

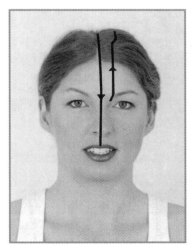

GOVERNING, BLADDER MERIDIANS

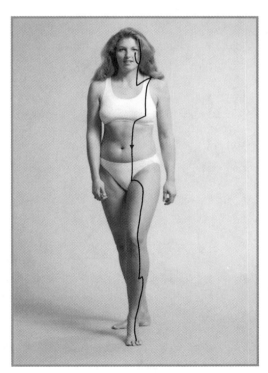

STOMACH MERIDIAN

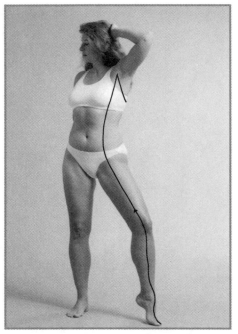

SPLEEN MERIDIAN

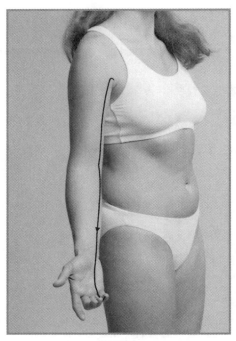

HEART

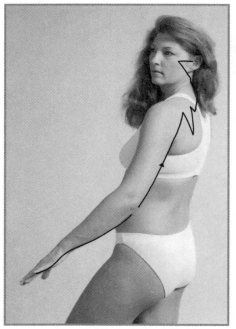

SMALL INTESTINE

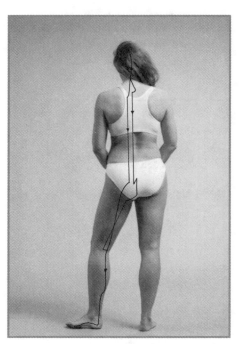

BLADDER

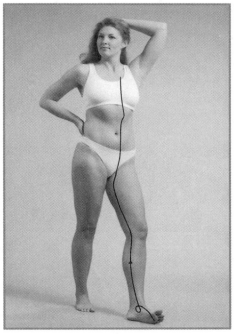

KIDNEY

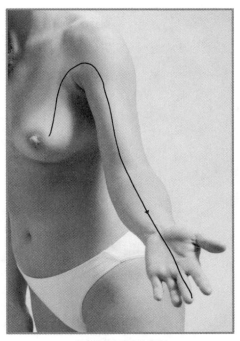

CIRCULATION-SEX

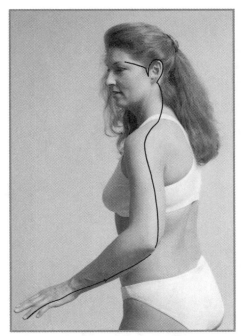

TRIPLE HEATER

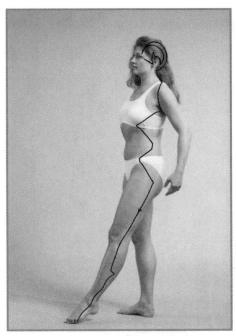

GALL BLADDER

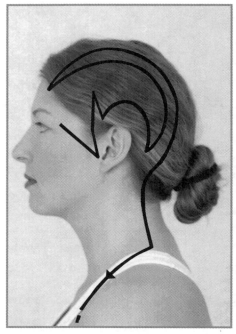

GALL BLADDER

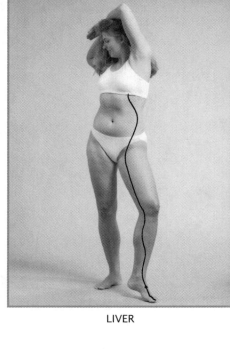

LIVER

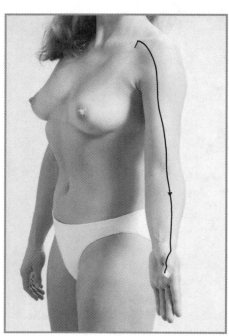

LUNG

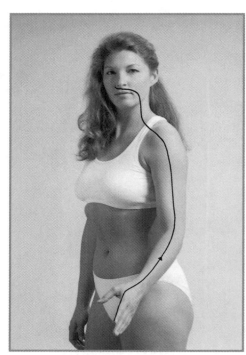

LARGE INTESTINE

Diagnosis of the Reaction to Substances and Other Stimuli

Muscles may test weak due to a lack of particular nutrients. Nutrition that can strengthen each muscle is listed in the section on muscle tests (pages 153–231). To test if nutrients can strengthen a weak-testing muscle (or make a hypertonic muscle normotonic), the examiner has the patient place some of the nutrient substance in the mouth, chew it, taste it and retain it in the mouth. Then the muscle is retested.

Non-toxic substances that are typically ingested orally should also be tested in the mouth. Substances that have an odor may be tested nasally by sniffing them. Smelling nutritional substances that have a distinctive odor will usually produce the same reliable reaction as tasting them. Controlled studies have revealed that the testing of nutritional substances by placing them in the hand is not as reliable. Taste (and smell) are the only accepted and proven Applied Kinesiology (ICAK) methods for testing nutritional and other non-toxic substances. The ICAK-D also recognizes hand-held testing, but only of energetic substances such as homeopathic remedies and flower essences.

Examiners using AK often use prepared organ or gland tissue for dysfunctions in the same organs (or glands) of the human body. To test such organ or gland extracts, herbs, medicines or other healing substances used for improving the function of the organs, the examiner uses a weak-testing muscle associated with the ailing organ or gland. The substance that, when chewed and retained in the mouth, makes the weak-testing muscle normotonic may aid the function of the associated organ or gland. However, if the substance strengthens the muscle but brings it into a hypertonic state, it should not be used!

The exact mechanisms of nutritional or other substance testing are unclear. A weak-testing muscle may be strengthened within seconds of placing the proper nutrition into the mouth. Clearly there is not time for the substance to be absorbed and transmitted to the brain via the bloodstream. Possibly the route for the observed change is via the nerves involved in taste.

When we taste foods, we know immediately if we like them or not. It is likely that when we taste a food substance, the brain knows the chemical content and its possible benefit for specific organs and glands. Perhaps this recognition causes the energy patterns of the positively affected regulation systems (including organs, glands and associated muscles) to immediately improve as observed by muscle testing.

Evidence indicates the existence of another pathway (besides taste) between the mouth and the brain. Radioactive food was placed in the mouth of rats. Only several seconds later, they were frozen in liquid nitrogen. Then slices of the brain were studied and found to contain some of the radioactive food. How it got into the brain so fast remains unexplained. But this experiment makes it clear that foods placed in the mouth are present in the brain within seconds.

The nutritional substance that will help a dysfunctioning organ will also reduce any tenderness in the organ or in the related neurolymphatic areas. This will occur immediately after placing some of the substance in the mouth and tasting it. If more than one substance strengthens the weak-testing muscles, the one that (when in the mouth) most reduces the related tenderness is the one to recommend (Leaf, 1995). But the examiner should also give anything else clinically needed to support the problem as long as it doesn't weaken a strong-testing indicator muscle or make it hypertonic.

For example, the best AK test result for osteoporosis may be magnesium. This may reduce pain more than any other remedy. But rebuilding bones also requires calcium (calcium orotate, calcium gluconate, calcium ascorbate, etc.) and vitamin D3, so these should be given too. These substances should be given in a form that is at least tolerated. They should neither weaken a strong indicator muscle nor make it hypertonic. The examiner doesn't even need to test if calcium or vitamin D3 makes a weak-testing muscle normotonic or takes the pain away because magnesium was already found to do so.

Improper nutrition can cause disturbances to the regulating systems. This can be easily detected with AK testing. The same procedure may be used to detect negative effects of any substance (or other stimulus) upon the regulating systems. However, when an allergic reaction is suspected, or the substance is somewhat toxic, it should be greatly diluted and/or presented in only a minute quantity for testing. Highly toxic substances should not be ingested in any quantity. The examiner should follow the old rule, "Primum nihil nocere!" or, The first thing is don't poison (injure) the patient. The examiner should neither provoke an allergic reaction nor injure the patient in any way.

It is a good idea to present stimuli in the way that the patient normally contacts them. Flowers, perfumes, auto exhaust or anything with an odor should be smelled. A face cream, lipstick or other cosmetic should be freshly applied (and smelled). Music (or noise) should be listened to. To test the effect of cigarettes or alcohol, it is best to test the first cigarette inhalation or drink of the day.

In most cases, substances that have a negative effect upon one regulating system will create a weakening of muscles from all regulating systems. Thus almost any muscle may be chosen for an indicator muscle in nutritional testing. However, some substances only have a negative effect upon muscles from specific regulating systems. For example, excess alcohol is known to have deleterious effects upon the liver. To determine if a client's liver has problems with alcohol, the examiner would be wise to choose an indicator muscle such as pectoralis major sternal from the liver regulating system.

Combinations of foods may be similarly tested. For example, protein and carbohydrates may each test normotonic when tested separately. However, they often cause the indicator muscle to test weak or hypertonic when placed together in the mouth. This technique can be used to create a personal nutritional plan defining which foods to eat together at one meal.

Almost any possible stimulus can be similarly tested. The effect of hot or cold is best tested by direct application to the area of the body in question. For example, immediately after a sports injury, the application of cold (ice) is recommended. After a day or two the application of warmth is recommended. To test which will help, TL the injury and test an indicator muscle. This should make the indicator muscle test weak. Now continue the weakening TL and apply cold to the injury. Retest the indicator muscle. Repeat this test with the application of warmth. The stimulus of cold or warmth that makes the indicator muscle normotonic is the correct one to apply.

For further discussion of these topics, see "Challenge" (pages 67–72).

1. Locate an organ that has a known dysfunction. Palpate the organ and its neurolymphatic points for tenderness.

2. Test the muscles related to the organ or gland. Find at least one that tests weak. If none can be found, TL the organ. If this weakens an indicator muscle, the TL plus indicator muscle combination can be used for subsequent tests.

3. Place a nutritional or medicinal substance known to have a positive effect upon this organ or gland into the patient's mouth and have her chew and taste it.

4. Retest the related muscle. If the previously weak-testing muscle now tests strong, retain the substance in the mouth, TL or tap the sedation point (or apply another weakening technique), and test again. If the muscle does not weaken, the substance has made the muscle hypertonic. Such a substance should not be taken! If touching the sedation point makes the muscle test weak, the muscle is now normotonic and this nutrition or medicine will be useful for correcting the dysfunction in the associated organ regulating system.

5. If more than one substance makes the muscle normotonic, the one that (when held in the mouth) most reduces the tenderness in the organ or its neurolymphatic point is the one to recommend to the patient. Also give anything else clinically needed to solve the problem as long as it doesn't weaken a strong-testing indicator muscle or make it hypertonic.

TESTING FOR POSSIBLE POSITIVE EFFECTS OF STIMULI

1. To determine if some stimulus has a positive effect upon some problem, find a muscle that tests weak because of the problem.

2. If no muscle can be located that tests weak because of the problem, use therapy localization or challenge to provoke the problem. In the following test, continue to apply the TL or challenge that causes an indicator muscle to test weak.

3. Apply the stimulus.

4. Test the previously weak-testing indicator muscle. If the indicator muscle only tested weak with TL or challenge, apply that weakening TL or challenge during this and the following step as well.

5. If the indicator muscle now tests strong, attempt to weaken it. (Tap the sedation point, pinch the spindle cells, stroke the associated meridian backward or apply the north pole of a magnet to the belly of the muscle.) If the muscle can be weakened, it is in a normotonic state. This indicates that the applied stimulus may be used and will have a positive effect upon the problem tested.

6. If the indictor muscle cannot be weakened, the stimulus has put it into a hypertonic state. This stimulus should not be used to correct the tested problem.

TESTING FOR POSSIBLE NEGATIVE EFFECTS OF NUTRITION OR OTHER NON-TOXIC SUBSTANCES

1. Consider which regulating system(s) may likely be affected by the substance in question.

2. Find a normotonic indicator muscle from the regulating system to be tested.

3. Place the nutritional substance into the patient's mouth and have her chew and taste it. Or, if the nutritional substance has an odor, have her smell the substance.

4. Retest the indicator muscle. If it now tests weak, or if it tests strong but cannot be weakened (hypertonic), then this nutritional substance has a negative effect upon the regulating system tested.

Hidden Problems

Sometimes an organ or gland has an obvious problem, but the associated muscles all test strong. And the muscles are not hypertonic but rather normotonic, i.e., they can be weakened by spindle cell pinching, touching or tapping their sedation points, stroking the corresponding meridian backward, or placing the north (south seeking) pole of a magnet upon the tested muscle's belly. It seems that in such cases, the body has compensated for the problem. Some "Robbing Peter to pay Paul" has occurred and the original problem is no longer visible via testing of the related muscles.

Often in such cases, the muscle will test weak when reflex points to the muscles and/or the ailing organ or gland are simultaneously therapy-localized. The exact neurological basis for this seeming compensation is not yet understood. When this procedure reveals a weakness, it is corrected by applying the proper type of stimulation for the reflex point touched. After correction, the muscle may be retested with the same therapy localization to confirm the correction.

FINDING HIDDEN PROBLEMS

1. Test muscles and perform all needed corrections.

2. Observe, examine and question the patient to determine any additional problems.

3. Test muscles known to be associated with any dysfunctioning organ or gland. If an area of the body has a problem, but no specific muscle is known to be associated with that area, have the patient therapy-localize the area and test an indicator muscle. If the patient has to get into a particular position to provoke the problem, have the patient get into this position and touch the problem area.

4. If the chosen muscle or indicator muscle in #3 tests weak, use standard techniques to locate and perform the needed corrective measures to strengthen the muscle. If, however, the muscle or indicator muscle remains strong, use the following technique to locate the cause of the hidden problem:

5. Test this muscle (or an indicator muscle) while stimulating the problem as in #3 while touching reflex points or other associated points, one at a time.

6. If a point is found that makes the muscle test weak, the proper corrective technique for this point will help to correct the cause of the hidden problem.

Correction:

1. Perform the correction procedure appropriate for that point.

Confirm the correction:

2. Retest the muscle (or indicator muscle plus TL or position) while touching the point that made it test weak.

3. If the muscle now remains strong, the correction is confirmed.

4. Return to #6 above and repeat the process until no points can be located which weaken the muscle/indicator muscle.

For further techniques to reveal hidden problems, see the following section on right hemisphere-left hemisphere brain activity. Muscles may also only test weak after multiple tests, after being stretched, or after other muscles contract first. For these topics, see the sections on repeated muscle testing (page 125), muscle stretch response (page 126), and reactive muscles (page 131).

To do everything possible to improve the function of a particular muscle, or to positively influence the function of the associated organ or gland, the muscle should be tested in all of the above ways and any detected imbalances should be corrected.

Activation of the Right and Left Halves of the Brain

The two hemispheres of the brain have different tasks. Hidden problems may emerge and be testable only when the brain is involved in a one-sided activity. The mechanisms involved are unknown. The most popular hypothesis is that by "activating" one half of the brain, the brain is somehow in better touch with the problem, which then shows up with muscle testing.

When skin sensation is lacking, therapy localization generally does not function. Goodheart found that in some cases of paralysis with lack of skin sensation, activating one half of the brain made therapy localization function. In classic Goodheart style, he took this finding and developed the following important therapeutic application. He reasoned that if unilateral brain activity could produce therapy localization when it was previously absent, then the brain-body connection was improved. To check this hypothesis, he asked a paralyzed patient to attempt to lift his right leg while reciting the multiplication tables. Mental math is a left-brain activity. The left brain controls the right side of the body. When the man reached 2 x 39, his leg lifted! Furthermore, humming (a right-brain activity) while attempting to lift the left leg produced movement in the leg after only two minutes of effort. This technique has helped many paralyzed individuals to move again.

A problem with the regulating system associated with a particular organ may be evident, but the associated muscles may all test strong. Even touching the reflex points of a muscle associated with the regulating system (as discussed above in the section on hidden problems) may not weaken the muscle and thus may not reveal the existence of the suspected problem. When further hidden problems are suspected, the patient is directed to activate the left hemisphere of her brain by performing some mathematical activity like reciting the multiplication tables. While she does so, she again therapy-localizes the various reflex points for the muscle while the examiner tests it. This is repeated while she activates the right hemisphere of the brain by humming an improvised tune (one without words that she thinks up on the spot). Although neither the therapy localization nor the humming (or mental math) alone weaken the indicator muscle, both together may well do so. When the combination of humming or mental math plus TL to a reflex point weakens the indicator muscle, the therapy-localized reflex point is then treated. Afterwards, the muscle is retested with therapy localization to the reflex point plus the brain hemisphere activity that caused the muscle to test weak. If the muscle no longer weakens, the correction is confirmed.

DETECTING HIDDEN PROBLEMS
THROUGH ACTIVATING
THE RIGHT AND LEFT HALVES OF THE BRAIN:

1. Test muscles and perform all needed corrections.

2. Consider the still-existent problems and deduce which muscles may be involved.

3. Have the patient therapy-localize reflex points for the suspect muscle and retest it. If this produces an active TL, treat the hidden problem as described in the previous section. If this fails to produce an active TL, retest the indicator muscle while performing the activities in 4 and 5 below:

4. TL each of the reflex points for this muscle again while the patient recites the multiplication tables.

5. TL each of the reflex points for this muscle again while the patient hums an improvised melody.

6. If the muscle tested weak with either math or humming, the muscle has a hidden problem.

Correction:

1. Perform the appropriate correction for the therapy-localized reflex point.

Confirm the Correction:

1. Have the patient again therapy-localize plus perform the brain activity that previously weakened the muscle, and test the muscle again.

2. If the muscle no longer weakens with the simultaneous therapy localization plus brain activity, the correction is confirmed.

Repeated Muscle Testing

At times, a muscle will test strong, none of its reflex points have an active TL, but it fails after repeated use. This is often a problem with athletes who begin their sport very well but tire out before they finish. Goodheart first observed this in a competitive skier who could not remain in his tightly tucked position throughout the downhill run. When he muscle-tested this skier, all of his leg muscles tested strong. Since the problem only emerged at the end of the race, Goodheart experimented with testing each muscle again and again, imitating the constant demand placed upon the muscles by the sports activity. This is an example of a basic principle of Applied Kinesiology: to test the patient in conditions duplicating the situation in his life that causes problems. When he tested the skier's hamstring muscles, one side remained strong during repetitive testing, but the other side weakened after being tested about five times. Goodheart was fascinated and remarked, "I have an answer, but I haven't asked a question." (Walther, 1984, p. 230.)

Goodheart next looked for something that would abolish this repetitive muscle test weakening. He had the client therapy-localize a neurolymphatic point for the hamstrings and again tested the weak hamstring muscles repetitively. This time they remained strong. Note that in this case, the muscle tested strong and therapy localization of the neurolymphatic points did not weaken it. The muscle only tested weak after repeated testing. Therapy localization of the neurolymphatic points for that muscle allowed the muscle to continue contracting repeatedly without weakening. Goodheart experimented and found that prolonged massage of the muscle's neurolymphatic points caused the muscle to remain strong in subsequent repeated testing. Based upon this successful therapeutic finding, he reasoned that the muscle weakness upon repeated testing was due to the lymph system not functioning properly. He suspected that this problem is due to lack of adequate lymphatic circulation through the muscle tissues.

Goodheart, of course, knew that all muscles consist of both fast and slow fibers. Fast fibers can only contract a few times before they tire. Since in repetitive muscle testing, the muscle tests strong for the first few contractions, he reasoned that the fast fibers must be functioning correctly. The skier's problem must then logically lie with the slow fibers, which were failing in their job of sustaining continuous or repeated contractions over a long duration.

Both the fast and the slow fibers are fueled by glucose. The body makes glucose from glycogen, the storage form of sugar in the body, as the need arises. Since the fast fibers stopped contracting, the supply of available glucose (already transformed from glycogen) appeared to be used up. It is then logical that the red slow fibers would also not have adequate glucose available for fuel.

The slow fibers can also use fat for fuel. When they cease functioning after several contractions of the muscle, their fat supply must logically be in deficient supply. The fat they use is delivered to them by the blood capillaries and the lymph system. The lymph system is not only a waste transport system. It also absorbs nutritional fats through the finger-like "lacteals" of the small intestine and delivers this fat into the bloodstream, which delivers it to the muscles for fueling of the slow fibers.

If the lymph is not circulating adequately, the fluids that leak out of the blood capillaries plus the waste products released from the cells build up in the interstitial spaces (between the cells). Since in such conditions of lymphatic congestion, there is little movement of the lymph fluids, the cells absorb the sugars and fats that are immediately next to the cell wall, and are then not supplied with further fuel.

The fast fibers can contract and thereby give the muscle strength for a few strong contractions before they are exhausted. Since for energy, the fast fibers split sugar quite uneconomically, they run out of fuel quickly. Even under the best of conditions, white (fast) fibers cannot be supplied with fuel fast enough to sustain repeated strong contractions. Thus, it is natural that they become exhausted rapidly. The slow fibers oxidize sugar completely. This very economical process creates many times the amount of energy from the same amount of sugar. They can also use fats for fuel. As long as oxygen and fuel are adequately supplied, slow fibers can support repeated contractions for extended periods of time. However, if lymph circulation is poor, slow fibers quickly use up their available fuel. Under these circumstances, the fuel is not replaced rapidly enough to sustain repeated contractions. If for these reasons, the red (slow) fibers cannot continue to contract, the muscle unlocks during repeated testing. This is Goodheart's hypothesis of why muscles may weaken with repeated use.

Another possible explanation lies in the chemistry within the muscle fibers. The white muscle fibers are anaerobic and produce the energy needed for contraction by splitting glucose into lactic acid. When the lymph system does not remove lactic acid from the muscle tissues fast enough, they become acidic (their pH level sinks.) It is the presence of lactic acid in the muscular tissues that causes the discomfort felt in fatigued muscles. When the pH level in a muscle is too low, the muscle fibers cease to contract. This protects the muscle from producing more lactic acid and further sinking the pH to levels so acidic that the muscle fibers could be destroyed. Thus elevation of the lactic acid levels may also be a reason why a muscle fails after several initial contractions.

Whether lactic acid buildup or Goodheart's hypothesis is the explanation for why a muscle fails after several contractions, inadequate lymphatic circulation is the logical cause in both cases. In order to stimulate the sluggish lymph system in the area of the muscle, the muscle's associated neurolymphatic reflex points require lots of stimulation. Extended stimulation of the neurolymphatic points (2–4 minutes or even longer) will give such a muscle the ability to remain strong upon repeated testing. This may need to be repeated by the patient at home for several weeks to bring a sluggish lymphatic system into proper activity.

The Australian Touch for Health teacher Joan Dewe (cofounder of the Professional Kinesiology Practitioner system, PKP) related the following story: In an Australian bar, the men practiced a competitive sport. They strapped an iron weight onto their shoe. With this weight they extended their leg as many times as they could. The strongest man there performed 16 extensions. Joan asked to try. They laughed because a woman wanted to attempt their test of strength. She asked if they were afraid of being bettered by a woman. They let her try. With the weight on her shoe, she crossed her arms over her chest. This allowed her to use her fingers surreptitiously to massage under the anterior edge of her rib cage (the neurolymphatic areas for the quadriceps muscles including rectus femoris, which extend the leg). The men stared with disbelieving eyes and gaping mouths as she exceeded sixteen repetitions. Through her massage of her quadriceps neurolymphatic reflex areas, her quadriceps muscles were supplied with fuel and the waste products of muscular contraction were more swiftly carried away, allowing her to perform better than all the men present.

In some cases, the weakness upon multiple testing is due to poor vascular circulation in the tissues of the muscle. This is more often the case with muscles that contain a higher concentration of fast fibers. In these cases, therapy localization of the neurovascular points will abolish the test weakness encountered after repetitive muscle tests. And stimulation of the neurovascular points will eliminate the problem. Some cases may require both neurolymphatic and neurovascular stimulation before the repeated muscle testing weakness is eliminated.

Aerobic red muscles contract more slowly than anaerobic white muscles. Mirroring this natural difference in function, muscles that contain a predominance of aerobic red fibers are tested slowly and rhythmically about 10 times in 10 seconds. Muscles with a higher concentration of fast fibers contract faster and should be tested faster. Such anaerobic white muscles should be tested about 20 times in 10 seconds. These tests are performed more rapidly than normal Applied Kinesiology muscle testing. The patient clearly does not have adequate time to build the tension up to a maximum level during each swift contraction. A *sub-maximal* level of contraction is adequate for repeated muscle testing.

Many times, lasting correction of repetitive muscle weakness requires nutritional supplementation. Iron is used for muscles that have a predominance of slow fibers. Pantothenic acid is the choice for predominantly fast-fiber muscles. When patients have many different muscles that all test weak upon multiple testing, they may not have enough quality nutritional fats to fuel their slow red muscle fibers. In such cases, fatty acids such as oil, evening primrose oil, sesame oil and/or fish oils are often needed.

In muscles that show weakness during multiple testing as above, check whether therapy localization of the neurolymphatic and/or neurovascular points for the muscle eliminates the weakening. The points that negate the weakening are those needed for the application of corrective treatment.

When muscles show weakness in repeated testing, the application of the above techniques will increase their capacity for endurance significantly. Anyone can benefit from increased endurance. This will benefit the elderly who tire before reaching the top of the stairs. This can also greatly assist athletes to attain their highest performance potential.

REPEATED MUSCLE TESTING TECHNIQUE

Test:

1. Test the muscle. If it tests weak, strengthen it before continuing.

2. Test aerobic (postural) muscles about 10 times in 10 seconds, or

3. Test anaerobic (phasic) muscles about 20 times in 10 seconds.

If you don't know which type the muscle is, try both types of testing.

4. If the muscle unlocks during the repeated testing, have the patient "insalivate" (chew, mix with saliva and retain in the mouth) a source of iron, then pantothenic acid, then fatty acid.

5. Perform the repetitive muscle testing after insalivation of each substance. If one of these abolishes the repetitive muscle weakness, recommend that the client include it in her daily diet. Have her rinse her mouth and check that the muscle again weakens with repetitive testing before proceeding.

6. Have the patient touch a neurolymphatic reflex point for the muscle.

7. While she touches the NL point, perform the repeated testing again.

8. Have the patient touch a neurovascular reflex point for the muscle.

9. While she touches the NV point, perform the repeated testing again.

10. If the muscle can contract ten times during repetitive muscle testing (with therapy localization of the NL or NV) without weakening, perform the following correction.

Correction:

1. If NL contact strengthened the test, deeply rub all the neurolymphatic points for the muscle for 2–4 minutes.

2. If NV contact strengthened the test, lightly hold (and tug in the direction of maximal pulsation) the neurovascular points for the muscle for at least 1 minute.

Confirm the correction:

3. Repeat the repeated muscle test (without touching the reflex points). If the muscle no longer weakens, the correction was successful.

Fascial Release or Chill and Stretch Techniques for Muscle Stretch Reaction

Normally, when a muscle is gently stretched, its level of tone will temporarily increase. For example, in muscle testing one applies an increasing force upon the limb tested, which stretches the neuromuscular spindle cells and signals the need for increased tension to hold the limb steady under the increasing force. When a muscle tests strong, but tests temporarily weak after gentle stretching, it is said to have an abnormal stretch reaction. For example, a ball thrower reaching back in preparation to throw the ball stretches the muscles used in the action. This should facilitate them. If the stretch reaction is present, these muscles will be inhibited just when they are most needed, resulting in less than optimal strength and coordination in the throwing motion.

To test for muscle stretch reaction, the muscle is first tested in the clear. If weak, standard AK techniques are applied to strengthen it. When it tests strong, the muscle is fully extended and given a slight tug or push toward further extension to stretch the fibers. The examiner must be careful not to give a powerful stretch as this will temporarily weaken any muscle. The muscle is immediately retested. If it tests weak after this stretching, the muscle has an abnormal stretch reaction.

Postural muscles such as the sacrospinalis, hamstrings, and quadriceps that work most of the time need to be stretched rather slowly to demonstrate the abnormal stretch reaction. Muscles that are usually inactive and contract for swift action (phasic muscles) need to be stretched rather swiftly to reveal an abnormal stretch reaction when one is present. When the muscle type is unknown, test after a fast stretch and again after a slow stretch.

To correct the abnormal stretch reaction, Goodheart recommends two techniques: the fascial release, and the chill and stretch (both explained in detail below). Fascial release seems to be the best choice when the associated gland or organ has dysfunction.

Chill and stretch is indicated when there is pain in or near the muscle tested.

Around every muscle and organ is a thin, strong, connective tissue (fascia) sack. The fascia is a slightly elastic membrane that allows organs and muscles to slide smoothly against one another. Ideally, the fascia sack should be the same length as the muscle and free to slide smoothly along other tissues. After injury to a muscle, the fascia may shorten and thicken like any scar tissue in the body. Injury and certain inflammatory illnesses can cause the fascia membranes to stick to one another. This limits the range of motion of the muscles involved and likely inhibits the free circulation of blood and lymph fluids.

Nerves and stretch receptors embedded in the fascia and in the muscle may cause pain when stretched, incorrectly signaling the nervous system to react by contracting and thus further shortening the muscle. When for any reason a muscle isn't stretched for a long period of time, the fascia around it shortens. This structurally limits the range of muscle lengthening. Self-applied attempts to stretch it typically produce only limited success and a lot of discomfort. For this reason, one who habitually slumps may find it difficult and painful to assume upright posture.

When the fascia around a muscle is shortened or adheres to other fascial tissues, the function of the organ or gland associated with the muscle is often disturbed. Applying the fascial release technique can help the organ or gland to return to normal function.

For example, the teres minor muscle is associated with the thyroid gland, which is involved in temperature regulation. If teres minor needs and receives fascial stretch, the body temperature may change swiftly and measurably. When patients with hypothyroid activity (which often causes low body temperature) receive fascial stretch to the teres minor, thyroid activity increases, and a rise in body temperature of 0.5–1.5° C within minutes is usual. This is an example of how fascial stretching of a muscle can affect the associated organ or gland.

AK testing confirms that when there is an abnormal stretch reaction, the neurolymphatic reflexes are active, indicating the need for increased drainage of the lymph fluids. Before performing the fascial release technique, it is advisable to increase the circulation and drainage of the affected areas. Otherwise the pressure applied upon the tissues swollen with excess lymph could stretch and damage the lymph vessels. For this purpose, the neurovascular and neurolymphatic reflexes to the affected muscle should be checked and corrected as necessary. Furthermore, the tissues should be drained of excess fluids mechanically. To do so, the examiner uses the whole surface of the hand to squeeze the proximal (toward the heart) end of the muscle firmly for 20–30 seconds. At the same time, he moves his hand toward the heart as far as the excursion of the skin allows. As the fluids are squeezed out, the tissues can be felt to slightly shrink. Then the examiner moves his hand along the muscle distally (further away from the heart), squeezes and moves his hand toward the heart again. This moves the fluids toward the heart end of the muscle. After holding this second hand position for about 10 seconds, he continues to maintain it and also squeezes the first position again. Then he moves to a third position more distal than the second and repeats the process. He continues squeezing the fluids toward and through the heart end of the muscle until the entire muscle feels more soft and pliable. Performing this maneuver first helps to prevent injuring the tissues when applying the more aggressive fascial release technique.

To perform the fascial release, the body is first brought into a position that gently stretches the muscle. The muscle is kept stretched during the whole procedure. Oil is spread on the skin above the tissues to be manipulated. To avoid rupturing small blood and lymph vessels, the examiner begins at the end of the muscle away from the heart. The examiner presses his fingers, thumbs, or knuckles into the muscle and slides with pressure along the muscle toward the heart. The flat surface of a fingernail or the side of the thumbnail may be used for a deeper, more aggressive effect. The movement is like ironing in that it smooths out the kinks and irregularities in the fascial

Draining a Muscle (the Rectus Femoris) in Five Steps

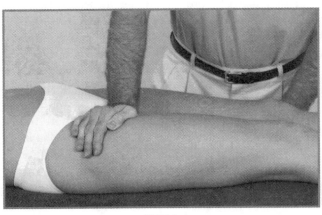

STEP 1

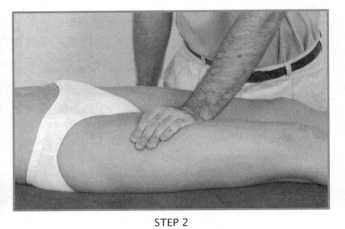

STEP 2

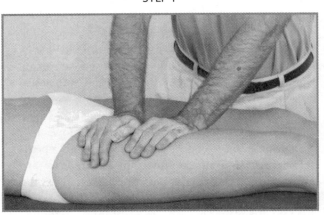

STEP 3

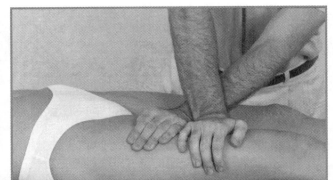

STEP 4

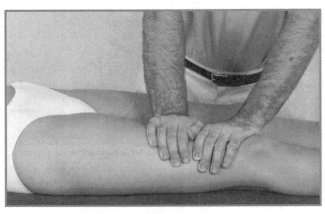

STEP 5

tissues. The examiner massages, kneads, and slides his hands along the muscle several times. Often the smoothing out of the fascial tissues can be felt during the process. The last step of the treatment is to stimulate the neurolymphatic and neurovascular reflexes for the muscle.

The abnormal stretch reaction may also be caused by palpatory hypertonic muscles. In this case, small, extremely sensitive "trigger" points may be located in or near the muscle. Trigger points for specific muscles have been well mapped by Travel and Rinzler (1952, 1976). For illustrations of the location of trigger points, the reader is referred to this source or to Walther, 1981, pp. 171–180 and Gerz, 1996, pp. 132–138. From the patient's report of the areas of pain, and comparison with illustrations of the areas of pain related to trigger points, the specific active

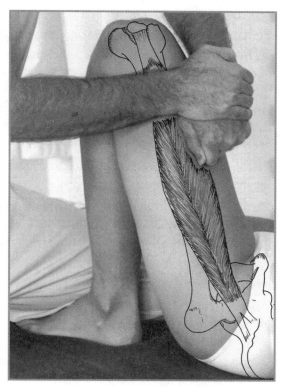

THE FASCIAL RELEASE TECHNIQUE

trigger point may be deduced. Pressure on active trigger points produces a predictable pattern of pain near and sometimes rather distant from the trigger point itself. Muscles with active trigger points are usually shortened and overly tense (palpatory hypertonic). One cannot fully extend such muscles without difficulty and pain. If a muscle with active trigger points is gently tensed and then plucked like the string of a musical instrument, it will quickly contract. This is called the "jump sign." Further analysis of trigger points will not be pursued in this text. Pain upon extension of a muscle and the jump sign are the diagnostic indicators for use of the following treatment:

The treatment of hypertonic muscles with trigger points involves applying cold to the muscle while gently stretching it. The spraying of a chilling fluid for this technique (as recommended in the AK literature) should be left to those professionally trained in its use. Goodheart refers to this technique as "spray and stretch." Its improper use can cause damage to the tissues by freezing them. Sliding along the affected tissue toward the heart with an ice cube (while stretching the muscle) is a relatively safe way to achieve the same effect. A convenient tool for this purpose can be made by freezing a wood dowel into a paper cup full of water (like a popsicle).

The fascia will often lengthen during the application of the ice. As it does so, the examiner takes up the slack and continues to extend and stretch the muscle further. This "chill and stretch" technique is capable of blocking and eliminating pain, even when underlying causes have not been corrected. Therefore, this technique should not be used repeatedly. When pain returns after such treatment, other causes should be diagnosed and corrected.

After the application of these techniques as required, stretching a muscle should no longer cause it to test weak. Combined with manipulation of the Golgi tendon organs and neuromuscular spindle cells, the fascial release technique (or "chill and stretch" as required) can swiftly return full extension to a shortened muscle. Application of these techniques may remove pain, increase the range of motion and, of special interest for athletes, dancers, etc., significantly improve performance.

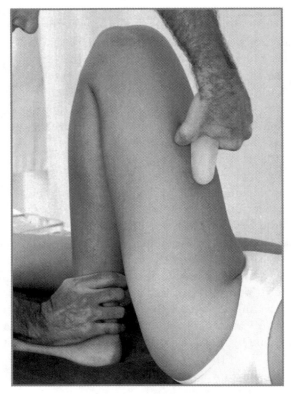

THE CHILL AND STRETCH TECHNIQUE

TESTING FOR MUSCLE STRETCH RESPONSE

1. Test the muscle and if weak, strengthen it.

2. Extend the muscle completely and gently stretch (extend) it a bit further. Slowly stretch postural muscles. Quickly stretch phasic muscles. Try both if you don't know which type the muscle is.

3. Retest the muscle. If it now tests weak, it has an abnormal stretch response.

4. If the associated gland or organ has a dysfunction, use the fascial release technique.

5. If it is difficult and painful to extend the muscle, have the patient gently contract the extended muscle. Then "pluck" it like the string of a musical instrument. If the muscle responds by "jumping," it needs the chill and stretch technique. (In this case, pressure on the trigger points will cause a predictable pattern of pain.)

6. Whether the muscle needs the fascial stretch or the chill and stretch, first drain it of excess fluids as outlined below.

DRAINING EXCESS FLUIDS FROM A MUSCLE

1. Grasp the heart-end of a muscle with the whole surface of one hand (two hands may be used for large muscles.) Squeeze the muscle firmly (0.5–5 kilos pressure). Begin with light pressure. If this fails to produce the desired effect (softening of the muscle after the treatment), begin again with increased pressure.

2. Without sliding along the skin, move the squeezing hand toward the heart as far as the excursion of the skin allows. Hold and continue squeezing for 20–30 seconds. Release.

3. Grasp immediately distal (further from the heart) to the first position, squeeze and push toward the heart again for 20–30 seconds again.

4. Continue to hold the second position and squeeze the first position again.

5. Move further distally along the muscle and repeat the process, pressing the fluids through and out of the muscle toward the heart. The muscle should now feel softer and more pliable.

PERFORMING THE FASCIAL RELEASE TECHNIQUE

1. When fascial release is required (see "Muscle Stretch Response" above), first drain the muscle of excess fluids.

2. Bring the body into a position that gently stretches the muscle. Keep the muscle stretched during the process.

3. Put oil on the whole surface of the muscle.

4. Begin at the distal end of the muscle (away from the heart). Use the fingers, thumb or knuckles to press in and slide along the tissues of the muscle toward the heart. Massage, knead and "iron" out any irregularities in the fascia.

5. Repeat this process, covering the whole area of the muscle, always sliding parallel to the fibers of the muscle.

Confirm the correction:

6. Repeat the muscle stretch. Retest the muscle. The muscle should no longer weaken.

7. Stimulate the neurolymphatic and neurovascular reflexes for the muscle.

PERFORMING THE CHILL AND STRETCH TECHNIQUE

1. Determine if this technique is needed (see "Muscle Stretch Response" above.)

2. Drain the muscle of excess fluids.

3. Extend and gently stretch the muscle and hold it in this position.

4. Slide ice slowly across the muscle from its distal end toward the heart.

5. As the muscle lengthens, continue to extend and stretch it further.

6. Continue to slide the ice firmly until the whole surface of the muscle has been covered. Do not excessively chill the muscle.

Confirm the correction:

7. Retest the muscle stretch response. Stretching should no longer cause the muscle to test weak. Range of motion should be better. Pain should be absent.

8. Cover and warm the muscle.

9. If the pain returns, do not repeat the chill and stretch technique. Determine and correct the underlying causes. If the muscle stretch response returns, there is likely an organ or gland involved and the muscle will require the fascial release technique.

Reactive Muscles

Elevated tonus in a muscle causes a change of tonus in other muscles. It is physiologically normal that certain muscles are inhibited *while* other muscles are activated (reciprocal facilitation and inhibition). When contraction of one muscle causes the *subsequent* weakening of another muscle, an undesirable reactive condition exists. In AK, one says that the muscles that are inappropriately stimulated to react are in a "reactive state" or there is a state of "reactive muscles." The muscle with elevated tonus that is causing the reactivity is called by Bruce Dewe (former ICAK member) in his PKP program the "reactor." This is an accurate description but is not generally accepted in the ICAK. In *You'll Be Better,* Goodheart called this muscle "hypertonic," "over-reactive," "the first muscle," "primary muscle" or simply "primary." This gay array of terms has caused much confusion to students of AK. In this book, the term "primary muscle" will be used. The primary and the reactive muscles are called a reactive muscle pair or a reactive muscle group if there is more than one reactive muscle involved. The reactive muscles are reactive to the primary muscle.

Because reactive muscles may test strong in the clear, they may be overlooked by an examiner using AK. When pain exists after a session, or when problems recur (such as a muscle again testing weak) soon after treatment, an examination for possible reactive muscles should be performed.

Reactive muscles are often a problem for athletes. Consider the case of a baseball pitcher. In throwing, the pectoralis major and anterior deltoid muscles are the prime movers. In preparation for throwing, the antagonists tighten to pull the arm back. This lengthens and stretches the prime movers in preparation for their action. As contraction of the antagonists (teres major, teres minor, trapezius, middle and posterior deltoids, rhomboids, etc.) becomes complete, reciprocal facilitation of the prime movers occurs. Thus, reaching back should immediately increase the tension in the muscles used for throwing forward. These mechanisms help the muscles to quickly apply full power. However, if the pectoralis or deltoid muscles are reactive to the rhomboid muscles (located between the shoulder blade and the spine) or other muscles involved in pulling the arm back, reaching back (activating the antagonists) will temporarily weaken the throwing action. Just when the athlete needs the greatest strength, he does not have it! A similar case may exist for any ball throwing or striking action such as in baseball batting, golf "driving" or playing tennis.

Primary muscles have usually received some form of prior injury, perhaps due to overexertion, sudden stretching, sudden contraction, a direct blow, or other trauma to the muscle. Asking a patient about such injuries can help the examiner locate possible primary muscles. Having the patient take the position he was in when an accident occurred can be especially helpful in identifying suspect primary muscles. The muscles that were traumatized by an accident are suspect primary muscles.

Primary muscles are not only created by accidents. Any muscle that is held constantly tight tends to become over-tensed, hard and painful. This continual tension causes the muscle to become a primary muscle and certain other muscles to become reactive to it. A classic example is the upper trapezius muscles which lift the shoulders and, when contracting on both sides at the same time, pull the head back. Most people carry their heads far forward of the line of gravity through their trunk. This improper posture puts continual stress upon the upper trapezius, which must hold the head back to prevent it from nodding forward. In this poor but typical posture, were the upper trapezius to relax, the chin would fall upon the chest.

Furthermore, most people raise their shoulders every time they do anything with their hands. This also places repeated unnecessary stress upon the upper trapezius muscles. As a result, at the end of each working day, most people complain of tension and pain in the upper trapezius muscles. Note that this is not a natural result of the daily work activities performed. The extra strain is produced by unnecessary postural errors.

By reason of poor alignment of the head upon the spine and excess lifting of the shoulders, the upper trapezius muscles are continually tightened. This excess tension causes the upper trapezius muscles to become primary muscles, which then turn off their main antagonists, latissimus dorsi. This is one explanation for the common experience of examiners using AK techniques that latissimus dorsi tests weak in almost every patient and is again weak at the start of every new session. This problem is easy to demonstrate. After strengthening the latissimus dorsi, the patient lifts her shoulders up to her ears (which tightens the upper trapezius) and then relaxes. Within the next 10 seconds, her latissimus dorsi is tested. If there is a primary-reactive relationship between these two muscles, latissimus dorsi will again test weak. Until the excess tension in the upper trapezius is eliminated (by reactive muscle treatment *and* by improved patterns of posture and use), the weakness of latissimus dorsi will continue to return.

The exact neurophysiology of reactive muscles is still unknown. It is suspected that the level of nerve signaling of proprioceptors (neuromuscular spindle cells or sometimes the Golgi tendon organs) in the primary muscle is inappropriately high. Thus normal contraction of the primary muscle causes the proprioceptors to send strong signals into the central nervous system, which causes the continued inhibition (weakening) of the reactive muscles. Since treatment of the proprioceptors in the primary muscle often corrects the reactive muscle condition, this hypothesis is likely correct.

When looking for reactive muscle groups, first

locate a possible primary muscle. A suspect primary muscle is one that is palpatory hypertonic, painful, stiff, shortened and/or was involved in an accident. Next, consider which muscles work in opposition to it. Reactive muscles are most often the antagonists to a primary muscle. Synergists can also be reactive to a primary muscle. Sometimes a muscle on one side of the body is reactive to the same muscle on the other side. This is often the case with the upper trapezius (located on top of the shoulder between the shoulder and the neck). In this case, the shoulder will be elevated on the side with the primary upper trapezius muscle. An interesting primary-reactive muscle relationship may exist between corresponding muscles in the two diagonal extremities. For example, the biceps (the flexor of the arm) on the right side may be reactive to the biceps femoris (hamstrings, the flexor of the leg) on the left side. This relationship is called muscle interlink.

Before testing for reactive muscles, the suspected primary and reactive muscles must test strong in the clear. If not, appropriate strengthening techniques are applied as needed until they do test strong. Next, the possible primary muscle is tested and the suspected reactive muscles are then tested within the next 10 seconds. If a muscle tests weak immediately after testing the suspected primary muscle, it is reactive to the primary muscle.

Treatment of a reactive muscle most often requires sedation of the neuromuscular spindle cells located in the belly of the primary muscle. When the level of signaling from the neuromuscular spindle cells is too high, the muscle itself (its synergists and stabilizers) will be overly facilitated and palpatory hypertonic. It may also be hypertonic (tests strong but cannot be weakened). In either case, some or all of its antagonists and perhaps other muscles will be overly inhibited and thus reactive to the overly facilitated main muscle.

However, when the level of signaling from the Golgi tendon organs is too high, the muscle itself will be inhibited. This will facilitate its antagonists, but its

synergists and stabilizers may be overly inhibited. In this case, it is the synergists and stabilizers that are the suspects for reactivity. Reactivity as a result of the improper signaling of the Golgi receptors is less common but should be considered, especially when activation of a muscle subsequently causes its synergists to weaken.

Synergists may also weaken due to dysfunctioning neuromuscular spindle cells in the prime mover. Perhaps the logical explanation for this unexpected phenomenon is the following: When one muscle is tightening more than is necessary to perform an activity, its synergists (though theoretically facilitated) do not need to contract to aid in the action and so remain relatively relaxed. Their job of contraction has been usurped by the overly tight agonist. So when a muscle causes one or more of its synergists to become reactive, check both the neuromuscular spindle cells and the Golgi tendon organs to determine which one is dysfunctioning.

Often therapy-localizing the affected proprioceptors in the primary muscle will eliminate its effect upon the reactive muscles. If so, this may be used to determine the exact location of the involved neuromuscular spindle cells or Golgi tendon organs requiring treatment. To do so (after identifying a primary-reactive pair of muscles), test the primary muscle and immediately test the reactive while therapy-localizing the belly of the reactive muscle (for the neuromuscular spindle cells) and then each end of the muscle (to test the Golgi tendon organs). If therapy localization to one of these areas of the muscle prevents the reactive muscle from weakening, the proprioceptors that need treatment are located there. Use the fingertips for more specific therapy localization to identify the exact position of the problematic proprioceptor(s).

One can often feel the affected proprioceptors as fibrous lumps in the muscle. Treatment is applied to the neuromuscular spindle cells (of the primary muscle) by squeezing them together in the direction of the muscle fibers, which are usually parallel to the length of the muscle. The Golgi tendon organ treatment (less frequently required) is effected by pulling the Golgi tendon organ away from the belly of the muscle toward the attachment of the tendon to the bone at one end of the muscle. Notice that two-point contact is necessary to push the neuromuscular spindle cells together whereas only one point of contact is needed to pull the Golgi tendon organ away. If the Golgi tendon organs at both ends of the muscle are involved, treat first one and then the other end of the muscle to avoid stretching the neuromuscular spindle cells in the belly of the muscle.

Sometimes, years after an injury, reactive muscle conditions may still cause pain. Treatment of the affected proprioceptors in the primary muscle will often eliminate such long-standing pains. Proper treatment of reactive muscle conditions can also result in an immediate increase in the possible range of movement of the affected body parts. Postural analysis comparison before and after reactive muscle treatment will often reveal positive improvements.

Often the muscles that "could have saved you if they had tightened enough" remain tight (and painful) even after the injured tissues have healed. This phenomenon is known as "muscle memory." In case such an accident should ever happen again, these primary muscles are already tensed and ready to protect you. And they may remain tensed and ready for years after the original incident!

Here's an example from my own family: At age 67, my father had an accident body surfing in Santa Monica, California, with high surf at low tide. With tons of water driving him forward and down, he saw sand with little water below him. He turned to take the blow on the back of his shoulder. The impact broke his shoulder blade as well as three ribs on the opposite side of his chest. One year later, his deltoid muscles on the side of impact were still extremely hard and painful. Had his deltoid muscles performed the superhuman task of lifting his elbow strongly enough to hold his body off the sand during the accident, he would theoretically not have broken his shoulder and

ribs. His deltoid muscles "remembered" the incident and remained tight to protect him from such an accident happening again. The continual tension in the deltoid muscles caused the rhomboids to be reactive. This excess tension also perpetuated the pain. As a result, during the whole year after the incident, he had continual pain and was unable to lift his arm above the level of his shoulder.

In the example of my father's body surfing accident, a single reactive muscle treatment restored the range of motion of his shoulder joint and eliminated most of the pain. However, the next day he said, "What did you do to me?" He complained his shoulder had about 10% of the same terrible pain he had when the accident occurred. This seems to be the effect of muscle memory being released by the reactive muscle treatment. Two further reactive muscle corrections of the same muscles were required to eliminate all of the pain. This re-emergence of the original pain does not always occur, but it is a good idea for the examiner to mention the possibility. The client should know that it is a positive sign, indicating the release of the original trauma, and that if it does occur, the muscles may need another treatment or two before they will remain in balance and pain-free.

Fluid buildup (edema) in the primary muscle (often present in the acute stages soon after an injury) may cause improper signaling from proprioceptors. In such cases, massage, lymph drainage, or neurolymphatic massage point stimulation should be employed to drain the excess fluid from the muscle tissue. Scar tissue in a primary muscle may cause improper proprioceptor signaling in chronic cases long after an injury. Or poor posture may have allowed the fascial sack around the muscle to shorten. Attempting proper posture may then stretch the fascial sack again, causing improper proprioceptor signaling. In these cases, deep stretching massage techniques (see "Muscle Stretch Reaction," page 126) may be needed to break up the adhesions and lengthen the fascial sack.

Very large or very tight muscles may require lots of neuromuscular spindle cell treatment. As the effect of spindle cell weakening may only last about 15 seconds, it is wise to reset the reactives (by testing or simply having the patient tighten them) after each 10–15 seconds of spindle cell weakening of the primary muscle. The best technique is neuromuscular spindle cell pinching of the primary muscle, test the reactive to reset it, and repeat this cycle several times. This is effective for large muscles like sacrospinalis primary-abdominals reactive (see case history #1 in Appendix VIII). For these two groups of muscles, it is easiest to do the neuromuscular spindle cell weakening of sacrospinalis and the tightening of abdominals with the patient lying on the side. Otherwise, the patient must lie on the stomach for the neuromuscular spindle cell work and roll over each time for abdominal testing. For abdominal activation on the side, the patient can press the knees against the examiner's leg while the examiner pushes upon the patient's chest. In the same position, the examiner can reach over the back and do the neuromuscular spindle cell pinching.

After the reactive muscle treatment, test the primary muscle and then immediately test the reactive muscles. If treatment has been appropriate and adequate, the former reactive muscles should now remain strong.

THE REACTIVE MUSCLE TECHNIQUE

Indication:

Any overly-tight muscles may be primary muscles. Suspect the existence of reactive muscles when any strengthened muscles become weak after certain activities. After the patient has had her weak-testing muscles strengthened, ask her to walk around, bend over, climb stairs and especially to perform any activities that she knows may cause her problems. Then recheck the muscles. If some muscles again test weak after activity, there is likely one or more primary muscles responsible for turning off the reactive muscles (making them test weak subsequent to the action of the primary muscles).

Test:

1. Individually test the suspect primary and reactive muscles. If any test weak, strengthen them.

2. Test the primary and immediately (within 10 seconds) test the suspect reactive muscle. If it now

Treatment of the Primary Sacrospinalis Muscle to Reactive-Abdominals

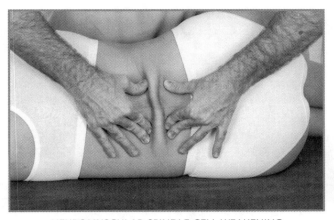

NEUROMUSCULAR SPINDLE CELL WEAKENING OF THE SACROSPINALIS

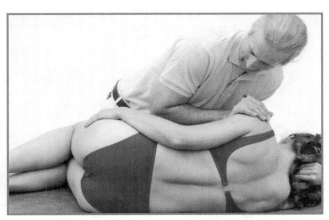

POSITION FOR TENSING TO RESET THE ABDOMINALS

tests weak, the primary-reactive muscle relationship exists.

3. Test the primary muscle and immediately test the reactive muscle while therapy-localizing the belly of the reactive muscle. If this causes the reactive muscle to remain strong, a neuromuscular spindle cell in this area requires treatment. Therapy-localize smaller areas to determine its exact position.

4. If no neuromuscular spindle cell can be located, test the primary muscle and immediately test the reactive muscle while therapy-localizing the Golgi tendon organs at each end of the muscle. If this causes the reactive muscle to remain strong, treatment of the Golgi tendon organ is required.

5. If TL to neither neuromuscular spindle cells nor the Golgi tendon organs causes the reactive muscle to remain strong, assume that neuromuscular spindle cells are at fault.

Correction:

1. Pinch the neuromuscular spindle cells of the primary muscle together to weaken it. If the exact location could not be determined, pinch them together over the whole range of the belly of the muscle. If Golgi tendon organ treatment to weaken the muscle is required, pull the affected Golgi tendon organ away from the belly and toward the end of the muscle. Optional: Test the primary muscle to confirm that it has been weakened.

2. Immediately test the reactive muscle to activate it. Or more easily, have the patient tighten the reactive muscle strongly.

3. Repeat steps 1 and 2 several times.

Confirm the correction:

Perform the test step 2 again. If you have corrected the primary-reactive relationship, the formerly reactive muscle will now test strong.

No list of reactive muscles is complete. Any muscle that was active when the body received a trauma may become involved in a primary-reactive muscle relationship. The list given below is only a guide to help the examiner look for possible reactive muscles. Some muscles that are not illustrated in this book are listed here for examiners familiar with these additional muscle tests. When looking for primary-reactive muscle pairs, also test contralateral muscles (muscle interlink) and all antagonists and synergists to the main muscle.

PRIMARY MUSCLE REQUIRING SEDATION	SUSPECTED REACTIVE MUSCLE
Adductors	Tensor fascia lata, Iliopsoas, Piriformis, Gluteus medius and maximus
Biceps femoris (hamstrings)	Sacrospinalis, Quadriceps, Popliteus, Latissimus dorsi (contralateral)
Deltoid, anterior	Deltoid (posterior)
Deltoid, ant. mid. & pos.	Rhomboids, Pectoralis majors and minor, Latissimus dorsi, Subscapularis
Gluteus medius	Rectus abdominis (contralateral), Adductors
Gluteus maximus	Sacrospinalis, Pectoralis major clavicular, Iliopsoas, Rectus femoris, Sartorius, Piriformis, Adductors, Tensor fascia lata
Infraspinatus	Pectoralis majors, Deltoid (anterior), Infraspinatus itself (superior and inferior fibers)
Iliopsoas	Adductors, Diaphragm, Gluteus maximus, Contralateral anterior neck flexors (SCM), Hamstrings, Quadratus lumborum, Sacrospinalis
Latissimus dorsi	Trapezius (upper),Hamstrings (contralateral), Supraspinatus, Deltoids, Levator scapula
Pectoralis major clavicular	Teres major, Teres minor, Latissimus dorsi, Trapezius (middle), Deltoid (pos.), Rhomboids, Supraspinatus, Gluteus maximus
Pectoralis major sternal	Supraspinatus, Trapezius (upper and lower), Deltoid (posterior), Serratus anticus, Rhomboids
Pectoralis minor	Serratus anticus, Supraspinatus, Deltoids, Trapezius, Rhomboids
Peroneus tertius	Tensor fascia lata, Tibialis anterior and posterior, Peroneus longus and brevis
Peroneus longus and brevis	Peroneus tertius, Tibialis anterior and posterior
Piriformis	Splenius capitis (contralateral), Gluteus medius, Tensor fascia lata, Adductors, Hamstrings (medial)
Popliteus	Gastrocnemius, Quadriceps, Hamstrings (lateral),Trapezius (upper), Rectus abdominis Quadriceps, Gluteus medius (contralateral), Sacrospinalis, Rectus femoris, Sartorius, Quadratus lumborum

PRIMARY MUSCLE REQUIRING SEDATION	SUSPECTED REACTIVE MUSCLE
Rectus abdominis, lower	Rectus abdominis, upper
Rectus abdominis, upper	Rectus abdominis, lower
Rectus femoris	Gastrocnemius, Rectus abdominis, Hamstrings, Sartorius, Gluteus maximus, Adductor magnus
Rhomboid major and minor	Deltoid, Serratus anticus, Supraspinatus, Latissimus dorsi, Pectoralis majors and minor Trapezius (upper, middle and lower)
Sacrospinalis	Rectus abdominis, Gluteus maximus, Hamstrings
Sartorius	Quadriceps, Gluteus medius and maximus, Adductors, Tensor fascia lata, Tibialis anterior Peroneus tertius
Sternocleidomastoideus (SCM)	Neck extensors, Trapezius (upper), Pectoralis major, clavicularis, opposite Sternocleidomastoideus
Serratus anticus	Rhomboid, Pectoralis major sternal, Pectoralis minor, Trapezius (middle)
Subclavius	Sternocleidomastoideus
Subscapularis	Teres minor, Infraspinatus, Deltoids, Supraspinatus
Supraspinatus	Rhomboids, Pectoralis minor, Teres major, Teres minor, Latissimus dorsi
Tensor fascia lata	Adductors, Peroneus tertius, Hamstrings, Gluteus maximus
Teres major	Pectoralis majors, Deltoid (anterior), Teres minor, Infraspinatus
Teres minor	Subscapularis, Latissimus dorsi, Deltoid, Supraspinatus.
Trapezius, lower	Pectoralis majors, Pectoralis minor, Levator scapula, Trapezius (upper)
Trapezius, middle	Pectoralis majors, Pectoralis minor
Trapezius, upper	Latissimus dorsi, Biceps, Subscapularis, Trapezius (upper—contralateral), Latissimus dorsi, Neck flexors (SCM)

Exercise

For health and optimal functioning, the body requires an adequate quantity of the right quality of movement. In his AK courses, Goodheart often said that as long as the muscles of the body test strong in AK muscle tests, normal daily activities will provide for adequate fitness. Goodheart himself played tennis for up to three hours several times per week! With his level of "normal daily activity" further exercise was not needed.

However, most of us need more exercise than we get. The need for exercise for training muscle strength is becoming an increasingly popular topic in AK. The following is a short description of how to perform the type of movements needed for health and for correction of typical postural problems.

BASIC FORMULA FOR AN EXERCISE ROUTINE

1. Warm up

2. Stretch

3. Exercise (whether light aerobic exercise such as running, or heavy anaerobic exercise such as weight-lifting)

4. Stretch

5. Cool down

Basic Formula for Exercise

1. If you have or suspect any physical problems, inquire of a doctor or sports therapist as to which exercises you may do, and how to perform them without danger of injury.

2. Warm up your body with light aerobics such as bicycle riding or easy gymnastics. Wait until you begin to sweat before continuing.

3. Stretch the muscles you intend to exercise. Do not bounce your weight upon a stretched muscle but rather take a position that gently stretches the muscle and places some body weight upon it. Then wait and breathe deeply until the muscle and other tissues let go and your extension increases. Be sure you are warmed up and stretched before performing any exercises that require strength.

4. Be sure that the muscles test strong when muscle-tested. Exercises produce less benefit, and may cause damage if they are performed with weak-testing muscles. If you have no one to test you, at least contract the muscle, rub its neurolymphatic points, and contract the muscle again before beginning with the exercises for this muscle. To strengthen the abdominals, also pull the sagittal suture open (see "Rectus Adominis," page 192).

5. Only perform motions that follow the natural motions of the joints and respect the structures of the body.

The bones of the neck are designed to bend forward and backward, lean right and left, and rotate to the right and the left. Other motions such as circles with the head should not be performed! Also, do not lean the head backward while standing. Due to years of the ubiquitous but incorrect posture of pulling the head back upon a neck that is slumped forward and down, the cervical intervertebral discs are thinner on the back side of the body. Pulling the head back places extra pressure on the already compromised posterior portion of these discs. Even when stretching with no added weight, only perform this movement when on the hands and knees or bending forward to remove the weight of the head from pressing upon the thin portion of these discs.

The lumbar vertebral discs are usually pinched posteriorly like the cervical discs. To avoid placing weight upon these already compromised discs, avoid leaning extremely backward while standing. To stretch this area, arch the back while on the hands and knees upon the floor (the yoga posture of the cat). To protect this often-injured area, normal sit-ups should also be avoided.

6. Begin gently and over a period of weeks gradually increase the weights used (if you exercise with weights) and the number of sets of each exercise.

7. After exercising, again stretch the muscles that were used. Also thoroughly stretch all shortened muscles, especially those of the pectoralis group.

8. Gradually cool down (i.e. walk after running).

BASIC FORMULA FOR MUSCLE INJURIES: "RICE"

1. Rest
2. Ice
3. Compression
4. Elevation

If you injure a muscle, first of all rest it. Don't continue with your workout. Place ice (wrapped in a towel and then in a plastic bag) upon the injured muscle. Apply compression such as wrapping it gently in an elastic bandage to prevent swelling. Elevate it above the level of your heart. This will also help prevent swelling. After a day or so, TL the injured area and muscle-test an indicator muscle. If this weakens the indicator muscle, test whether the application of cold or warmth makes the indicator test strong, and apply this kind of stimulus. Other possible treatments can be tested in the same way. Enzymes such as found in fresh pineapple and in the many digestive and metabolic enzyme products available without a prescription are recommended to dissolve the blood released into the tissues by the injury. The following day, when you again start calisthenics involving that muscle, begin slowly. If such calisthenics do not invoke pain at the time, and these can be performed without provoking pain or swelling the following day, the intensity of the exercises can be gradually increased. When you proceed to your usual weight-exercise, use less weight than normal and perform less strenuous maneuvers. Gradually build up to your normal workout over a period of several days or weeks as needed for recovery.

TWO TYPES OF EXERCISE: AEROBIC AND ANAEROBIC

1. Aerobic exercises are easy-to-do exercises that are repeated for extended periods of time. Light weight lifting, running, swimming, bicycling, trampoline springing, and dancing are typical aerobic exercises. Since many people don't make time for exercise at all, and exercise is necessary for health, some English doctors have recommended enthusiastic love-making as a good aerobic exercise. Aerobic exercises are performed near but not over a heart rate of 180 minus your age. If you are out of shape, lower this number even further. If you are very fit, your aerobic heart rate may be safely chosen a bit higher than 180 minus your age. This type of exercise uses oxygen to burn fat for fuel. It results in more slender muscles capable of sustained activity. It is wise to build up aerobic fitness before including anaerobic exercises in your routine. For aerobic fitness, at least 20 minutes of exercises in the target heart beat range (180 minus age for the maximum, 15–20 below this rate for a minimum) is recommended. An electronic heart monitor makes this easy to control. This device makes one sound when the heart goes over the desired maximum and another sound when it goes under the desired minimum. Aerobic exercises can be performed with good results 4–6 days per week.

2. Anaerobic exercises are strenuous exercises that one cannot perform for more than 12 repetitions before exhaustion of the muscles used occurs. Weight lifting near maximum weights, chin-ups, dips, and hand-stand push-ups are typical examples. Anaerobic exercises push the heart rate up higher than aerobic exercises. The body cannot burn fat with oxygen this rapidly so it breaks down blood sugar for fuel. This lowers the amount of sugar circulating in the blood, which may produce intense hunger. Anaerobic exercise produces thicker muscles capable of exerting great force for short periods of time. Rest between anaerobic

exercises. Avoid elevating the heart rate excessively. Aerobic exercises may be performed the next day, but one should rest one day to allow the muscles to recuperate before again performing anaerobic exercises.

Muscle and Fitness magazine reported research in which half of the subjects lifted weights but did not have to lower them. The other subjects only had to lower the weights but not lift them. Lowering the weight is called "negative" exercise. Surprisingly, lowering the weights produced a greater increase in strength and muscle mass than lifting the weights. Considering this finding, be sure to lower the weights slowly to get the greatest benefit from weight lifting, or from exercises in which you lift your own body weight.

IMPROVING POSTURE

1. A depressed attitude is reflected in a slumped posture. And a slumped posture predisposes toward depression. The two mutually influence one another. Change the underlying attitudes—the mental posture—and the physical posture may follow. But body habit can be strong enough to pull you back. Change your physical posture, and your mental/emotional attitudes will change. Specific mental-emotional states are only achievable from specific postures. For example, you cannot feel depressed without collapsing your chest downward.

2. Perform exercises to strengthen the muscles needed to support upright posture.

3. Stretch the muscles whose prior shortening have pulled the body into poor posture.

4. The procedures of Alexander Technique likely provide the best training in posture and movement. Private sessions with a qualified teacher are recommended. In such lessons, you will learn to release the tight muscles at the back of your neck to allow the head to come forward and up, the back to lengthen and widen.

5. Because AK muscle testing and balancing both improve posture and change the subjective sense of what feels right, better posture and patterns of use are automatically assumed without having to consciously attend to them.

TYPICAL POSTURAL DIFFICULTIES

In the upper torso, almost everyone has stronger muscles on the front than the back. We are oriented forward and down toward our desks, sinks, automobiles, etc., so naturally the muscles on the front of the chest are more fit than those on the back. In these and other activities we mostly perform motions that inwardly rotate the shoulders. Even sport and fitness enthusiasts typically do more bench presses than rowing movements. So they too have stronger pushing muscles (pectoralis major clavicularis, pectoralis major sternal, pectoralis minor, anterior deltoid, middle deltoid, triceps, coracobrachialis, etc.) than pulling muscles (rhomboids, trapezius, posterior deltoids, latissimus dorsi, teres major, teres minor, supraspinatus, infraspinatus, biceps, etc.). This is easily seen in the deltoid (shoulder) muscles. The deltoid is typically large in the anterior and middle sections but quite small in its posterior portion. For various reasons, even athletes who consciously exercise their pulling muscles, tend to ignore the external rotators of the shoulder. Although latissimus dorsi and teres major are used in popular pulling motions like chin-ups and rowing, they are also internal rotators of the shoulder.

As a result of these imbalanced activities, the most-used muscles of the chest (the pectoralis group) and the inward rotators of the shoulders tend to be comparatively over-strong and shortened. This is called "adaptive shortening." Their opponents tend to be weak, to muscle-test weak and be overly lengthened. The shortened pectoralis muscles and internal rotators pull the shoulders forward and down, rotate them inward and round the back. These changes establish a new and incorrect norm of balance between these sets of muscles. The weakness in the external rotators of the shoulders predisposes them to the common "rotator cuff" injuries. The rotator cuff muscles hold the humerus into the shoulder joint. Actually, the shoulder joint is structurally quite unstable. It is like a ball pulled onto an open pan by the four rotator cuff muscles: the supraspinatus, infraspinatus, teres minor and subscapularis. These little muscles need to be strong to protect the shoulder from injury. To correct these postural problems, specific exercises are needed to strengthen, and thereby shorten the neglected muscles and also to stretch the incorrectly shortened muscles.

Specific Exercises for the Most Commonly Neglected Muscles

The following is in no way intended to be a complete exercise plan but rather a list of specific exercises for the muscles often ignored and most in need of exercise. Performing these exercises as described will improve posture, prevent injuries and relieve many pains.

Low back pain is the most common physical difficulty that causes discomfort and makes people unable to work and function well. Typically people have overly contracted low back muscles combined with weak abdominal muscles. This produces a "swayback" with eventual pinching of the discs. Making the abdominal muscles test strong with AK techniques will usually temporarily remove the pain. Performing the reactive muscle technique with the primary sacrospinalis and reactive abdominals will provide a longer-lasting correction (see page 135). But in most cases, for lasting freedom from pain, the abdominal muscles also need to be physically stronger.

Sit-Ups

Rectus abdominis, the muscle that appears like a "washboard" on the abdomen, is the main abdominal muscle. More than any other muscle, the abdominals often not only muscle-test weak but are functionally weak. To better support the low back and protect it from pain and disc damage, strong abdominal muscles are needed. However, the typical "sit-up" exercises mostly strengthen the iliopsoas muscles, which connect the inner femur with the lumbar vertebrae and the pelvis. These cannot pull the ribs to the pubic bone like the abdominal muscles do. If iliopsoas is short or overly tense, it pulls the lumbar vertebrae forward, creating a hollow low back. Overly exercising the iliopsoas may increase low back problems. Plus, sit-ups put tremendous pressure on the intervertebral discs and can damage them and/or pinch the nerves that exit the vertebral column between the lumbar vertebrae.

Before exercising the abdominals, first test and correct them with Applied Kinesiology techniques so that they test strong. Then to exercise the abdominals safely, lie on the back, bend the knees and sit up only until the scapulae leave the floor. The function of the abdominals is only to pull the lower edge of the front of the rib cage toward the pelvis. When doing sit-ups, this motion is complete before the low back leaves the floor. The rest of the normal sit-up motion is accomplished by the hip flexors such as iliopsoas. Doing sit-ups this modified way only changes the angle between all the lumbar vertebrae by a total of about 3°, thus minimizing any pinching of the discs. As an easy control, reach with the hands as you sit up until the hands are beside the knees. Do not sit up further than this. In order to avoid the typical poor postural habit of collapsing the chest, some authorities recommend doing sit-ups with the shoulders held back and the shoulder blades pulled together. Begin with 5–10 repetitions and increase the number as your strength increases. When doing 25 repetitions becomes easy, put the hands behind the neck for more resistance and decrease the number of repetitions. Do this exercise both with the feet supported (held down to the floor) for more lower abdominal activity and unsupported for more upper abdominal activity.

For the neglected upper body muscles, perform exercises of the external shoulder rotators and those that pull the arm and shoulder back (posterior). Take

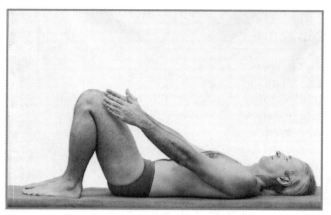

SIT-UPS: BEGINNING POSITION

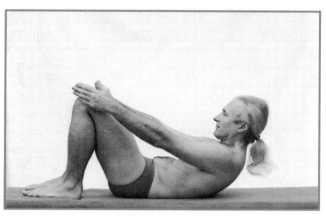

SIT-UPS: FINISHING POSITION

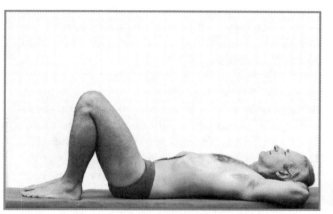

SIT-UPS: WITH HAND BEHIND HEAD
BEGINNING POSITION

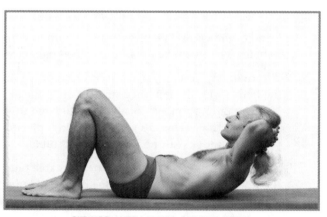

SIT-UPS: WITH HAND BEHIND HEAD
FINISHING POSITION

care that the arm is not raised to the front or side higher than 60° (measured between the body and the arm) with internal rotation ("hunching" the shoulders forward). This can cause impinchment syndrome (of the tendons of supraspinatus, biceps or the bursa of the joint) and lead to tendinitis in the shoulder. There is not much space between the head of the humerus and the acromion of the shoulder joint. External rotation of the shoulder (pulling the shoulders back) allows the tendons and bursa to more easily clear the roof of the shoulder when the arm is raised.

Most of the external rotators of the shoulder (listed below) are rather small and functionally not very

strong muscles. Exercise them with small weights (1–6 pounds) and gradually work up to no more than 20 pounds. Lift and lower the weights slowly with absolutely no jerking movements.

Lying L Flyes

The term, "lying L flyes" refers to the posture in which the elbow is bent 90° and a movement like flying or flapping the wings is performed. Lying L flyes are an excellent exercise for the teres minor, a true external rotator muscle of the shoulder. To perform them, lie on a bench on your right side. Support yourself with your right arm folded under your head or extended

Exercise	Main Muscles Active
Lying L (butter)flyes	Teres minor, infraspinatus
Sitting or standing L flyes	Infraspinatus, teres minor
Bent over flyes	Posterior deltoid, external rotators, middle trapezius
Lying flyes	Posterior deltoid, external rotators, middle trapezius
Lying supraspinatus flyes	Supraspinatus, deltoids
Bent rowing	Teres major, trapezius, rhomboids, posterior deltoids, biceps
Chin-ups standing on a stool	Latissimus dorsi, lower trapezius, biceps

down upon the floor. Choose one of the following three initial positions:

1. Bend both legs and place your left leg upon your right leg. Place your head on your folded right arm.

2. Alternatively, you may place your left foot flat on the bench with the left knee straight up in the air. In this position, you may rest your right hand over your right thigh. This is a good position if placing your arm under your head is uncomfortable.

3. Extend your right arm down below the table onto the floor on holding on to the leg of the table for support. You may hook your right foot over the edge of the bench for increased stability.

Which ever of these three initial positions you choose to assume, next bend your left elbow 90° and prop it upon a firm pillow on your left side. Bring your forearm down across your chest. Begin with a very light weight (~1 pound) in your left hand. Rotate the weight up as high as it is comfortable to do, keeping the elbow in place. If you are rehabilitating an injury to the shoulder, only lift the weight to slightly above horizontal. Lower the weight and repeat the movement for 6 to 8 repetitions. Repeat on the other side. Do not allow the elbow to slip off to the side or the back to rotate with the motion. Keep the elbow bent 90° and down upon the side. As your strength increases, increase the weight but never use more than 15 pounds with this exercise.

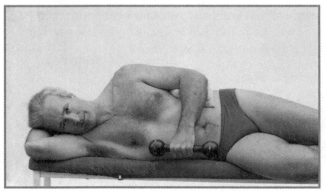

LYING L FLYES: WITH THE ARM UNDER THE HEAD

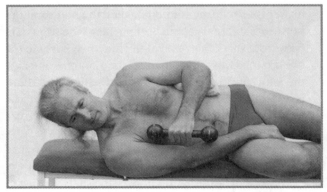

LYING L FLYES: HOLDING THE THIGH

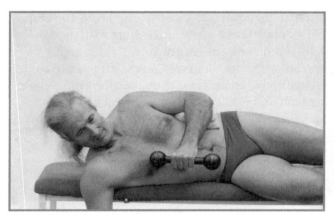

LYING L FLYES
USING THE ARM DOWN FOR SUPPORT

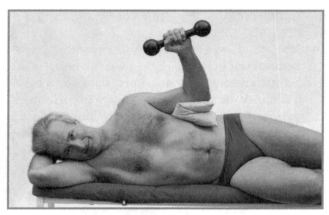

LYING L FLYES
END POSITION

Standing or Sitting L Flyes

Standing or sitting L flyes are an excellent exercise for the other true external rotator of the shoulder, the infraspinatus. The posterior deltoids are active in this exercise as well. For this exercise, you will need to support the elbow at a level just below armpit height. Stand or sit with your chest diagonal to the support to enable free rotation of the forearm around the elbow. Hold a light dumbbell (1–20 pounds maximum) in your right hand with your right elbow bent 90°. The angle between your trunk and your right shoulder should be less than 90° (oriented slightly downward from shoulder to elbow). These adjustments of angle are necessary to avoid impinchment at the shoulder joint. Support your right elbow upon the back or in the palm of your left hand. Keep the 90° angle of the elbow and lower the weight to an angle just below horizontal. Gently reverse the direction with no jerking and raise the weight to the starting position. Perform 6 to 8 repetitions. Repeat with the left arm.

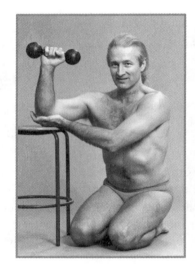

STANDING OR SITTING
L FLYES
BEGINNING POSITION

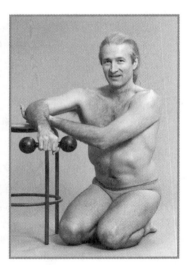

STANDING OR SITTING
L FLYES
END POSITION

Bent-Over Flyes

Bent-over flyes put the main work of contraction into the posterior deltoids. These are small muscles that are often ignored in training programs, so go lightly at first with the weight (1–5 pounds). To perform this exercise, bend forward at the hips until the back is near horizontal. Keep the knees gently bent to reduce stress to the low back. Use two dumbbells (or soup cans or bottles of water, etc.). Start with the arms hanging downward. Begin to lift the weights by spreading the arms and continue to lift them to horizontal and in line with the ears. Keep the elbows gently bent and rotate the arms externally a bit as you raise them. When you use heavier weights, support your chest on a narrow bench.

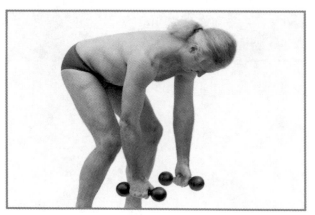

BENT-OVER FLYES: BEGINNING POSITION

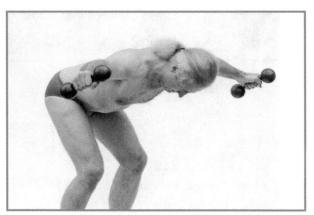

BENT-OVER FLYES: END POSITION

Lying Flyes

Lying flyes put even more activity into the posterior deltoids than bent-over flyes. Also, this exercise includes the first 90° of the motion of the posterior deltoids that is missed by the bent-over flyes. Strength in this range of the motion is important in various sports: An example is the tennis backhand stroke. Begin in the same lying-on-the-left-side position as for lying L flyes. Hold a very light dumbbell down toward the floor in your right hand with your palm facing inward toward the bench. Begin with 1–4 pounds and work up to no more than 10 pounds. The posterior deltoid has poor leverage in this position so don't overload it! Keep the elbow gently bent throughout the motion. Slowly lift the weight until your arm is nearly vertical. Do not roll back as you lift the weight. Slowly lower the weight and do 6 to 8 repetitions. Repeat with the weight in the left hand.

Lying Supraspinatus Flyes

Lying supraspinatus flyes target the supraspinatus muscle. Like the lying flyes, this exercise includes the first 90° of supraspinatus and deltoid motion that most other exercises of these muscles omit. Performing this exercise with the arm externally rotated puts more work into the anterior and middle deltoids. With the arm internally rotated, the supraspinatus and posterior deltoids are more active. To perform this exercise, lie in the same position as for the lying L flyes and the lying flyes. Use a very light dumbbell. Begin with the weight held in the nearly straightened arm down toward the floor. Lift the weight slowly, parallel to the bench, first toward your feet and then on up to about 60° above horizontal. With internal rotation, never raise the arm more than 60° above horizontal! Slowly lower and repeat for 6 to 8 repetitions. Repeat with the other arm.

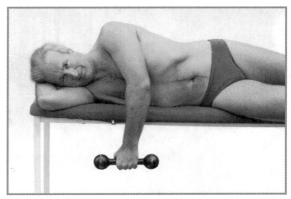

LYING FLYES: BEGINNING POSITION

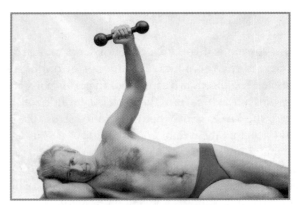

LYING FLYES: END POSITION

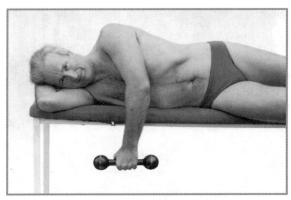

LYING SUPRASPINATUS FLYES: BEGINNING POSITION WITH INNER ROTATION

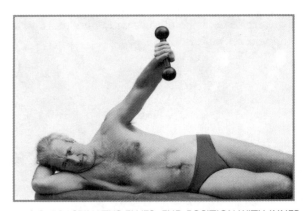

LYING SUPRASPINATUS FLYES: END POSITION WITH INNER ROTATION

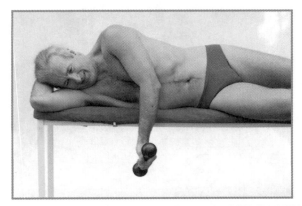

LYING SUPRASPINATUS FLYES: BEGINNING POSITION WITH OUTER ROTATION

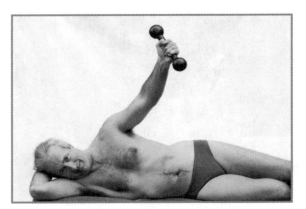

LYING SUPRASPINATUS FLYES: END POSITION WITH OUTER ROTATION

Bent Rowing

Bent rowing is a good exercise for teres major, the trapezius, the rhomboid, and the posterior deltoid muscles. The biceps are active too. To perform it, bend forward at the hips until the back is near horizontal. Keep the knees gently bent to reduce stress to the low back. Pull the weight up to the side as if you were rowing a boat. When you use heavier weights, support your chest on a bench. If you have a narrow bench, you can row with both arms at once. If your bench is wide, support yourself with the one hand or forearm on the bench and row with the other arm. Reverse sides and repeat. Be sure to pull the shoulder back as well as the hand toward the shoulder. Doing this exercise with the elbows wide puts more work into the teres major muscle.

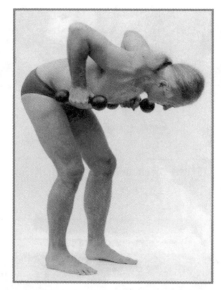

BENT ROWING: END POSITION

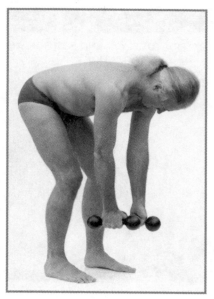

BENT ROWING: BEGINNING POSITION

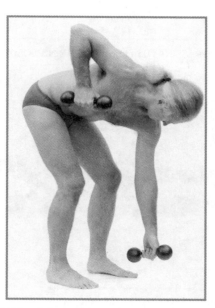

BENT ALTERNATE ROWING: END POSITION

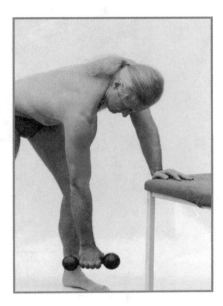

BENT ROWING WITH ONE SUPPORTING ARM BEGINNING
POSITION

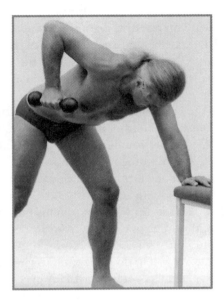

BENT ROWING WITH ONE SUPPORTING ARM END
POSITION

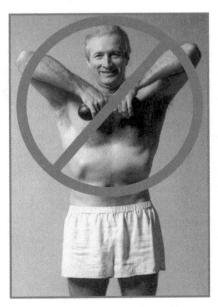

AVOID UPRIGHT ROWING!

When you do this exercise with both arms simultaneously, squeeze the shoulder blades together when the weights are maximally elevated. When you lift each weight alternately, first lift the weight to maximal elevation with no rotation of the back, and then rotate the back to lift the weight a bit higher.

Upright rowing is not advised. This exercise places the shoulder in extreme inward rotation with the arms held high. Three is the danger of impingement in the shoulder joint and subsequent tendinitis or bursitis. You may not feel any pain until hours or days later and therefore may not know which exercise was the problem.

Chin-Ups

Chin-ups are too difficult for many people so it is here advised that you perform them while standing upon a stool. That way the legs can take some of the weight. Also, having the feet on a stool keeps the legs bent at the hips, which is less of a strain upon the low back than hanging straight.

Allow the arms enough of the weight so that you reach exhaustion and can't do more than twelve repetitions. As long as you have no pain or joint problems, make the full range of the movement. Pull up from fully extended arms all the way to chest touching the bar. Do chin-ups with your palms facing toward you and again with your palms facing away. To change the angle of exercise from vertical to horizontal, put your feet on someone's shoulders. This position allows you to do horizontal rowing without the strain of leaning over forward. However, this exercise requires lots of strength and a very sure grip on the bar, so it is recommended only for the advanced.

Stretching the Pectoralis Muscles

After performing these and/or other exercises, be sure to stretch the muscles used. Then stretch the pectoralis muscles. One easy way is to lie on your back on a narrow bench or a large exercise ball. Hold two light dumbbells in your hands and spread your arms wide. Allow the weight to pull your hands and shoulders down toward the floor, stretching your pectoralis muscles and other inner rotators of the shoulders.

Alternately, you can stand in a doorway with your upper arm parallel to the floor and your forearm against the door jamb. Step and lean forward until the door jamb pulls your arm and shoulder posteriorly. Remain in this position about 20 seconds. Repeat with the elbow higher than the shoulder. Repeat both positions with the other arm.

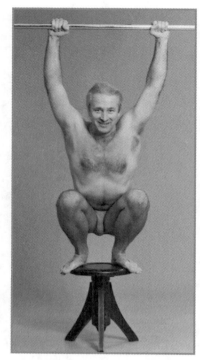

CHIN-UPS STANDING ON A STOOL,
PALMS FORWARD: BEGINNING POSITION

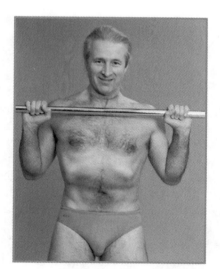

CHIN-UPS STANDING ON A STOOL,
PALMS FORWARD: END POSITION

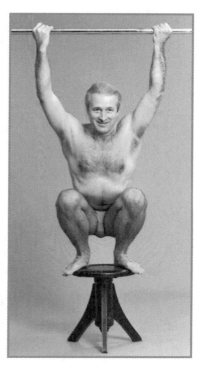

CHIN-UPS STANDING ON A STOOL,
REVERSE GRIP: BEGINNING POSITION

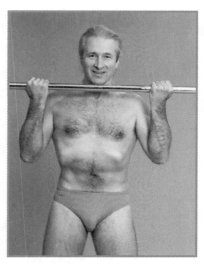

CHIN-UPS STANDING ON A STOOL,
REVERSE GRIP: END POSITION

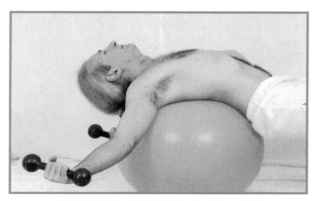

STRETCHING THE PECTORALIS MUSCLES
LYING OVER A BALL

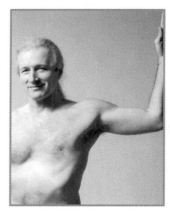

STRETCHING THE
PECTORALIS MUSCLES

STANDING IN A DOORWAY
WITH HORIZONTAL ARM
POSITION

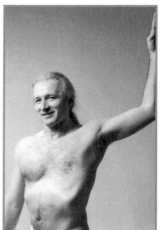

STRETCHING THE
PECTORALIS MUSCLES

STANDING IN A DOORWAY
WITH DIAGONAL ARM
POSITION

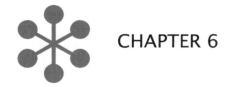 **CHAPTER 6**

Muscle Tests

This chapter contains abbreviated information about thirty-three muscles, how to muscle—test, and how to correct them. All anatomical terms used here are defined in Appendix I: Glossary. Abbreviations for the vertebral segments: Cervical = C, Thoracic = T, Lumbar = L, Sacral = S. The *origin* and *insertion* describe where the two ends of the muscle attach to bone, tendons or ligaments. The *action* is motion produced by contraction of the muscle. The *position* describes the initial parameters of the muscle test. If *stabilization* is required to test the muscle, it is described. The *muscle test* describes how the examiner applies pressure in the test. The *front neurolymphatic, back neurolymphatic and neurovascular points* are described and graphically presented. The *sedation point* is shown graphically. The typical *reactive muscles* are listed. The *meridian* and *organ/gland* correspondences for each muscle are given. *Nutrition* that may strengthen specific muscles is presented. A *discussion* of the muscle, and what weakness of the specific muscle may imply, follows.

Adductors

Origin: On the anterior and lateral surfaces of the pubic bone and the ischial tuberosity.

Insertion: Along the whole length of the medial side of the femur.

Action: Pulls the legs together (hip adduction). The various adductor muscles are also somewhat active in medial rotation, hip flexion and hip extension.

Position: Patient lies on the side with the legs straight and in line with the torso. The examiner lifts the top leg up from the table and stabilizes it under the knee. Then examiner lifts the leg that is initially upon the table up past the midline of the body and toward the other leg and places his hand on the medial side of this leg near the knee.

Stabilization: The patient can help stabilize the trunk by holding onto the edge of the table.

Muscle Test: The examiner presses the lower leg toward the table. No rotation of the pelvis is allowed.

Front Neurolymphatic: Behind the nipple. To avoid pain, make contact immediately lateral to the nipple and then push in carefully toward the ribs. If preferable, instruct the patient to massage these points herself.

Back Neurolymphatic: Just distal to the inferior tip of the shoulder blade.

Neurovascular: On the middle of the lambda suture located between the back of the ear and the posterior fontanelle.

Reactive Muscles: Iliopsoas, piriformis, tensor fascia lata, gluteus medius and maximus.

Meridian: Circulation-sex

Organ/Gland: Reproductive organs and glands. During the female climacterium, changes in the hormone system including the thyroid, pituitary, and adrenal glands—and problems with the liver and reproductive organs—may also be involved in weakness of the adductors. Conversely, testing and correcting the adductors can help to reestablish a better balance of hormones during the climacterium.

Nutrition: Vitamin E, niacin, zinc.

Discussion: The adductors may also be tested supine. To do so, the examiner must stabilize one leg while attempting to abduct the other. The adductors are the leg muscles a rider uses to grip the horse. The constant pressures that riding produces upon the adductors may make them chronically weak, leading to the "O" legs often seen in cowboys. One-sided weakness will cause the pelvis on the same side to sink. Weakness in the adductors is often the cause of shoulder pains and "tennis elbow." This may be due to the fact that tennis playing produces much side-to-side motion requiring dynamic adductor activity. The neurolymphatic reflex points for the adductors also stimulate the lymphatic drainage from the shoulder and arms, which can help promote healing in these areas.

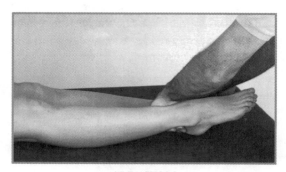

ADDUCTORS
TESTED SUPINE

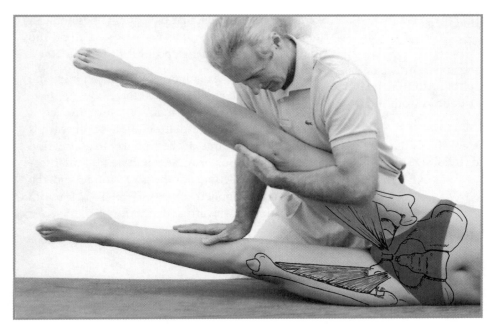

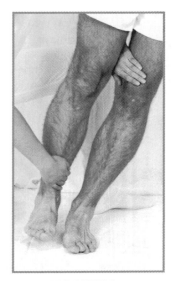

ADDUCTORS
TESTED STANDING

ADDUCTORS, TESTED LYING ON THE SIDE

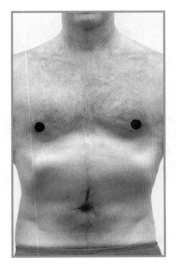

ANTERIOR NL

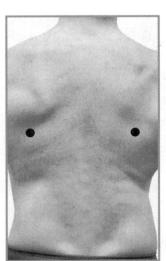

POSTERIOR NL

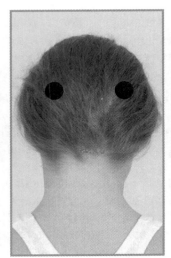

NEUROVASCULAR POINT

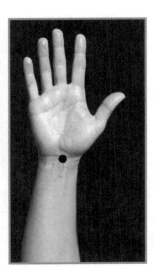

SEDATION POINT, CIRCU-
LATION-SEX 7

Deltoids: Anterior, Middle, and Posterior

Origin: Middle deltoid from the upper surface of the acromion process. Anterior deltoid from the lateral third of the clavicle. Posterior deltoid from the lateral inferior scapular spine.

Insertion: All three divisions of the deltoid insert into the deltoid tubercle on the lateral side of the mid-humerus.

Action: Anterior deltoid—abduction, flexion and medial rotation of the humerus.

Middle deltoid—pure abduction of the humerus.

Posterior deltoid—abduction, slight extension and lateral rotation of the humerus.

Position: With the patient sitting or standing, the arm is abducted 90° and the elbow is flexed 90°. This flexion of the elbow allows the examiner to observe for any rotation of the humerus, which should not be allowed during the test. For the anterior deltoid, laterally rotate the humerus about 45° (which places the hand higher than the shoulder) and slightly flex the shoulder (which brings the elbow around toward the front of the body). For the middle deltoid, the forearm remains parallel to the floor. For the posterior deltoid, position the humerus with a slight internal rotation and slight extension (elbow slightly posterior).

Stabilization: For the anterior deltoid, stabilization is posterior on the shoulder tested. Stabilization may not be required for the middle deltoid test. However, if the patient has the tendency to elevate the shoulder, the examiner should place his hand over the shoulder to prevent this. For the posterior deltoid, stabilization is anterior on the shoulder tested.

For all deltoid tests, the scapula must be fixed. If the muscles that do so (the upper and middle trapezius, serratus anticus, pectoralis minor and the rhomboids) test weak, the examiner must either strengthen them first or stabilize the scapula during the tests. The examiner should watch that the patient does not lean the trunk, rotate the humerus, bend or extend the elbow or otherwise change position during the tests.

Muscle Test: The examiner makes contact upon the distal aspect of the humerus near the elbow. For testing all three deltoids, the main pressure applied is adduction. For anterior deltoid, the test pressure is applied along the line of the forearm in a direction downward and posterior. For middle deltoid, pressure is pure adduction. For the posterior deltoid, the test pressure is applied along the line of the forearm in a direction downward and anterior.

Front Neurolymphatic: Between ribs 3 and 4 near the sternum.

Back Neurolymphatic: Between the transverse processes of thoracic vertebrae 3 and 4.

Neurovascular: Upon the bregma.

Reactive Muscles: Rhomboids, pectoralis majors and minor, latissimus dorsi, subscapularis.

Meridian: Lung.

Organ/Gland: Lung.

Nutrition: Vitamin C, RNA, beta-carotene, water.

Discussion: Bilateral weakness in any division of the deltoids may indicate a vertebral fixation at the junction of the cervical and thoracic vertebrae. This may be confirmed by having the patient place one hand there while the weak-testing deltoid division of the other arm is again tested. If therapy localization of this area strengthens the deltoid, the fixation is confirmed. In this case, chiropractic correction of the fixation may be needed to obtain a lasting correction of the deltoid.

A lower trapezius bilateral weakness can hide a bilateral weakness in any division of the deltoids. For this reason, the lower trapezius should be tested and corrected before testing the deltoids.

Sometimes the anterior deltoid will be palpatory hypertonic while the middle and posterior divisions test weak. For this problem, the examiner should utilize the proprioceptor techniques (neuromuscular spindle cell or Golgi tendon organ), the fascial release, or the chill and stretch techniques upon the palpatory hypertonic anterior deltoid as indicated by the specific case.

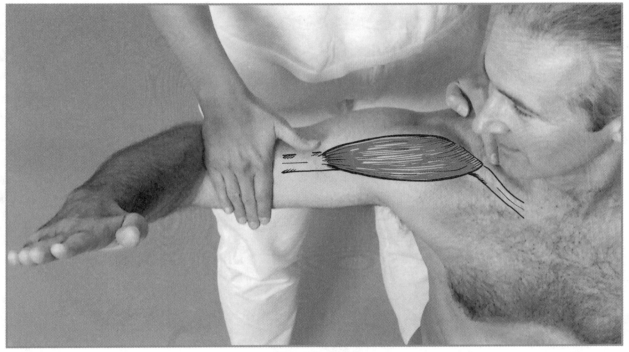

ANTERIOR DELTOID

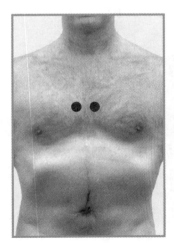

ANTERIOR NL

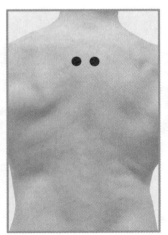

POSTERIOR NL

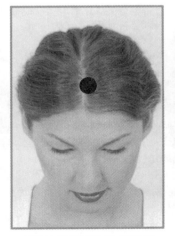

NEUROVASCULAR POINT

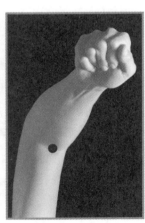

SEDATION POINT
LUNG 5

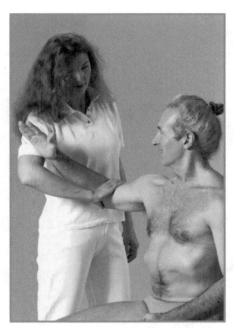

ANTERIOR DELTOID

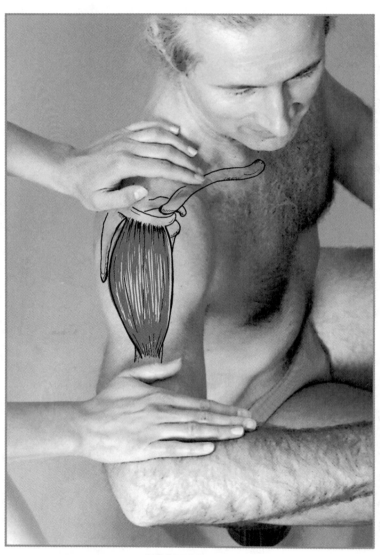

MIDDLE DELTOID

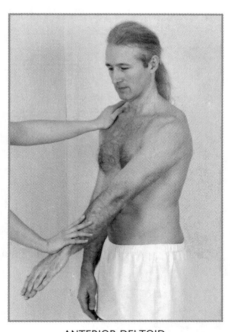

ANTERIOR DELTOID,
TESTED STANDING

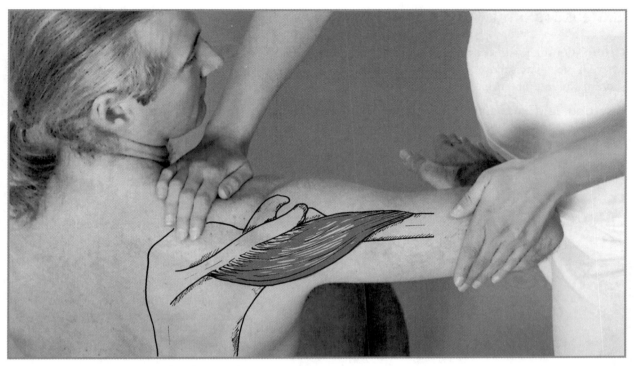

POSTERIOR DELTOID

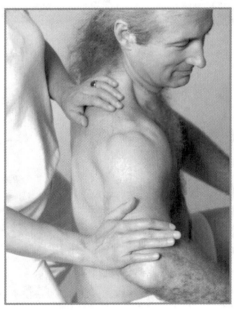

POSTERIOR DELTOID

Gluteus Maximus

Origin: On the posterior medial edge of the ilium where it meets the sacrum and on the dorsal surface sacrum and lateral margin of the coccyx.

Insertion: Into the lateral posterior superior part of the femur plus into the iliotibial tract (long flat tendon/ligament) of the fascia lata.

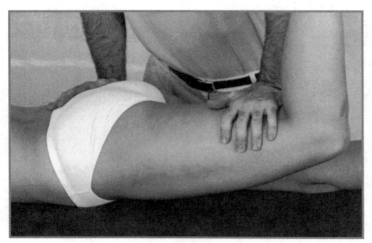

GLUTEUS MAXIMUS

Action: Extends and helps rotate the thigh laterally. When the hip is fixed as in standing, the gluteus maximus extends the pelvis on the thigh.

Position: The patient lies prone, bending his leg at least 90° and extending his hip (by lifting his leg from the table) maximally.

Stabilization: The examiner stabilizes the opposite hip down against the table. Do not allow the patient to straighten the leg (which allows the hamstrings to get involved) or rotate the pelvis during the test.

Muscle Test: With a hand near the back of the knee, the examiner pushes the leg down toward the table (toward flexion of the hip).

Front Neurolymphatic: A wide stripe along the whole length of the anterior lateral surface of the thigh.

Back Neurolymphatic: In the depressions between L5 and the PSIS.

Neurovascular: On the middle of the lambda suture located between the back of the ear and the posterior fontanelle.

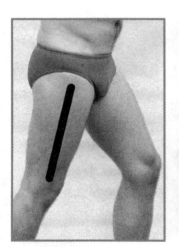

ANTERIOR NL

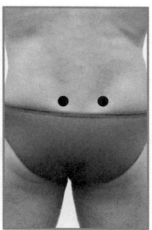

POSTERIOR NL

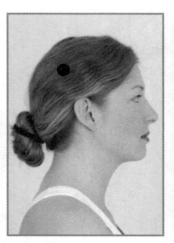

NEUROVASCULAR POINT

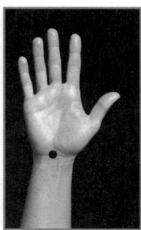

SEDATION POINT, CIRCU-
LATION-SEX 7

Reactive Muscles: Sacrospinalis, pectoralis major clavicular, iliopsoas, rectus femoris, sartorius, piriformis, adductors, tensor fascia lata.

Meridian: Circulation-sex.

Organ/Gland: Reproductive organs and glands.

Nutrition: Vitamin E, niacin, zinc.

Discussion: One-sided weakness of gluteus maximus will cause the pelvis to sink and rotate forward on the side of weakness. When gluteus maximus is weak on both sides, there will be a sway back and difficulty with walking. This double-sided weakness may be the result of a fixation of the upper cervical spine. If gentle rotation of the head and neck does not free this fixation, it may require chiropractic correction. Gluteus maximus is often weak on one side and palpatory hypertonic on the other. Strengthen these muscles as

usual. However, if the palpatory hypertonic muscle does not release with the usual techniques, lean the heel of the hand heavily upon the tight gluteus maximus until it is felt to relax.

Suspect gluteus maximus weakness when the patient complains of difficulty climbing stairs. Gluteus maximus weakness may be associated with a lack of sexual drive and problems with the sexual organs.

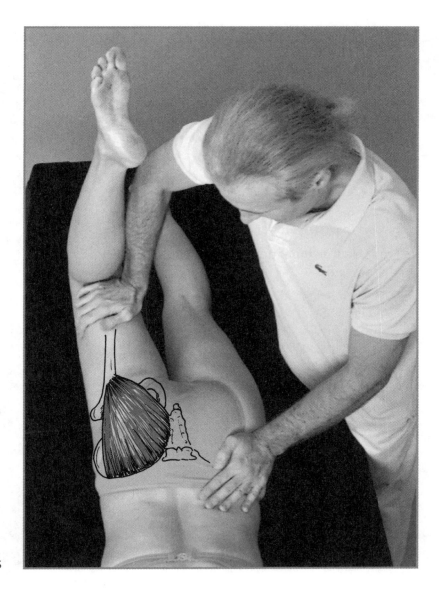

GLUTEUS MAXIMUS

Gluteus Medius

Origin: A wide attachment of the posterior ilium on the anterior three-quarters of the iliac crest.

Insertion: Into the lateral surface of the greater trochanter.

Action: Abduction and medial rotation of the thigh. Stabilizes the pelvis laterally.

Position: On the side, supine or standing. The leg is fully extended and held out laterally and slightly posterior.

Stabilization: The examiner must see that the pelvis remains stable. Typically when gluteus medius tests weak, the patient will attempt to roll toward the side tested to have fascia lata take over as the prime mover. When testing supine, the examiner must stabilize the opposite ankle.

Muscle Test: Press the leg in medially toward the other leg. In the supine position, the patient should lie near the side of the table so that the leg tested can be positioned a bit lower than the level of the table.

Front Neurolymphatic: Top edge of the pubis symphysis.

Back Neurolymphatic: In the depressions between L 5 and the PSIS.

Neurovascular: On the posterior part of the parietal eminences.

Reactive Muscles: Contralateral rectus abdominis, adductors.

Meridian: Circulation-sex

Organ/Gland: All the reproductive organs and glands, male and female.

Nutrition: Vitamin E, niacin, zinc.

Discussion: Weakness in gluteus medius may only be observable when tested upright with weight on the opposite leg. When gluteus medius is weak on one side, the pelvis, shoulder and head will be higher on the same side. When walking, the opposite pelvis side will hang down and the leg on this side will swing forward more laterally than usual, creating a limp typical of one-sided gluteus medius weakness.

Imbalances of gluteus medius are often associated with endocrine problems, especially of the reproductive glands. These include menstrual cramps, breast pains, prostate problems and impotence (see case history #5 in Appendix VIII).

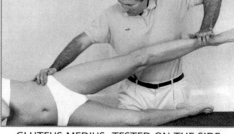

GLUTEUS MEDIUS, TESTED ON THE SIDE

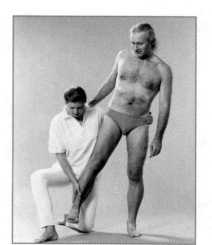

GLUTEUS MEDIUS

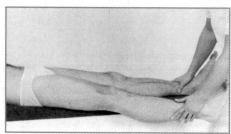

GLUTEUS MEDIUS, TESTED SUPINE

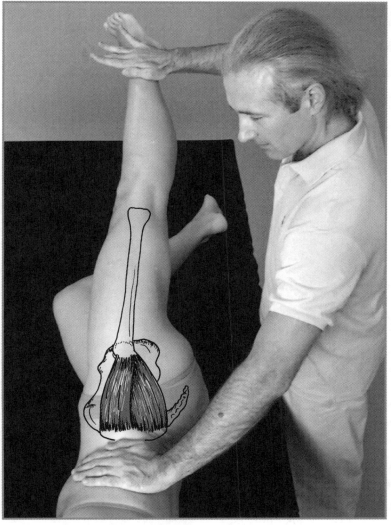

GLUTEUS MEDIUS

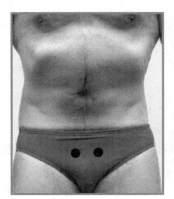

ANTERIOR NL

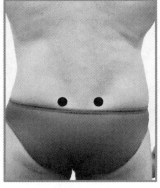

POSTERIOR NL

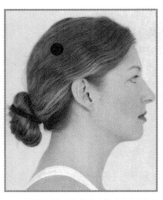

NEUROVASCULAR POINT

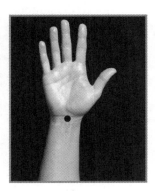

SEDATION POINT, CIRCU-
LATION-SEX 7

Hamstrings: Medial and Lateral

Origin: On the ischial tuberosity (sit bones).

Insertion: The medial hamstring (Semitendinosus) inserts into the lateral and posterior surfaces of the tibia just below the knee. The lateral hamstring (Biceps femoris) inserts into the lateral and posterior sides of the fibula just below the knee.

Action: Both hamstrings work together to flex the knee, and to extend and adduct the thigh.

Position: The patient lies prone. The knee is flexed no more than 60° up from the table. The greater flexion of the knee, the greater the tendency for the hamstrings to cramp when tested.

Stabilization: The examiner grasps the bellies of the hamstrings and leans his body weight upon them to hold the thigh down upon the table and to help prevent the hamstrings from cramping during the test.

Muscle Test: With hand contact on the leg just proximal to the heel (but not on the Achilles tendon), the examiner presses the leg down toward the table (toward extending the knee). Pressing down and laterally tests the medial hamstrings. Pressing down and medially tests the lateral hamstrings.

Front Neurolymphatic: Proximal to the lesser trochanter of the femur.

Back Neurolymphatic: In the depression between the transverse processes of L-5 and the PSIS.

Neurovascular: On the sagittal suture 2.5 cm anterior to the lambda.

Reactive Muscles: Sacrospinalis, contralateral latissimus dorsi, quadriceps, popliteus.

Meridian: Large Intestine.

Organ: Rectum.

Nutrition: Vitamin E and F. If cramping of the hamstrings is a problem, calcium or nutrients that work with calcium such as magnesium and betaine hydrochloride may be needed.

Discussion: Because the hamstrings are pelvic and knee stabilizers, they should be checked whenever there are problems with the pelvis or knees. The hamstrings are the main posterior stabilizers of the pelvis. When they are weak, the pelvis will tilt forward, increasing the curve of the low back (lumbar lordosis). The medial hamstrings can be somewhat isolated by pressing the leg toward extension and slightly lateral. The lateral hamstrings can be somewhat isolated by pressing the leg toward extension and slightly medial.

The hamstrings make a convenient indicator muscle when the patient is lying prone. With the knee only slightly bent, the tendency for hamstrings to cramp is reduced. Alternately, an assistant can provide pressure upon the belly of hamstrings to prevent it from cramping during testing.

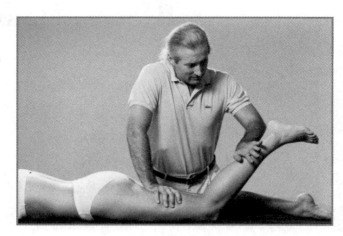

HAMSTRINGS

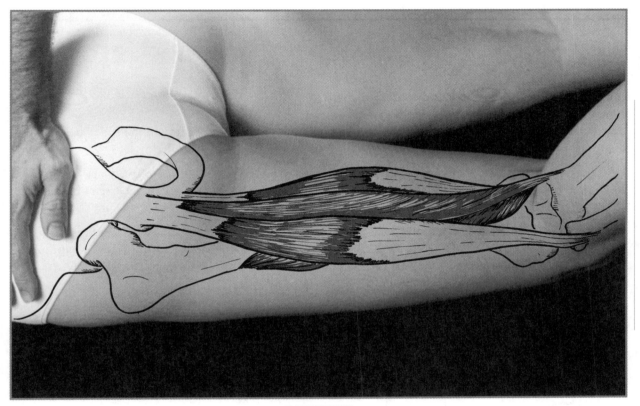

HAMSTRINGS

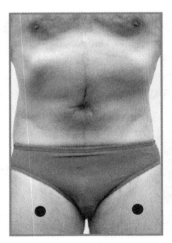

ANTERIOR NL

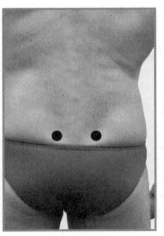

POSTERIOR NL

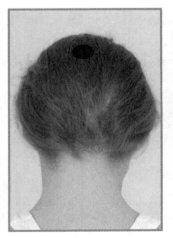

NEUROVASCULAR POINT

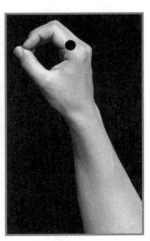

SEDATION POINT, LARGE
INTESTINE 2

Iliopsoas

Origin: Psoas on the anterior side of the transverse processes L1–L5, lateral side of the vertebral bodies and discs from T12 to L5. Iliacus on the upper two-thirds of the inner side of the ilium (the largest muscle-to-bone attachment in the body), to the ala (wings) of the sacrum and to the anterior sacroiliac, lumbosacral and iliolumbar ligaments.

Insertion: Psoas and iliacus both insert into the lesser trochanter of the femur.

Action: Psoas and iliacus have the same insertion and nearly the same action. They flex the thigh, weakly rotate it laterally and abduct it slightly. When the leg is fixed, one-sided contraction leans the back laterally. Iliopsoas, here considered functionally as one muscle, is the most active muscle in sitting up from a supine posture. It is the primary muscle that brings the leg forward when walking or running.

Position: The patient lies on the back, lifts one leg up (flexes the hip), abducts the leg slightly and rotates the leg laterally as much as possible. Observe that the lateral rotation is from the hip and not only from the ankle. Walther suggests lifting the leg up high and abducting it out wide to better isolate the iliacus from the synergistic psoas.

Stabilization: The examiner must fixate the opposite hip to prevent the body from rotating toward the side tested.

Muscle Test: The examiner pushes the leg down toward the table (extension of the hip) and out to the side (abduction). The direction should be diagonal, between the direction of contraction of rectus femoris and the adductors. The examiner needs to be gentle and avoid applying excess pressure when performing this test.

Front Neurolymphatic: 2.5 cm above the navel and 2.5 cm to each side.

Back Neurolymphatic: In the space between the transverse processes of T12 & L1.

Neurovascular: In little indentations 4 cm to each side of the occipital protuberance, the little bump at the back base of the skull.

Reactive Muscles: Adductors, diaphragm, gluteus maximus, contralateral anterior neck flexors, hamstrings, quadratus lumborum, sacrospinalis.

Meridian: Kidney.

Organ/Gland: Kidney.

Nutrition: Vitamins A, E, water.

Discussion: The iliopsoas is an important postural muscle pair, active in maintaining upright posture. Excess bilateral tension increases the lumbar "swayback" curve. Bilateral weakness causes a loss of the normal lumbar curve. One-sided weakness causes the foot to turn in or the hip to sink on the weak-testing side. Conversely, walking with one or both feet turned in can make iliopsoas test weak. Iliopsoas supports the sacroiliac. When iliopsoas is too tight, it can jam the sacrum and ilium together in a fixation. When iliopsoas is too loose, the sacroiliac is unstable and can go out of alignment (subluxate). Iliopsoas function should be examined in any low back pain or disc problems.

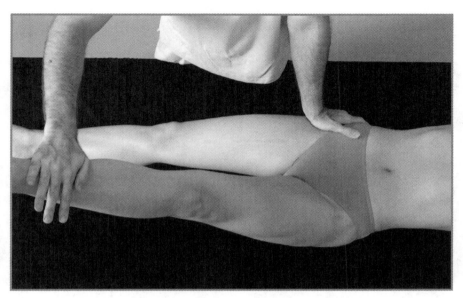

ILIOPSOAS, TEST BEGINNING POSITION

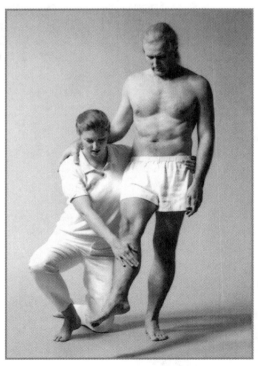

ILIOPSOAS, TESTED STANDING

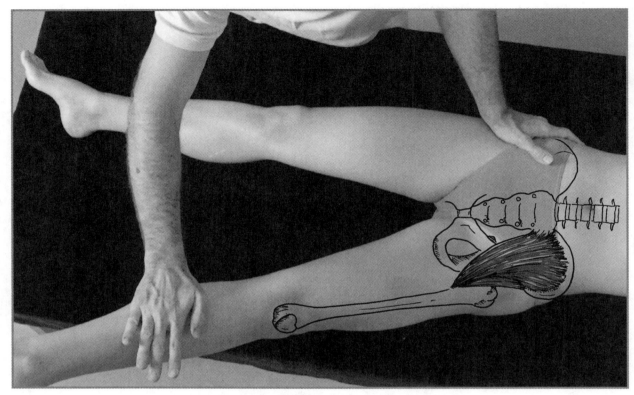

ILIACUS, END POSITION WHEN IT TESTS WEAK

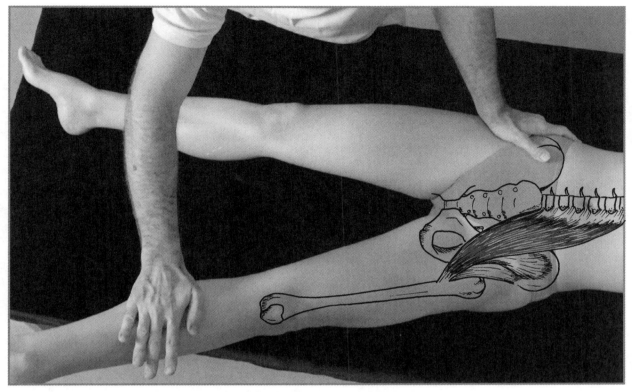

PSOAS, END POSITION WHEN IT TESTS WEAK

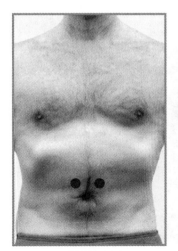

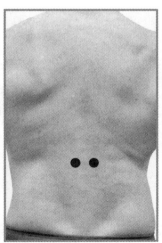

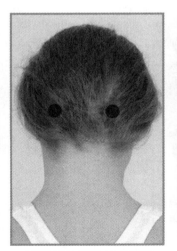

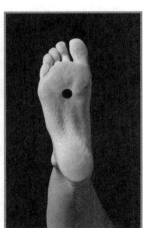

ANTERIOR NL

POSTERIOR NL

NEUROVASCULAR POINT

SEDATION POINT, KIDNEY 1

Infraspinatus

Origin: Along the middle two-thirds of the medial, dorsal border of the scapula (below the spine of the scapula).

Insertion: Over and into the lateral top of the humerus and the capsule of the shoulder joint.

Action: Stabilizes the head of the humerus into the glenoid cavity. Laterally rotates the humerus (synergistic with teres minor). The superior fibers aid in abduction. The inferior fibers aid in adduction.

Position: The humerus is raised 90° out to the side and externally rotated as much as possible. The elbow is flexed 90°.

Stabilization: The humerus should not move during the test. The examiner stabilizes the humerus to detect any attempt to move it in any direction.

Muscle Test: Pressure is applied proximal to the wrist to rotate the forearm around and down toward the feet.

Front Neurolymphatic: Between ribs 5 and 6 where they meet the sternum on the right side. Goodheart confirmed the existence of extra neurolymphatic points for infraspinatus located under the pectoralis major sternal muscle at the level of the upper edge of the armpit with the arm raised horizontally from the side.

Back Neurolymphatic: T12 lamina.

Neurovascular: The lump about 5 cm down from the top of the sternum.

Reactive Muscles: Pectoralis major clavicular and sternal, anterior deltoid, superior and inferior fibers of the infraspinatus itself.

Meridian: Triple heater.

Organ/Gland: Thymus.

Nutrition: Organic iodine as found in kelp, zinc, copper, vitamin C, vitamin A.

Discussion: Infraspinatus is such a close synergist to teres minor that it is difficult to determine the differential function of these two muscles. Therapy localization plus comparison of the symptoms of thyroid versus thymus malfunction will help the examiner tell the difference. When weak, subscapularis will often be palpatory hypertonic as a result. The origin of infraspinatus is very wide. To test its various fibers, test various ranges of abduction of the humerus from 70° to 130°.

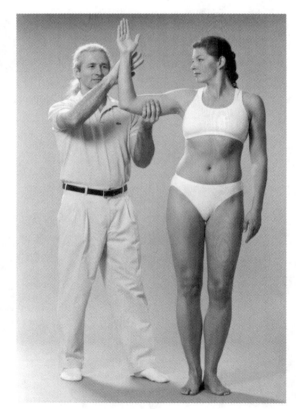

INFRASPINATUS

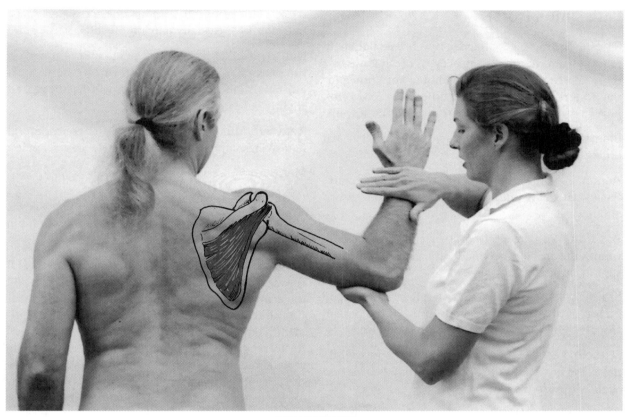

INFRASPINATUS

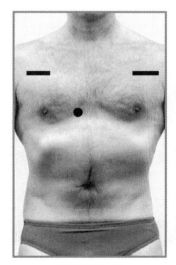

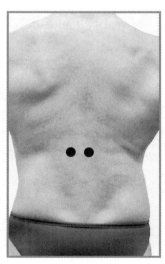

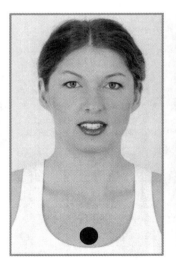

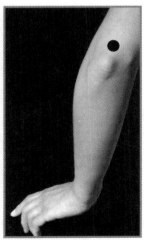

ANTERIOR NL

POSTERIOR NL

NEUROVASCULAR POINT

SEDATION POINT,
TRIPLE HEATER 10

Latissimus Dorsi

Origin: The muscle is attached by a broad, flat, sheet tendon from the spinous processes of the lower six thoracic vertebrae and all the lumbar vertebrae plus the posterior crest of the ilium, the lower 3 to 4 ribs, plus an attachment to the bottom tip of the scapula.

Insertion: Into the medial side of the humerus just under the shoulder joint.

Action: Pulls the arm (humerus) down and in, rotates the arm medially, pulls the shoulder blade downward and inward.

Position: With the elbow fully extended, the patient rotates the arm inward (medially) and holds the arm slightly away from the side.

Stabilization: The examiner stabilizes with a hand on top of the shoulder tested to prevent the patient from leaning sideways or lifting the shoulder.

Muscle Test: The examiner abducts and slightly flexes the arm (pulls the arm away from the side and slightly toward the front).

Front Neurolymphatic: In the junction of rib and cartilage in the depression between ribs 7 and 8, directly below the nipple on the left side only.

Back Neurolymphatic: In the intertransverse space between T7–8 (usually only on the left).

Neurovascular: Just above the squamosal suture on the parietal bone, slightly posterior to the vertical auricular line (about two finger-widths above and slightly behind each ear).

Reactive Muscles: Upper trapezius, contralateral hamstrings, supraspinatus, deltoids, levator scapula.

Meridian: Spleen

Organ/Gland: Pancreas

Nutrition: Vitamins A and F, betaine, zinc, selenium and chromium.

Discussion: These "wing" muscles are active in all rowing motions and especially in movements that pull the arms down (caudal) and in to the sides (adduction) like chin-ups. Medially rotating the arm optimally aligns the origin and insertion of latissimus dorsi for testing. However, this position makes it possible to bend the arm, allowing biceps to aid (synergize) in the action. For this reason, it is absolutely necessary for the examiner to make sure that the elbow remain completely extended during the test. If the patient can hyperextend the elbow (most common in women), the elbow must remain hyperextended during the test.

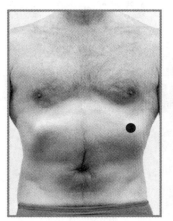

ANTERIOR NL

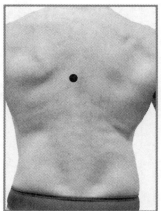

POSTERIOR NL

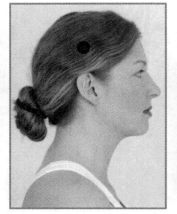

NEUROVASCULAR POINT

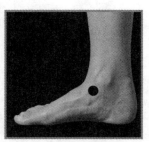

SEDATION POINT, SPLEEN 5

To prevent unwanted bending of the elbow, instruct the patient to imagine clamping a newspaper between the upper arm and the side of the chest. During the test, the examiner must avoid accidentally touching (challenging) the alarm points along the radial artery of the wrist.

Latissimus dorsi often test weak secondary to hypertonic upper trapezius on the same side. Until the hypertonicity of the upper trapezius is adequately reduced, the latissimus dorsi weakness will return; even after successful strengthening techniques have been applied (see "Reactive Muscles," page 133).

Latissimus dorsi is a good indicator of blood sugar imbalances and digestive problems. It often tests weak by reason of some malfunction in its associated gland, the pancreas. When so, a left-side weakness often indicates problems with insulin production. A right-side weakness often correlates with an imbalance in pancreas enzyme production.

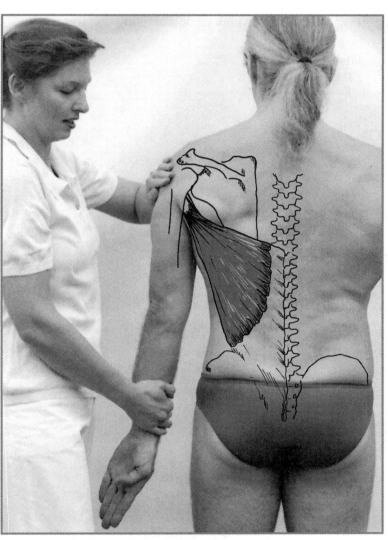

LATISSIMUS DORSI

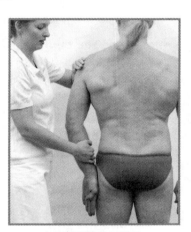

LATISSIMUS DORSI,
TESTED FALSE

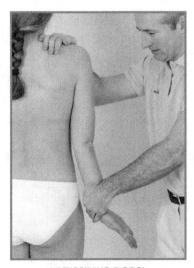

LATISSIMUS DORSI,
TESTED WITH THE ELBOW
HYPEREXTENDED

Pectoralis Major Clavicular

Origin: On the anterior surface of the sternal half of the clavicle.

Insertion: Into the anterior surface of the humerus, just below the shoulder joint.

Action: Flexes the shoulder and adducts the humerus horizontally toward the opposite shoulder (brings the arm up and in). It is the main flexor of the shoulder.

Position: The elbow must remain extended. The patient holds her fully straightened arm directly to the front of the trunk. The arm is maximally rotated inward, which points the thumb toward the feet. The shoulder is in a relaxed position and not elevated.

Stabilization: The examiner stabilizes the opposite shoulder to prevent the trunk from rotating toward the arm tested.

Muscle Test: To avoid causing pain, the examiner uses a full open-hand contact proximal to the patient's wrist. Pressure is then applied laterally and slightly inferior.

Front Neurolymphatic: Under the left breast in the arc between ribs 6 and 7 from the sternum to the mammillary line (usually only on the left).

Back Neurolymphatic: Between T6–7 near the laminae (usually only on the left).

Neurovascular: Bennett's "emotional reflex" points located directly above the irises on the frontal bone eminences.

Reactive Muscles: Teres major, teres minor, latissimus dorsi, rhomboids, latissimus dorsi, middle trapezius, posterior deltoid, supraspinatus, gluteus maximus.

Meridian: Stomach.

Organ/Gland: Stomach.

Nutrition: Vitamin B complex, especially B12, copper, zinc, betaine hydrochloride.

Discussion: Pectoralis major clavicular is related to emotional disturbances, which are known to cause problems with the stomach. Weakness when tested bilaterally (but strength on one or both sides when tested individually) may indicate a lack of adequate hydrochloric acid production in the stomach. This may be due to zinc deficiency. This may not show until a bilateral weakness of the lower trapezius is corrected. Many examiners only test this muscle bilaterally.

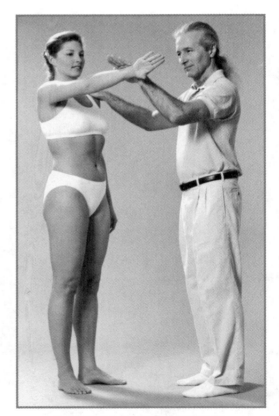

PECTORALIS MAJOR CLAVICULAR,
TESTED STANDING

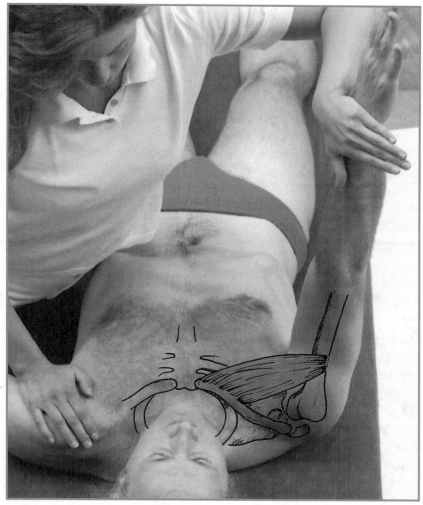

PECTORALIS MAJOR CLAVICULAR

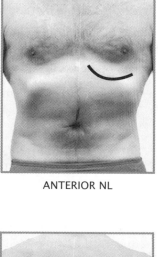

ANTERIOR NL

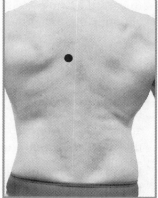

POSTERIOR NL

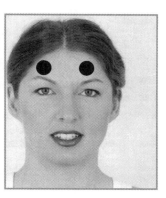

NEUROVASCULAR
POINT

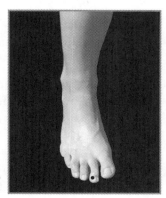

SEDATION POINT,
STOMACH 45

Pectoralis Major Sternal

Origin: Along the side of the sternum to the 7th rib.

Insertion: Into the anterior lateral surface of the humerus below the shoulder joint (distal to the insertion of the pectoralis major clavicular).

Action: Pulls the arm down and in (caudal and medial).

Position: The elbow must remain extended. The patient holds her fully straightened arm directly to the front of the trunk. The arm is maximally rotated inward, which points the thumb toward the feet.

Stabilization: The examiner stabilizes the opposite shoulder or hip to prevent the trunk from rotating toward the arm tested. If the hip is stabilized, the abdominal muscles must be able to fix the chest to the pelvis.

Muscle Test: To avoid causing pain, the examiner uses a full open hand contact proximal to the patient's wrist. Pressure is applied at a 45° angle up and away (cranial and lateral). The exact direction is best applied along a line from the middle of the origin to the middle of the insertion.

Front Neurolymphatic: Under the right breast in the arc between ribs 5 and 6 from the mammillary line to the sternum.

Back Neurolymphatic: Between T5–6 near the laminae, usually on the right side.

Neurovascular: Usually on the natural hairline about 4 cm above the frontal eminences, vertically above the outside edges of the eyes.

Reactive Muscles: Rhomboids, upper and lower trapezius, posterior deltoid, serratus anticus, supraspinatus.

Meridian: Liver.

Organ/Gland: Liver.

Nutrition: Vitamin A, bile salts, choline, inositol, methionine, taurine. (See case history #4 in Appendix VIII.)

Discussion: Pectoralis major sternal makes an excellent indicator muscle for liver function. Sometimes weakness is found in individuals who have a fear of light. In such cases, vitamin A is helpful with both the weakness and the fear of light. When pectoralis major sternal tests weak, the rhomboids will secondarily become hypertonic. Strengthen pectoralis first and, if need be, apply muscle stretch techniques or proprioceptor manipulation to reduce the tension in the rhomboids.

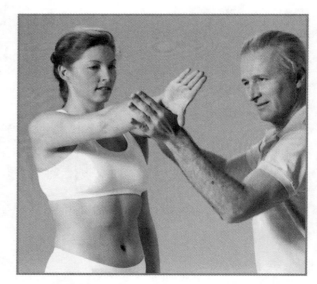

PECTORALIS MAJOR STERNAL, TESTED STANDING

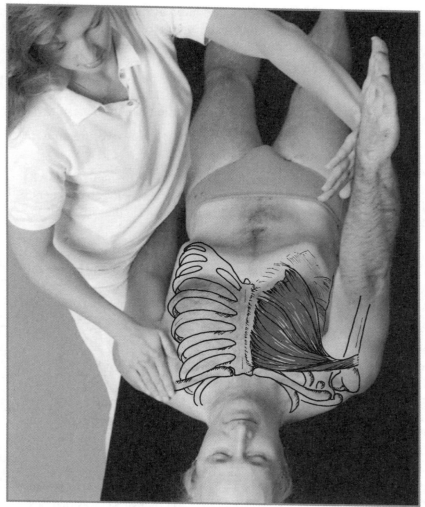

PECTORALIS MAJOR STERNAL

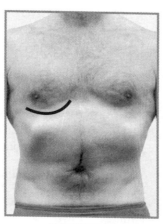

ANTERIOR NL

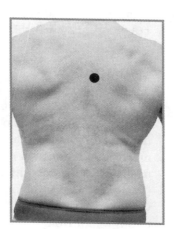

POSTERIOR NL

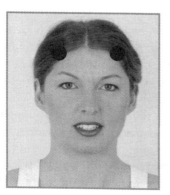

NEUROVASCULAR
POINT

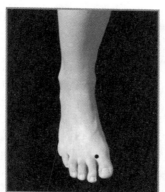

SEDATION POINT,
LIVER 2

Pectoralis Minor

Origin: From ribs 3, 4 and 5 near where the ribs turn into cartilage before meeting the sternum.

Insertion: Into the coracoid process of the scapula.

Action: Pulls the coracoid process anterior, medial and inferior, flexing the shoulder joint. Helps with the act of forced inspiration.

Position: The patient lies supine.

Stabilization: Walther and Frost: Hold opposite shoulder down upon the table. Leaf: Stabilize the shoulder on the side tested. The patient's abdominal muscles must be able to fix the rib cage to the hips. If the patient's abdominal muscles test weak and cannot be strengthened, the examiner must stabilize the rib cage.

Muscle Test: Walther has the patient lift the shoulder up off the table. The examiner presses the shoulder down toward the table (posterior, lateral and caudal) following the arc of the motion that the shoulder took in attaining the test position. Leaf recommends that the patient adduct the straightened arm to align with the opposite anterior superior iliac spine (front of the opposite hip). The examiner then elevates (abducts) the arm. Neither test isolates the pectoralis minor from the pectoralis majors (clavicular and sternal divisions). Palpation is the most important diagnostic procedure for pectoralis minor.

Discussion with Gerz led me to design a more effective test for pectoralis minor. The client lies supine with the arm straightened, abducted 120°, and extended at the shoulder as far as the weight of the arm will pull it down toward the floor. If the arm hangs below the level of the examiner's table, the pectoralis majors will be removed from synergizing in the test. In this position, the patient flexes the shoulder up off the table. More specifically, she flexes the pectoralis minor by pulling the coracoid process anterior, medial and inferior. The examiner presses the shoulder down toward the table exactly opposing the arc of the motion produced by the contraction of pectoralis minor (posterior, lateral and caudal). If the arm cannot hang down lower than the level of the table (which is very often the case), this test cannot be performed because the pectoralis majors and minor are shortened and held too tight. This observation is in itself an important diagnostic result.

Front Neurolymphatic: Just above the xiphoid process on the sternum.

Back Neurolymphatic: None recognized in AK. Research by other schools of kinesiology recommends T8–9, 9–10, 10–11 between where the ribs meet the vertebrae (Dewe, 1989).

Neurovascular: None recognized in AK. Dewe found that the same neurovascular point as used for the upper trapezius works for the pectoralis minor. This point is located above the cheekbone where the temporal and sphenoidal bones meet, about 3 cm posterior to the outer corner of the eye.

Reactive Muscles: Serratus anticus, supraspinatus, deltoid, upper trapezius.

Meridian: No meridian is recognized in AK. Dewe's research correlates pectoralis minor with the stomach meridian.

Organ/Gland: Stomach?

Nutrition: RNA, niacin, niacinamide, B-complex vitamins, zinc, water, herbs and other substances that positively influence the flow of lymph.

Discussion: Pectoralis minor is difficult to isolate for testing because pectoralis major sternal (synergist) usually assists it in its function. The pectoralis minor is an important anterior shoulder stabilizer. It is the only shoulder muscle that does not attach to the humerus. This makes it difficult to test because there are no long levers upon which to apply direct pressure. Gerz considers pectoralis minor to be the most important (and least tested) muscle in Applied Kinesiology (Gerz, 1996, p. 50). Pectoralis minor is most often shortened and tight. This may be felt by palpating the muscle perpendicular to the direction of its fibers. When it is shortened, the shoulders are pulled forward and inward (anterior and medial), producing a very common "slumped" postural appearance. A bundle of nerves and veins passes under the pectoralis minor muscle. When the muscle is tight, these get squeezed between the pectoralis minor and the rib cage. This may cause pain and stiffness in the shoulder joint. The thoracic duct and the right lymphatic duct empty the lymph gathered from the entire body into the junction between the subclavian and internal juggler veins. They both rise in an arch under the clavicle and return caudal before entering the veins. The pectoralis minor does not pass directly over these ducts. But all the structures of the neck are invested in connected fascia. The pull exerted upon the facial structures of the neck by a tight pectoralis minor can squeeze the lymphatic ducts, limiting the flow of lymph and thereby blocking the entire lymph drainage of the body.

Pectoralis minor is seldom found to be undertoned. This is because almost everyone has more developed muscles on the anterior side of their bodies than the posterior side. Just about everyone orients themselves toward their desks, steering wheels, etc. This gives their "pushing" muscles lots of activity. Few people, even weight lifters, give equal exercise to the pulling and rowing muscles of the back. This can be easily seen in the comparative size of the large and strong anterior deltoids (shoulder flexors) and the typically small and weak posterior deltoids (shoulder extensors). As a result, all the pectoralis muscles become overly trained, shortened and tight compared to their antagonists. For further discussion of this topic, see the section "Exercise" on page 141.

Pectoralis minor may be shortened in response to a bilateral weakness in the middle or lower trapezius muscles. If these muscles test weak, they must be strengthened first before reassessing pectoralis minor. Middle trapezius may be bilaterally weak due to a fixation of the thoracic and lumbar vertebrae, which requires chiropractic correction before any correction of pectoralis minor will hold.

To lengthen a shortened pectoralis minor, use proprioceptor manipulation of the neuromuscular spindle cells and Golgi tendon organs, fascial stretch technique, "chill and stretch," and reactive muscle work as indicated for the specific case.

For lasting correction of shortened pectoralis minor muscles, training to increase the strength of the shoulder extensors (teres minor, teres major, latissimus dorsi, trapezius, rhomboids, posterior deltoids, etc.) is usually required.

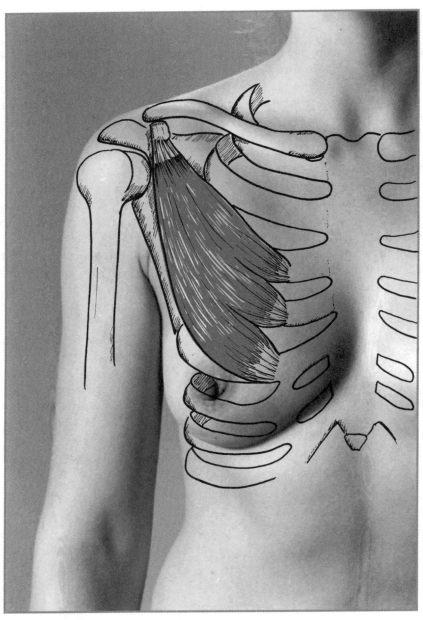

PECTORALIS MINOR

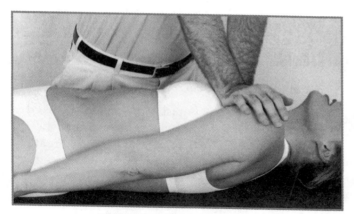

PECTORALIS MINOR (WALTHER)

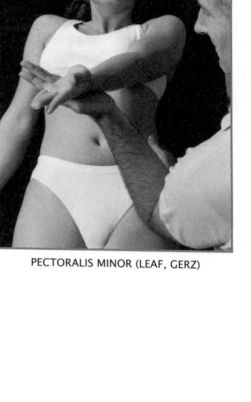

PECTORALIS MINOR (LEAF, GERZ)

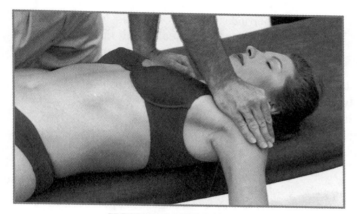

PECTORALIS MINOR (FROST)

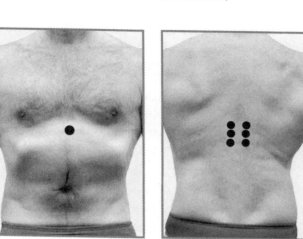

ANTERIOR NL

POSTERIOR NL

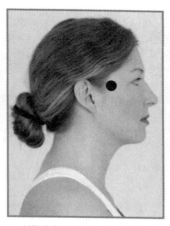

NEUROVASCULAR POINT

SEDATION POINT,
STOMACH 45

Peroneus Longus and Brevis

Origin-Longus: On the lateral head of the tibia, and on the head and upper two-thirds of the lateral surface of the fibula and on the intermuscular septa.

Brevis: On the distal two-thirds of the fibula on the lateral surface plus on the intermuscular septa.

Insertion-Longus: Wraps around the lateral side of the foot and affixes to the lateral side of the proximal end of the first metatarsal and the lateral side of the adjacent bone, the medial cuneiform.

Brevis: Into the lateral side of the proximal end of the 5th metatarsal.

Action: Flexes the sole of the foot (plantar flexion) and turns the foot outward. Also provides lateral stabilization to the ankle.

Position: The foot must be completely straightened (plantar flexed) and then turned out laterally (everted) as far as possible. With maximal plantar flexion, the range of motion to the side is small, perhaps 10–30°. The patient will attempt to extend the toes and dorsiflex the foot. If so, instruct him not to do so and start the test again. It may take several tries to get the test parameters right.

Stabilization: Upon the medial side of the leg just proximal to the ankle.

Muscle Test: With contact on the lateral side of the foot (and not against the toes), the examiner applies pressure to turn the foot back inward (in the direction of inversion).

Front Neurolymphatic: On the inferior edge of the pubic bone.

Back Neurolymphatic: Between L5 and the PSIS.

Neurovascular: On the frontal bone eminences.

Reactive Muscles: Tensor facia lata, tibialis anterior and posterior, peroneus tertius.

Meridian: Bladder.

Organ: Urinary bladder.

Nutrition: Calcium, potassium, B complex, avoid foods containing oxalic acid (coffee, cranberries, plums, etc.). If the patient cannot hold the breath longer than 30 seconds, repeat the tests (peroneus and holding the breath) with thiamine chewed and held in his or her mouth.

Discussion: Peroneus tertius, longus and brevis all stabilize the ankle laterally. As the heel leaves the ground, peroneus tertius is first active. When walking, if the peroneus tertius is weak, the heel and ankle will jerk laterally as the heel leaves the ground. As the heel rises high from the ground, peroneus tertius is inhibited and peroneus longus and brevis become active.

The peroneus brevis has the same action as the longus and is tested at the same time. Peroneus longus and brevis test weak in many patients. Many beginning examiners fail to find weakness in peroneus because of allowing dorsal flexion of the foot (in the peroneus longus and brevis test) and extension of the toes in either test. A screening test for peroneus weakness is to have the patient lie supine with knees directly up (no outward rotation at the hips) and hang the feet over the edge of the table. If the foot rotates in (inverts), peroneus will likely test weak. Recurrent spraining of the ankle is often due to weak-testing peroneus muscles. Peroneus longus and brevis are often reactive to the peroneus tertius, especially after peroneus tertius has been injured by spraining the ankle. Correcting this reactivity may be an important step in preventing further ankle sprains. (See case history #2 in Appendix VIII.)

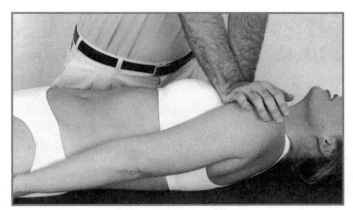

PECTORALIS MINOR (WALTHER)

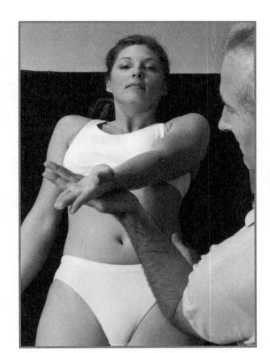

PECTORALIS MINOR (LEAF, GERZ)

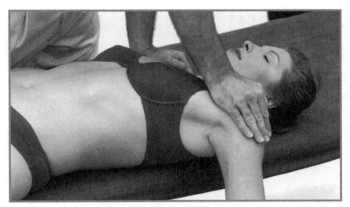

PECTORALIS MINOR (FROST)

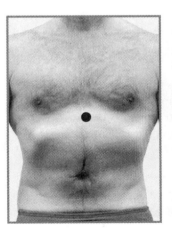

ANTERIOR NL

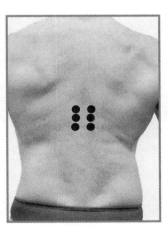

POSTERIOR NL

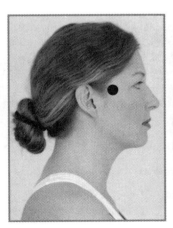

NEUROVASCULAR POINT

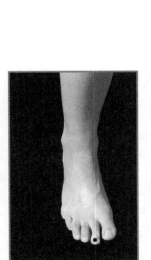

SEDATION POINT,
STOMACH 45

Peroneus Longus and Brevis

Origin-Longus: On the lateral head of the tibia, and on the head and upper two-thirds of the lateral surface of the fibula and on the intermuscular septa.

Brevis: On the distal two-thirds of the fibula on the lateral surface plus on the intermuscular septa.

Insertion-Longus: Wraps around the lateral side of the foot and affixes to the lateral side of the proximal end of the first metatarsal and the lateral side of the adjacent bone, the medial cuneiform.

Brevis: Into the lateral side of the proximal end of the 5th metatarsal.

Action: Flexes the sole of the foot (plantar flexion) and turns the foot outward. Also provides lateral stabilization to the ankle.

Position: The foot must be completely straightened (plantar flexed) and then turned out laterally (everted) as far as possible. With maximal plantar flexion, the range of motion to the side is small, perhaps 10–30°. The patient will attempt to extend the toes and dorsiflex the foot. If so, instruct him not to do so and start the test again. It may take several tries to get the test parameters right.

Stabilization: Upon the medial side of the leg just proximal to the ankle.

Muscle Test: With contact on the lateral side of the foot (and not against the toes), the examiner applies pressure to turn the foot back inward (in the direction of inversion).

Front Neurolymphatic: On the inferior edge of the pubic bone.

Back Neurolymphatic: Between L5 and the PSIS.

Neurovascular: On the frontal bone eminences.

Reactive Muscles: Tensor facia lata, tibialis anterior and posterior, peroneus tertius.

Meridian: Bladder.

Organ: Urinary bladder.

Nutrition: Calcium, potassium, B complex, avoid foods containing oxalic acid (coffee, cranberries, plums, etc.). If the patient cannot hold the breath longer than 30 seconds, repeat the tests (peroneus and holding the breath) with thiamine chewed and held in his or her mouth.

Discussion: Peroneus tertius, longus and brevis all stabilize the ankle laterally. As the heel leaves the ground, peroneus tertius is first active. When walking, if the peroneus tertius is weak, the heel and ankle will jerk laterally as the heel leaves the ground. As the heel rises high from the ground, peroneus tertius is inhibited and peroneus longus and brevis become active.

The peroneus brevis has the same action as the longus and is tested at the same time. Peroneus longus and brevis test weak in many patients. Many beginning examiners fail to find weakness in peroneus because of allowing dorsal flexion of the foot (in the peroneus longus and brevis test) and extension of the toes in either test. A screening test for peroneus weakness is to have the patient lie supine with knees directly up (no outward rotation at the hips) and hang the feet over the edge of the table. If the foot rotates in (inverts), peroneus will likely test weak. Recurrent spraining of the ankle is often due to weak-testing peroneus muscles. Peroneus longus and brevis are often reactive to the peroneus tertius, especially after peroneus tertius has been injured by spraining the ankle. Correcting this reactivity may be an important step in preventing further ankle sprains. (See case history #2 in Appendix VIII.)

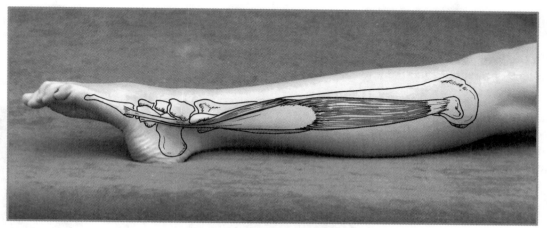

PERONEUS LONGUS AND BREVIS

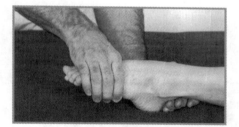

PERONEUS LONGUS AND BREVIS

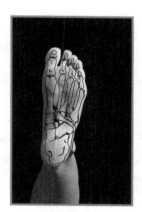

INSERTION OF THE
PERONEUS LONGUS

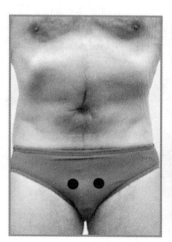

ANTERIOR NL

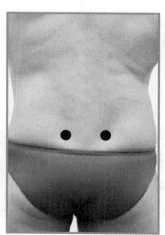

POSTERIOR NL

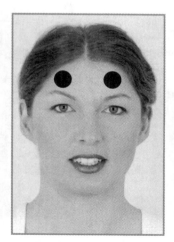

NEUROVASCULAR POINT

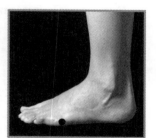

SEDATION POINT,
BLADDER 65

Peroneus Tertius

Origin: On the lower one-third to one-half of the anterior surface of the fibula and the intermuscular septum.

Insertion: Into the dorsal surface of the proximal end of the 5th metatarsal (the bone in the foot from which the little toe continues.)

Action: Flexes the foot dorsally and everts the foot.

Position: The patient lies supine (or sits). The foot is dorsiflexed and everted maximally. The toes are flexed to prevent extension of the toes.

Stabilization: The examiner stabilizes the leg above the malleoli (ankle bones). This is easier to do when the patient lies with the heel upon the table.

Muscle Test: Pressure is applied with a soft, broad contact upon the dorsal side of the 5th metatarsal in a direction toward plantar flexion and inversion.

Reactive Muscles: Tensor fascia lata, tibialis anterior and posterior, peroneus longus and brevis.

Meridian, Organ, and Nutrition: Same as for Peroneus Longus and Brevis.

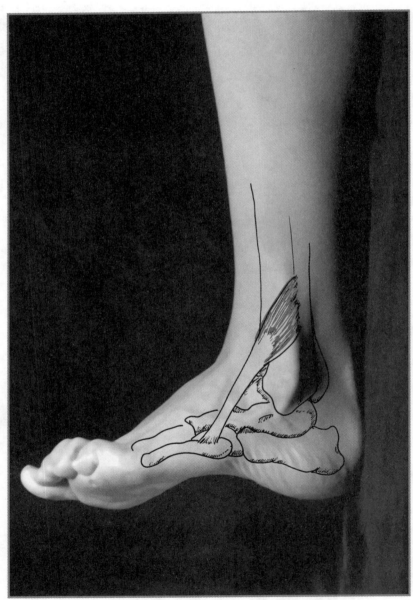

PERONEUS TERTIUS

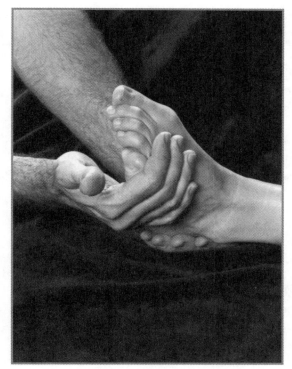

PERONEUS TERTIUS

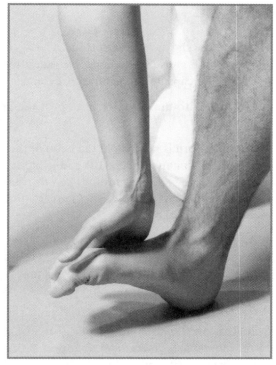

PERONEUS TERTIUS, TESTED STANDING

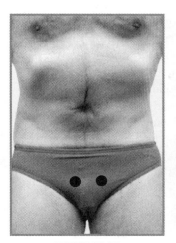

ANTERIOR NL

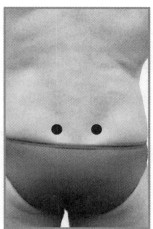

POSTERIOR NL

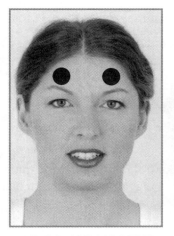

NEUROVASCULAR POINT

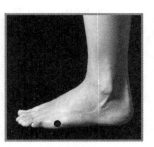

SEDATION POINT,
BLADDER 65

Piriformis

Origin: On the anterior surface of the sacrum between and lateral to the anterior sacral foramen and onto the capsule of the sacroiliac joint.

Insertion: Into the superior border of the greater trochanter.

Action: Piriformis helps hold the head of the femur into the acetabulum (hip joint). With the hip extended or flexed less than 90°, piriformis *laterally* rotates the thigh. With the hip flexed more than 90°, piriformis *medially* rotates the thigh.

Position: The patient lies supine with the knee flexed 90° and the hip flexed *less than* 90°. The thigh is rotated outward (laterally). Piriformis may also be tested with the patient prone and the knee flexed 90° and the thigh rotated outwardly.

Stabilization: The examiner stabilizes above the knee to prevent any medial or lateral motion of the thigh. When using piriformis as an indicator muscle, the examiner may stabilize the knee against his chest. This leaves his other hand free for TL or challenge.

Muscle Test: Supine or prone. The examiner presses above the ankle to rotate the thigh inwardly. The examiner stabilizes the thigh near the knee to prevent motion of the thigh during the test.

Front Neurolymphatic: On the superior aspect of the pubic bone.

Back Neurolymphatic: Between PSIS and the L5 spinous process.

Neurovascular: On the parietal eminence, above and posterior to the ear.

Reactive Muscles: Contralateral splenius capitis, gluteus medius, tensor fascia lata, adductors, medial hamstrings.

Meridian: Circulation-sex.

Organ/Gland: Reproductive organs and glands.

Nutrition: Vitamin E, vitamin A, niacin, zinc.

Discussion: Like iliopsoas, piriformis extends across the sacroiliac junction. These two muscles are therefore involved in stabilizing this important joint. Piriformis is involved in most problems of the pelvis and lumbar spine. When piriformis tests weak on both sides, there may be severe structural problems in the pelvis. However, it is more common to find bilateral weakness in piriformis in chronic cases of urogenital problems. This may take the form of sexual problems including pain on intercourse in females and male impotence. In such cases, if piriformis can be strengthened on both sides, the urogenital problems can usually be successfully treated. When piriformis is weak on one side only, the other side is very often extremely palpatory hypertonic. This can cause the ilium to be pulled and fixed against the sacrum on the hypertonic side. Sciatic nerve pain is often on the side of the palpatory hypertonic piriformis. In such cases of one-sided weakness, strengthen piriformis on the weak side first. If necessary, use standard Applied Kinesiology techniques (fascial release, chill and stretch, proprioceptor manipulation, reactive muscles) for the palpatory hypertonic side. This may free the iliosacral fixation without the need for chiropractic correction.

Piriformis is often used as an indicator muscle. To do so, the examiner stands to the side of the supine patient and tests the leg that is toward him. He stabilizes the patient's knee against his chest with the thigh rotated laterally. This allows him to have one hand free for therapy localization or challenge tests. To perform the test, he places his hand above the patient's ankle and pulls the patient's lower leg in an attempt to medially rotate the thigh.

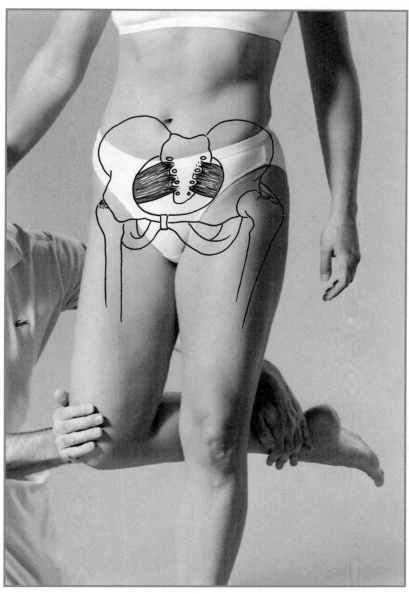

PIRIFORMIS

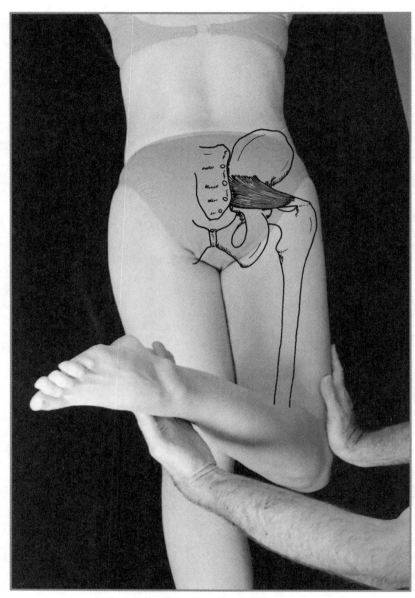

PIRIFORMIS, TESTED PRONE

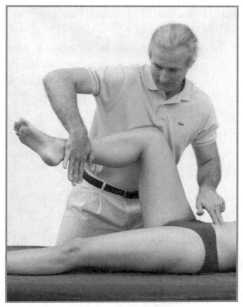

PIRIFORMIS AS AN INDICATOR MUSCLE

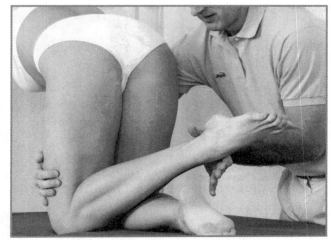

PIRIFORMIS, TESTED ON THE HANDS AND KNEES

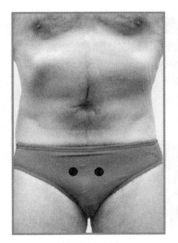

ANTERIOR NL

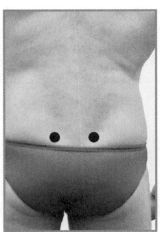

POSTERIOR NL

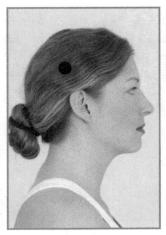

NEUROVASCULAR POINT

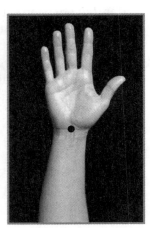

SEDATION POINT, CIRCU-
LATION-SEX 7

Popliteus

Origin: On the lateral distal end of the femur, on the posterior horn of the lateral meniscus, and on the head of the fibula.

Insertion: Into the posterior surface of the proximal end of the tibia.

Action: With the femur fixed, the popliteus rotates the tibia medially. With the tibia fixed, the popliteus rotates the femur laterally on the tibia. As the heel strikes the ground in walking or running, the popliteus contracts, which bends the knee and thus creates a shock absorber effect. When the knee is flexed, popliteus withdraws the lateral meniscus. Popliteus stabilizes the knee posteriorly.

Position: The patient lies prone or supine. The knee and the ankle are both flexed 90°. The tibia is rotated medially on the femur.

Stabilization: The patient must be able to fix the ankle and there must be no pain or problems in the foot, ankle or knee. The patient must also fix the femur to prevent rotation during the test. The examiner stabilizes the lateral aspect of the heel.

Muscle Test: Pressure is applied with a broad, soft, hand contact on the medial and under side of the foot near (but not upon) the toes. The opposite hand provides counter-pressure on the heel. The effort is to laterally rotate the tibia. Rotation of the foot may take place even without popliteus weakness. The actual motion during the test is very small. The indication of weakness of the popliteus is lateral rotation of the tibia during the test. This can be most easily detected by watching the head of the tibia (the tibial tubercle) and the head of the fibula. Since the fibula is attached to the tibia, they rotate simultaneously. If during the test, the tibial tubercle rotates and causes the head of the fibula to no longer protrude so far laterally, the popliteus tested weak.

Front Neurolymphatic: In the intercostal space between ribs 5 and 6 from the mammillary line to the sternum on the right side.

Back Neurolymphatic: Between the laminae of thoracic vertebrae 5 and 6 on the right.

Neurovascular: On the medial aspect of the knee (over the meniscus).

Reactive Muscles: Gastrocnemius, lateral hamstrings, quadriceps and upper trapezius.

Meridian: Gall Bladder.

Organ/Gland: Gall Bladder.

Nutrition: Vitamin A, betaine, essential fatty acids (vitamin F), gall salts.

Discussion: When popliteus is weak, the knee in standing is typically unstable and most often hyperextended (or bent more than usual). When the popliteus is weak, the lateral meniscus often has problems. If the popliteus tests weak bilaterally, therapy-localize the mid-cervical vertebrae. If this strengthens the popliteus, there is a mid-cervical fixation that may require chiropractic correction. Hyperextension injuries to the knee strain the popliteus.

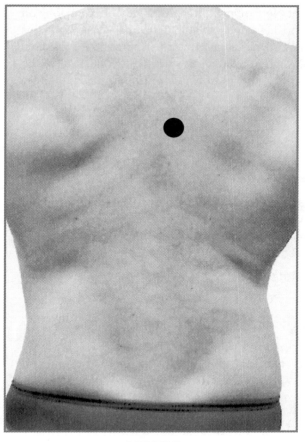

POPLITEUS

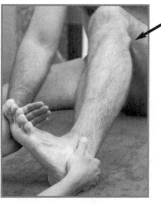

POPLITEUS TEST,
BEGINNING POSITION

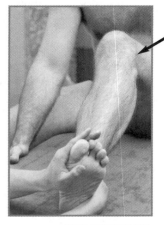

POPLITEUS TEST,
END POSITION WHEN IT TESTS WEAK

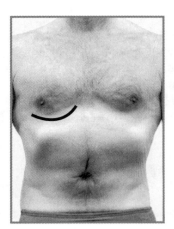

ANTERIOR NL

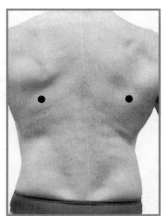

POSTERIOR NL

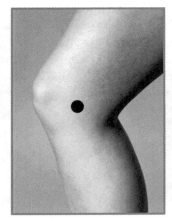

NEUROVASCULAR POINT

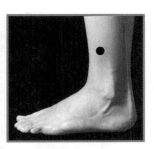

SEDATION POINT,
GALL BLADDER 38

Rectus Abdominis Group

Origin: From the symphysis pubis and the pubic crest.

Insertion: Into the cartilage of the 5th, 6th and 7th ribs near the sternum an on the lateral aspect of the xiphoid process.

Action: The rectus abdominis connects the ribs and the pelvis, thus holding abdominal organs in. With the help of gluteus maximus and the hamstrings, the rectus abdominis keeps the pelvis from tilting forward (anteriorly).

Position: The patient sits with extended legs, torso at 90° to the legs. Patient crosses arms upon the chest (with hands closed and elbows away from the chest to avoid TL to any active points). If any low back pain exists, the test should be performed with the knees and hips bent.

Stabilization: Patient's leg flexors must fix the hips to the legs. If they cannot, they must be strengthened before this test can be performed. Examiner must hold the patient's legs down toward the table.

Muscle Test: Examiner places one hand on the sternum and pushes the upper body away from the legs. Alternately, using one arm, the examiner places his elbow on one of the patient's shoulders and his hand on the other shoulder. During the test, a strong iliopsoas can hold the lumbar spine forward, giving the impression of strong abdominals. The examiner should observe carefully if the patient can stabilize the ribs toward the pubis. Any separation of the ribs from the pubis indicates weak-testing abdominals.

Front Neurolymphatic: A line about 10 cm long on the medial thigh just above the knee. Massaging this area produces an unpleasant electric shock sensation. It is advised to stand toward the feet and out of the reach of your patient to avoid being accidentally struck.

Back Neurolymphatic: In the space between L5 and the PSIS.

Neurovascular: Where the vertical auricular line crosses the parietal eminences.

Reactive Muscles: Quadriceps, contralateral gluteus medius, sacrospinalis, rectus femoris, sartorius, quadratus lumborum, between sections of rectus abdominis itself.

Meridian: Small intestine.

Organ/Gland: Small intestine.

Nutrition: Vitamin E, coenzyme Q10.

Discussion: If the patient has a history of low back disc problems, test with the knees bent to put less stress on the discs. To support the patient, the examiner must lean weight against the thighs near the knees to keep the patient's feet upon the table.

When the rectus abdominis tests weak, it cannot provide support to the pelvis, which then tips forward (tilts anteriorly), creating an excessive lordosis (hollow low back). This places a great stress upon the discs between the lumbar vertebrae.

When the patient has any chronic disturbances in the small intestine, the rectus abdominis will typically test very weak, and the neurolymphatic reflexes will be extremely tender. In such cases, dietary corrections, and other lymphatic corrections including the

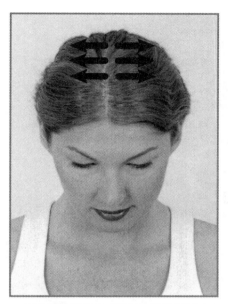

OPENING THE SAGITTAL SUTURE TO
STRENGTHEN
THE RECTUS ABDOMINIS

drinking of more water will be needed before the correction of the abdominis will hold.

Weak-testing abdominal muscles are found in conjunction with a jamming together of the sagittal suture. If this suture remains jammed, any correction of the abdominals will not hold. To test if the suture is involved with weakness of the abdominals, the patient TLs the suture while the examiner repeats the muscle test. If the rectus (or other) abdominis muscles now test strong, the sagittal suture is involved. Correcting this jamming of the sagittal suture is one of the simplest and safest of all cranial fault corrections. Using the fingertips on each side of the suture, the examiner pulls it apart as if trying to pull open the top back of the patient's head to the right and left. This is performed three or four times, and then the abdominal muscles are retested to confirm the correction.

Many times, the abdominals (which are spinal flexors) test weak as a result of excess tension in their main antagonist, sacrospinalis (a spinal extensor). After strengthening the abdominals, check if tensing the sacrospinalis makes them again weak. If so, apply the reactive muscle technique to lower the tension in the sacrospinalis and free the abdominals from its influence (page 135).

The various divisions of the rectus abdominis are individually enervated and may be reactive to one another. When the back is rounded (straightening the lumbar curve), the lowest division is tested. Beginning from this rounded posture, a step-wise straightening of the back before testing tests the various upper divisions sequentially from lower to higher.

(For instructions as to how to safely exercise the abdominals, see the "Exercise" on pages 142–143).

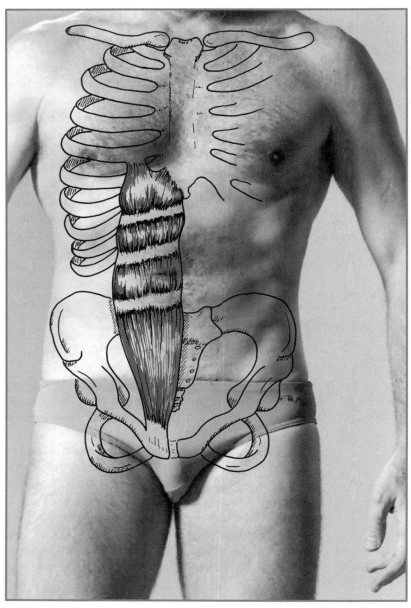

RECTUS ABDOMINIS

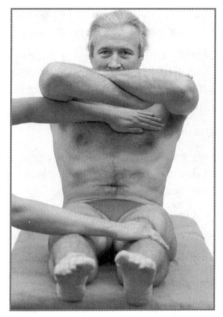

RECTUS ABDOMINIS,
WITH STRAIGHT LEGS

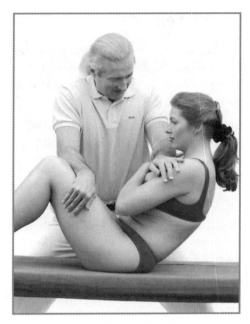

RECTUS ABDOMINIS,
WITH BENT LEGS

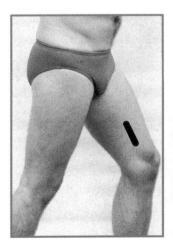

ANTERIOR NL

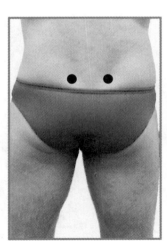

POSTERIOR NL

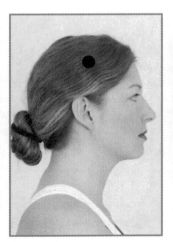

NEUROVASCULAR POINT

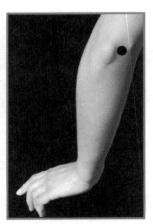

SEDATION POINT,
SMALL INTESTINE 8

Rectus Femoris

Origin: Two heads, one on the anterior inferior edge of the ilium (hip bone) and the other just below the first and attached to the superior edge of the hip socket.

Insertion: Into the top of the patella (knee bone) and on from the patella to the tibial tubercle just caudal to the knee.

Action: Extends the lower leg on the knee and flexes the thigh on the hip.

Position: The hip and knee are flexed 90° with no rotation. Rotation inward will bring fascia lata too much into play. Rotation outward will allow too much activity of iliopsoas and sartorius. These muscles are synergists and will be somewhat active in this test, even with no rotation.

Stabilization: With the patient sitting or supine, stabilization is not required. In standing, hold the patient's pelvis firmly and have the patient lean one hand upon the examiner's shoulder. The patient's abdominal muscles must be strong enough to prevent movement between the pelvis and the trunk.

Muscle Test: With a hand anterior and just proximal to the knee, the examiner pushes to extend the hip.

Front Neurolymphatic: Under the anterior inferior border of the rib cage. Be careful not to press directly below (caudal to) the sternum. The xiphoid process extends below the sternum and can be easily broken.

Back Neurolymphatic: T8–T11 laminae.

Neurovascular: Over the posterior part of the parietal eminence (on the side of the top of the head, above and behind the ear).

Reactive Muscles: Gastrocnemius, hamstrings, rectus abdominis, sartorius, gluteus maximus, adductors.

Meridian: Small intestine.

Organ/Gland: Small intestine.

Nutrition: Vitamin B complex, vitamin D, calcium, coenzyme Q10, acidophilus.

Discussion: Problems with the function of the small intestine can often be improved by extended stimulation of the neurolymphatic reflexes for quadriceps. Goodheart often calls rectus femoris "quadriceps" in the literature. Rectus femoris is one of the four

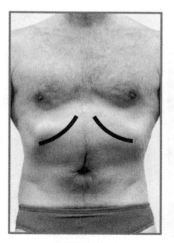

ANTERIOR NL

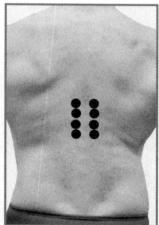

POSTERIOR NL

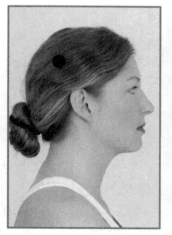

NEUROVASCULAR POINT

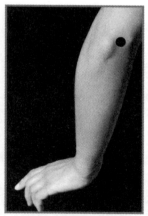

SEDATION POINT,
SMALL INTESTINE 8

quadriceps muscles, which all have the same reflex points. For a discussion of the use of the neurolymphatic reflexes to allow quadriceps to continue to contract at full power for extended lengths of time (useful to athletes!) see the section on repeated muscle testing (page 123).

In many athletic injuries, quadriceps is often found to be involved in reactive muscle relationship, either as the primary or a reactive muscle. Correcting this reactive muscle relationship can help the athlete to return more quickly and without pain to his or her sport.

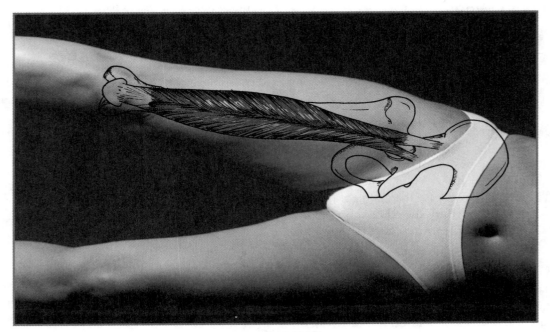

RECTUS FEMORIS

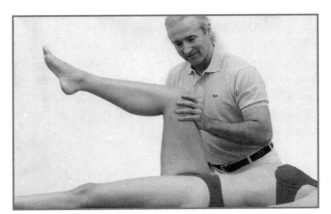

RECTUS FEMORIS, TESTED PUSHING

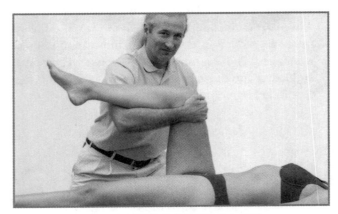

RECTUS FEMORIS, TESTED PULLING

Rhomboid Major

Origin: Both Walther and Leaf: from the spinous processes of T2–5. Other authorities say T1–5.

Insertion: Into the medial margin of the scapula.

Rhomboid Minor

Origin: Walther and Leaf-from the spinous processes of C7 and T1. Other authorities say C6 and C7.

Insertion: Into the medial margin of the scapula above rhomboid major.

Action of both: Adduction and elevation of the medial border of the scapula.

Position: The standing or seated patient adducts and elevates the scapula. If the patient cannot elevate the medial border of the scapula, the middle trapezius is being recruited to perform the adduction. The arm, which is used as a lever for testing the rhomboids, should be in a neutral or slightly externally rotated position.

Stabilization: The patient must be able to hold her arm down against her side. The examiner should stabilize the top of the shoulder on the side tested to prevent the patient from tipping toward this side during the test.

Muscle Test: The examiner pulls the elbow to abduct it away from the body. Movement of the elbow away from the body does not, in itself, indicate rhomboid weakness. The examiner should observe for any abduction and/or sinking of the scapula, which is the true indication of rhomboid weakness.

Front Neurolymphatic: On the left side between ribs 6 and 7 from the mammillary line to the sternum.

Back Neurolymphatic: Between T6–7 by the laminae on the left side.

Neurovascular: Walther lists the frontal bone eminences (used for pectoralis major clavicularis—the stomach meridian). Leaf lists the points above and more lateral to the frontal bone eminences (used for pectoralis major sternal—the liver meridian).

Reactive Muscles: Deltoid, serratus anticus, supraspinatus, latissimus dorsi, upper, middle and lower trapezius, coracobrachialis, pectoralis majors and minor.

Meridian: Liver (Stomach).

Organ/Gland: Liver (Stomach).

Nutrition: Vitamin A, choline, inositol, methionine.

Discussion: Goodheart has associated the rhomboids with both the liver and the stomach meridians. The rhomboids seem to respond to neurovascular and neurolymphatic stimulation of the reflexes for both the stomach and the liver. Therefore, if the desired effect is not achieved with treatment of the neurolymphatic reflex points on the left side, use those on the right as well.

When serratus anticus is weak, the antagonistic rhomboids will often become shortened and hypertonic. This is often observed in patients who have pain between the scapulae. In such cases, attempting to get the rhomboids to relax will usually not succeed until serratus anticus is first strengthened. Although antagonistic to the rhomboids in the motion of the scapula, serratus anticus is synergistic to the rhomboids in their combined action of fixing the medial border of the scapula down upon the rib cage.

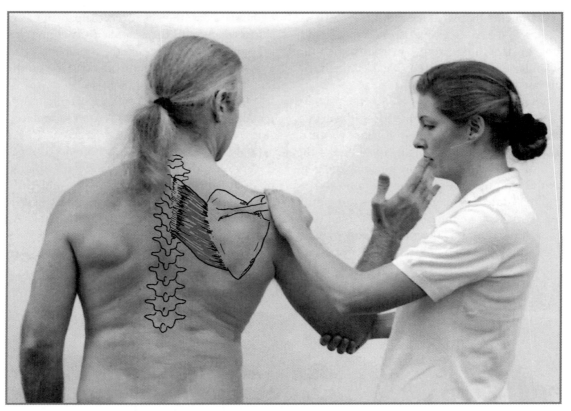

RHOMBOIDS, END POSITION WHEN THEY TEST WEAK

Leaf comments that weakness of the rhomboids allows the scapula to excessively rotate during elevation of the arm to the front. This can stretch the suprascapular nerve and thereby weaken the infraspinatus muscle.

The rhomboids are often involved as the primary or the reactive muscle in combination with various other shoulder muscles. Since in normal posture, there is little space between the medial edge of the scapula and the vertebral column, pinching the neuromuscular spindle cells of the rhomboids (as required to sedate a primary muscle) is difficult to perform. To make more room for such treatment, the examiner stands behind the patient and reaches under the armpit and then grasps the superior aspect of the shoulder. Then he levers the patient's arm anteriorly, which pulls the scapula away from the vertebral column. This lengthens the rhomboids, producing more space for the neuromuscular spindle cell manipulation.

When the rhomboids are overly tight, they inhibit the ability to extend the arms (and shoulders) anteriorly, as one would to give or receive a hug. Interestingly, in my work as a psychologist, I have often observed a correlation between hypertonic rhomboids and an inability to reach out—a fear of opening oneself to another person. This is just an anecdotal observation and does not (yet) form a part of Applied Kinesiology.

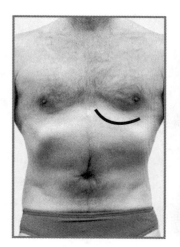

ANTERIOR NL

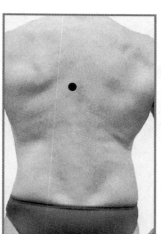

POSTERIOR NL

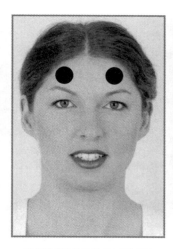

NEUROVASCULAR POINT

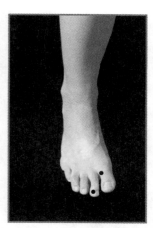

SEDATION POINT, LIVER 2 AND STOMACH 45

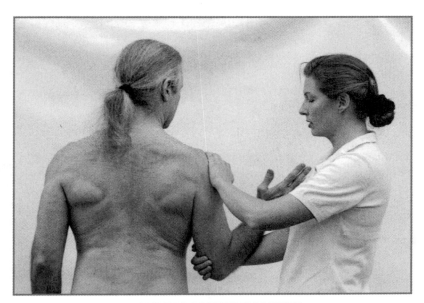

RHOMBOIDS, BEGINNING POSITION

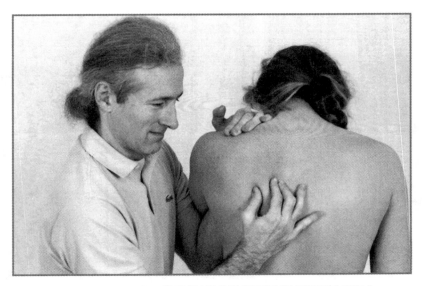

RHOMBOIDS, PINCHING THE NEUROMUSCULAR SPINDLE CELLS

Sacrospinalis Group

Origin: (Many separate muscles) upon the sacrum, iliac crest, spinous processes, transverse processes and ribs.

Insertion: Into the ribs, spinous processes, transverse processes and occiput.

Action: Extension, rotation and lateral flexion of the vertebral column, lateral motion of the pelvis.

Position: The patient lies prone and lifts one shoulder up from the table without using the hands.

Stabilization: The opposite hip is held down on the table.

Muscle Test: The examiner pushes the raised shoulder down toward the table.

Front Neurolymphatic: On the anterior surface of the pubic bone and 2.5 cm lateral to each side of the navel.

Back Neurolymphatic: L2, over the transverse processes.

Neurovascular: Frontal bone eminences.

Reactive Muscles: Gluteus maximus, hamstrings, abdominis.

Meridian: Bladder.

Organ: Urinary bladder.

Nutrition: Vitamins A, C, P, E and calcium.

Discussion: To get a general idea of the function of sacrospinalis, have the patient lean directly to each side (laterally flex the spine) with no tilt of the hips and no rotation of the spine. The patient will not be able to lean as far toward the side of sacrospinalis weakness.

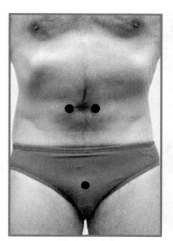

ANTERIOR NL

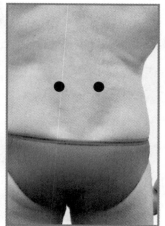

POSTERIOR NL

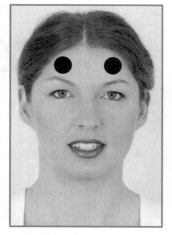

NEUROVASCULAR POINT

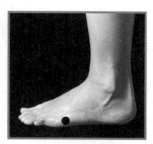

SEDATION POINT,
BLADDER 65

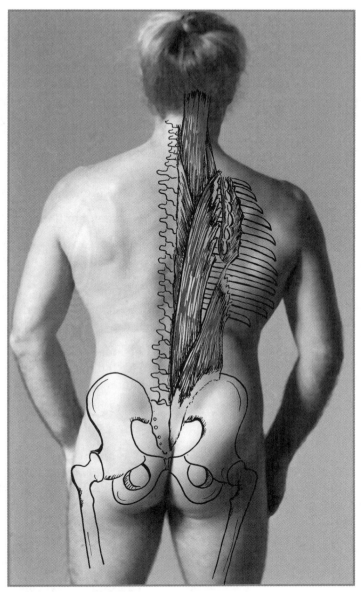

SACROSPINALIS

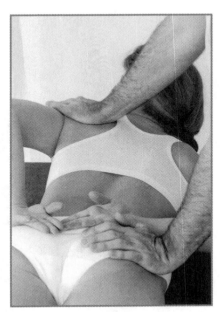

SACROSPINALIS

Sartorius

Origin: On the front top of the hip bone (anterior superior iliac spine).

Insertion: On the medial side of the shinbone (tibia) just below the knee.

Action: Sartorius extends over two joints and flexes the knee and the hip. It rotates the thighs laterally. It stabilizes the medial side of the knee and, when the knee is flexed, it rotates the tibia medially. When the leg is fixed, sartorius flexes the hip upon the thigh and stabilizes the pelvis anteriorly.

Position: The client lies supine, slightly flexes the knee and the hip joints, and rotates the thigh laterally (knee out).

Stabilization: Normally not required. If the client slips on the table, she may hold on to the sides of the table.

Muscle Test: With one hand, the examiner grasps the leg above the ankle and pulls to extend the knee.

The other hand pushes the knee in the direction of hip extension, thigh adduction and medial rotation. Both hands must act at the same time. Experiment with the exact direction of pressure to produce maximal contraction as observed in the contraction of the sartorius muscle.

Front Neurolymphatic: 5 cm above the navel and 2.5 cm to each side.

Back Neurolymphatic: T11, 12 near the lamina.

Neurovascular: Posterior fontanelle (lambda).

Reactive Muscles: Quadriceps and anterior tibialis.

Meridian: Circulation-sex and sometimes triple heater.

Gland: Adrenal.

Nutrition: Vitamin C, pantothenic acid, adrenal extracts, tyrosine, B6, B12, folic acid.

Discussion: The sartorius is the longest muscle in the body. It is an anterior pelvic stabilizer. Weakness in sartorius can cause the ilium on the side of

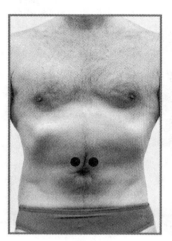

ANTERIOR NL

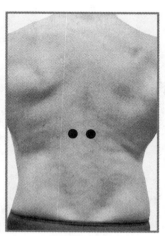

POSTERIOR NL

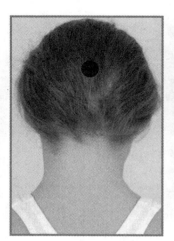

NEUROVASCULAR POINT

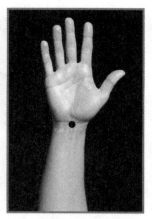

SEDATION POINT, CIRCU-LATION-SEX 7

weakness to subluxate posteriorly and can result in "knock knees." In these conditions, the sartorius' continual effort to stabilize the problem joints will make the origin and/or insertion of sartorius very tender. All functions and imbalances associated with the adrenals (low blood pressure, hypoglycemia or low blood sugar, hyper insulin production, allergies, and asthma) can influence sartorius function. Infections and adrenal exhaustion influence sartorius. Conversely, balancing the sartorius can positively influence the function of the adrenals including all the above-listed adrenal-related problems.

If the client is strong, the examiner may need to use rotation of his or her pelvis to deliver the force needed for the test. Sartorius often reveals weakness only when the patient is tested in sitting position.

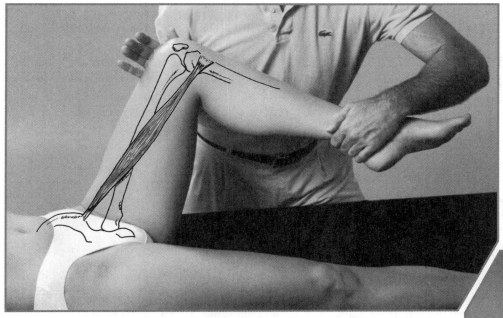

SARTORIUS

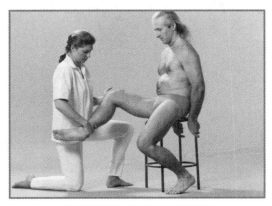

SARTORIUS, TESTED SITTING

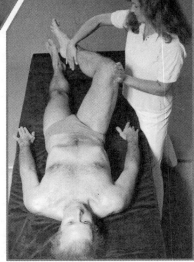

SARTORIUS

Serratus Anticus

Origin: The lateral superior surfaces of the first 8 or 9 ribs.

Insertion: Underneath the vertebral edge of the scapula.

Action: Pulls the scapula laterally and rotates it to place the shoulder joint more vertical. Holds the vertebral border of the scapula down upon the rib cage (as does its synergists in this activity, rhomboids and middle trapezius). With the scapula fixed, serratus anticus lifts the ribs and assists in forced breathing.

Position: The straightened arm is flexed at the shoulder to 100°-150° (various angles to test the various fibers of this muscle) and abducted about 30°.

Stabilization: Not generally needed for this test.

Muscle Test: The examiner presses the lateral edge of the inferior tip of the scapula medially and feels the medial edge with his fingers. With his other hand, he pulls down upon the forearm, proximal to the patient's wrist. If the scapula moves medially and the medial edge flares away from the rib cage, serratus anticus tested weak. The examiner must place his hand upon the scapula and/or observe the scapula for movement during the test. Most effective is for the examiner to press upon the lateral edge of the scapula during the test. If the scapula moves medially, the serratus anticus tested weak.

Front Neurolymphatic: Between ribs 3, 4 and 5 near where they meet the sternum.

Back Neurolymphatic: T3, 4 and 5 laminae.

Neurovascular: Anterior fontanelle (bregma).

Reactive Muscles: Rhomboid, pectoralis major sternal, pectoralis minor, middle trapezius.

Meridian: Lung.

Organ/Gland: Lung.

Nutrition: Vitamin C, water, beta-carotene.

Discussion: The test determines if serratus can stabilize the scapula. The arm is used as a lever. No movement should occur at the shoulder joint during the test. The deltoid and supraspinatus must be strong in order to test the serratus. When serratus anticus is weak, pushing with straight arms to the front is difficult. If a weight is held straight out to the front, the vertebral (medial) edge of the scapula will flare up away from the back.

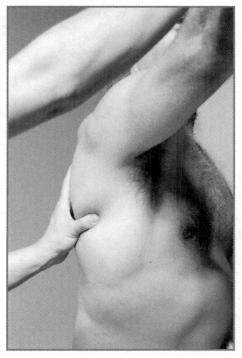

SERRATUS ANTICUS, THUMB GRIP

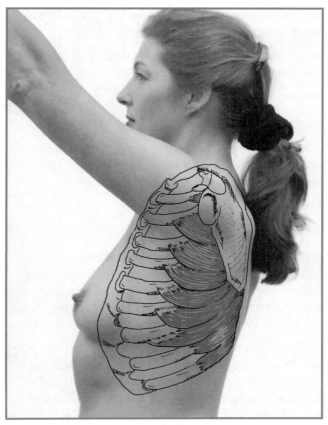

SERRATUS ANTICUS

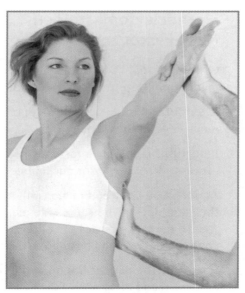

SERRATUS ANTICUS

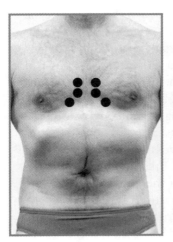

ANTERIOR NL

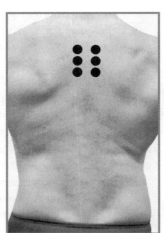

POSTERIOR NL

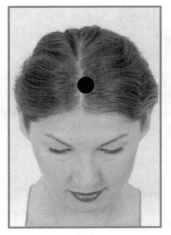

NEUROVASCULAR POINT

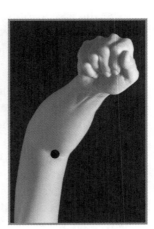

SEDATION POINT,
LUNG 5

Sternocleidomastoideus: Neck Flexors

Origin: Sternal head: on the anterior surface of the manubrium (top-front of the sternum).

Clavicular head: upon the upper surface of the medial half of the clavicle.

Insertion: Upon the lateral surface of the mastoid process and the superior nuchal line of the occiput.

Action: One-sided contraction pulls the head toward the shoulder on the same side as the muscle and rotates the head toward the opposite side. Bilateral contraction flexes the head upon the neck.

Position: The patient lies upon the back. The arms are flexed and lifted above the head to avoid pressing on the table during the test. To test bilaterally, the patient flexes (lifts) the head from the table. To test unilaterally, the patient fully rotates the head away from the side to be tested and lifts it from the table. The examiner places his other hand upon the table under the head to catch it in case of weakness.

Stabilization: Tested supine, the table provides the necessary stabilization. If this test is performed standing, the examiner must provide stabilization with one hand upon the upper back. When testing in this position, as soon as the muscle demonstrates any weakness, the test pressure must immediately cease. Great care must be observed to never push the head back and down, which could damage the neck.

Muscle Test: Bilateral: Using a broad area of contact, the examiner places his hand upon the middle of the forehead of the patient and presses posterior, carefully following the arc of the anatomical movement. Under no conditions should the pressure be straight down toward the table, which could injure the intervertebral discs. In the unilateral test, the examiner places his hand upon the parietal bone. The exact area of contact is defined by how far the patient can rotate his head. The direction of pressure is posterior and slightly lateral, in a curve following the anatomical arc of motion produced by the contraction of the muscle.

Front Neurolymphatic: 1st intercostal space, about 9 cm from the sternum

Back Neurolymphatic: C2 lamina.

Neurovascular: Ramus of the jaw below the zygoma.

Reactive Muscles: Neck extensors, upper trapezius, pectoralis major clavicularis, opposite sternocleido-mastoideus.

Meridian: Stomach.

Organ: Sinuses, lymphatic drainage of the head.

Nutrition: B6, B3 (niacinamide or niacin), organic iodine, herbal and homeopathic remedies for the sinuses, especially nosodes and lymph drainage remedies. Leaf recommends a 5-to-1 ratio of niacinamide or niacin to B6 as being most effective.

Discussion: The sternocleidomastoideus (SCM) is actually a group of several associated muscles. The contraction of the sterno-cleido-mastoideus is easily visible, springing out of the neck during the muscle test. Although quite useful as a general test, the bilateral test does not adequately isolate the SCM. In this test, the scalenes and several other neck flexor muscles are also active. To best isolate the SCM, the head should be maximally rotated, and the SCM of each side tested independently. The examiner observes for any attempt to reduce the angle of rotation during the test. This usually indicates a weakness of the SCM and an attempt to recruit the scalenes, which are most active at 10° of rotation. Inability to remain in the full rotation or pain upon doing so should be considered a sign of muscle weakness and treated without putting the patient into unnecessary stress or pain that could be caused by testing. Pressure is applied in the direction of the tangent of the arc produced by the anatomical motion of contraction of the SCM. Applying test pressure with a broad contact of the palm avoids possible tugging on the skin, which can produce a false weakness of the muscle test.

Patients with chronic sinus conditions or problems in the upper vertebrae of the neck may have extremely weak-testing neck flexors. In such cases, this test is only to be performed with very gentle test pressure.

The neck flexors are functionally much weaker than their opponents, the neck extensors. Due in part to the postural habit of holding the head far forward of the line of gravity, the neck extensors rarely relax. This often creates a pattern of (chronically tight) primary muscle-neck extensors to (chronically weak, inhibited) reactive muscle-neck flexors. If this condition exists, treatments to strengthen the neck flexors will only have temporary success until the treatment for reactive muscles is applied. To test for such reactivity, the neck flexors must first test strong or be temporarily strengthened, for example, by massage of the appropriate neurolymphatic reflex points. Then the neck extensors are contracted bilaterally. If the patient is supine, this may be easily accomplished by having the patient firmly pull the head back down upon the table.

Immediately following this contraction of the neck extensors, the neck flexors are bilaterally tested. If they now test weak, treatment for reactive muscles is indicated. In this case, such treatment consists of neuromuscular spindle cell pinching of the belly on the upper trapezius muscles and other neck extensors located parallel to the spine in the neck, parallel to the contracting length of the muscles. Areas of palpable hardness are repeatedly and deeply pinched. Support must be given to the forehead so the neck extensors are not contracted against the force required for the neuromuscular spindle cell pinching treatment. This may be accomplished by having the patient sit next to the table, place his elbows upon the table, and his forehead upon the heels of his hands. Alternatively, he can lie prone with his forehead upon his forearm or a hard pillow. It is important to pinch deeply into the muscle and not only upon the skin. Then the neck muscles are tested bilaterally to reset them. This process is repeated several times, focusing upon the areas of hardness and/or pain in the upper trapezius muscles and other neck extensors. After effective treatment, contraction of the neck extensors should no longer weaken the neck flexors.

Reactive conditions may also exist between unilateral SCM and upper trapezius muscles and also between the SCM muscles on each side. A noteworthy reactive condition may also be observed between the reactive SCM on one side and the contralateral psoas muscle. The author observed and treated this condition in a European soccer player. After hitting the ball very hard with one side of his head, he found that the SCM on that side became hypertonic. Subsequently, the insertion of the psoas on the opposite side of his body became extremely tender to the touch and painful when he stood or ran. Not only was the contralateral psoas insertion tender, it also tested weak on this side. The inhibition of the contralateral psoas muscle, created by the hypertonic SCM, also caused him to be out of balance and unstable when upright. Reactive muscle treatment directed toward the hypertonic SCM eliminated the pain and improved his balance and coordination.

Notice in this case how the activity of the unilateral SCM nearly mirrors the activity of the contralateral psoas. The contraction of the right SCM pulls the head forward and pulls the right ear toward the midline. The contraction of the left psoas lifts the left leg forward and pulls it toward the midline. Though the whole trunk lies between them, so considered, these two muscles may be seen as having a related and opposing function. This is an example of the complex relationship often observed between muscle pairs involved in reactive conditions.

Reactive muscle treatment should be long-lasting. However, the postural problem that caused the chronic contraction of the neck extensors needs to be corrected, for example, by lessons in Alexander Technique (training in optimal posture and movement of the body). Or, if the cause of the muscular imbalance was a trauma, emotional stress release methods may need to be performed. If these steps are skipped and the reactivity is only treated manually, the reactive condition with the associated patterns of tension, pain, and possible malfunction of the gait mechanism is likely to recur.

Malfunction of the neck flexors often causes peripheral nerve and vascular entrapments in the shoulders and arms. When this is suspected, have the patient lie supine and test the function of various arm muscles that should test strong. Then retest the same muscles with the head elevated and rotated to contract the neck flexors. If the muscles now test weak, have the patient expand and lift the rib cage. If this does not cause a strengthening of the formerly weak-testing muscles, a nerve entrapment has been located. These may be corrected with AK procedures such as chill and stretch or fascial release, carefully applied to the SCM.

The SCM is particularly interesting because it has double enervation from C2–C3 and from the tenth cranial nerve. The only other muscle in the body that has double enervation is the upper trapezius, which is the major neck extensor. These two muscles have a finely attuned simultaneous interaction without which the fine coordination of the walking (gait) pattern would not be possible. Goodheart suggests that the double enervation of these muscles is necessary for the correct function of the gait coordination. In walking or running, there should be a well-orchestrated facilitation and inhibition of the next flexors and extensors. When the left leg steps forward, the right shoulder moves forward. In order to keep the head facing forward, the right SCM as well as the left upper trapezius (and other left neck extensors) are inhibited. This is the normal walking or gait coordination. Goodheart devised a method to test for the normal facilitation and inhibition of these muscles:

The patient steps forward on his right foot and puts much of his weight upon it. Some weight is also upon the ball of the left foot with the heel raised as would be the case when taking a step in walking. In this position, the SCM and upper trapezius muscles are tested. If the gait mechanism is intact, in this position the left SCM and the right upper trapezius should be inhibited and therefore test weak. Since the upper trapezius is typically in a state of chronic tension, the weakness produced in this test may be difficult to ascertain.

Unilateral weakness of the SCM and/or upper trapezius muscles can produce a lateral tilt of the head, which may cause occipital or upper cervical subluxation and improper stimulation of the head-on-neck reflexes, with consequent disruption of the equilibrium mechanism. In cases of dizziness, this possible cause should be considered.

In my work as a psychologist, I have observed that bilateral weakness of the neck flexors is often coupled with a weakened ability to effectively overcome obstacles and push one's will through against the opposition of others. These muscles must be strong in order to "butt heads" effectively, as observed in dominance rituals in the animal kingdom. Weak-testing neck flexors may be associated with being a "pushover." These are only anecdotal observations and do not (yet) form an official part of Applied Kinesiology.

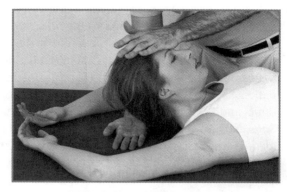

STERNO-CLEIDO-MASTOIDEUS,
BILATERALLY TESTED

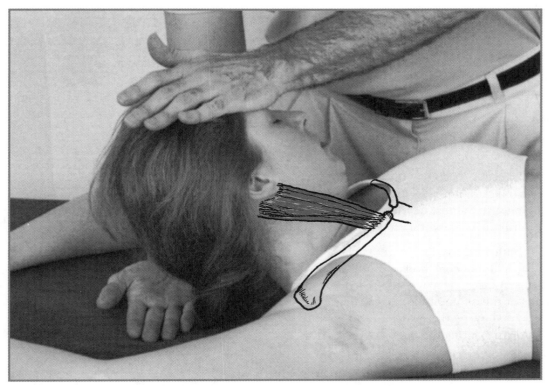

STERNO-CLEIDO-MASTOIDEUS, UNILATERALLY TESTED

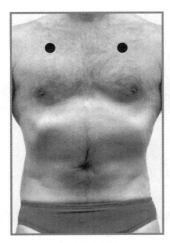

ANTERIOR NL

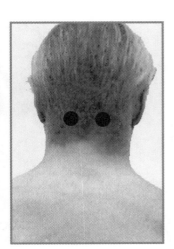

POSTERIOR NL

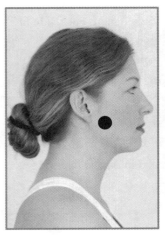

NEUROVASCULAR POINT

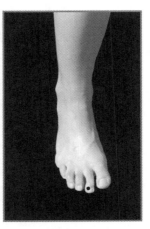

SEDATION POINT, STOM-
ACH 45

Subclavius

Origin: On the top of the first rib and its cartilage.

Insertion: Subclavius has a wide insertion under the middle of the clavicle.

Action: Pulls the clavicle anterior and interior and pulls it medially toward the sternal-clavicular joint.

Position: Walther says that this muscle is not directly testable. He tests indirectly by having the client TL subclavius while an indicator muscle is tested. Goodheart, Leaf and Gerz use the test devised by Alan Beardall with the arms held straight up to the ears.

Stabilization: If both arms are tested at once, no stabilization is needed. If only one arm is tested, the examiner stabilizes upon the trapezius on the side tested with fingers or thumb upon the clavicle. This has the advantage of allowing the examiner to feel if the subclavius is active during the test.

Muscle Test: The examiner applies pressure proximal to the wrist to bring the arm away from the head. The slightest motion of the clavicle indicates weakness of the subclavius.

Front Neurolymphatic: At the junction of the clavicle, sternum and first rib. Also just up from the bottom of the sternum (Dewe).

Back Neurolymphatic: One inch to each side of T1 (on the lamina). Also T10–11, two inches to each side of the spine (Dewe).

Neurovascular: Two finger-widths in front of the ear on a line just above where the top of the ear attaches to the head.

Reactive Muscles: Upper trapezius.

Meridian: None recognized in AK. Dewe's research says heart.

Organ: Heart?

Nutrition: Vitamin E, B-complex, C, heart, magnesium.

Discussion: Subclavius is usually involved in the "frozen shoulder" syndrome. In such cases, the client must lean sideways to lift the arm above horizontal. In 30% of such cases, strengthening of the subclavius immediately improves the ability to elevate the shoulder. AK recommends treatment applied directly to the muscle such as proprioceptor manipulation or fascial release.

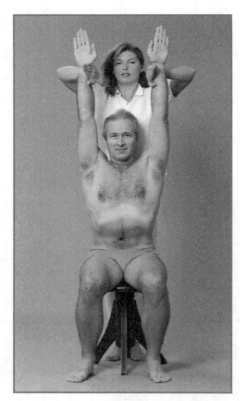

SUBCLAVIUS, BILATERALLY TESTED

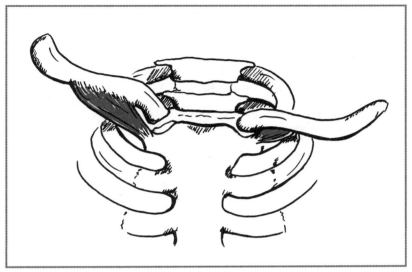

SUBCLAVIUS, RIGHT CLAVICLE ROTATED NON-ANATOMICALLY
TO REVEAL THE MUSCLE

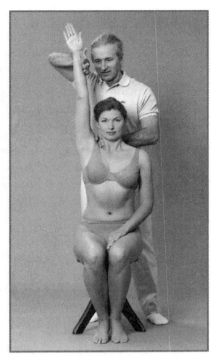

SUBCLAVIUS,
UNILATERALLY TESTED

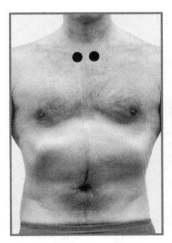

ANTERIOR NL

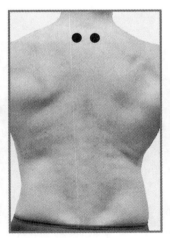

POSTERIOR NL

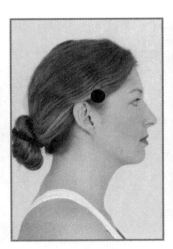

NEUROVASCULAR POINT

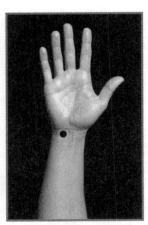

SEDATION POINT,
HEART 7

Subscapularis

Origin: On nearly the whole inner surface of the scapula.

Insertion: Into the anterior surface of the humerus at the level of the shoulder joint and into the inferior portion of the shoulder joint capsule.

Action: Rotates the humerus inwardly. Assists in adduction of the shoulder. Also pulls the head of the humerus forward and down when the arm is raised, which stabilizes the head of the humerus in the glenoid cavity.

Position: The humerus is at 90° to the side of the trunk. The elbow is bent 90°. The humerus is rotated medially, which brings the hand down toward the hip as far as possible without lifting the shoulder. The test may be performed standing, sitting, prone or supine.

Stabilization: The examiner stabilizes the humerus near the elbow to detect any attempt to move the upper arm, which should remain motionless during the test.

Muscle Test: The examiner presses proximal to the wrist to laterally rotate the forearm around the humerus and up toward the head.

Front Neurolymphatic: Between ribs 2 and 3 where they meet the sternum.

Back Neurolymphatic: Between the transverse processes of T2-3.

Neurovascular: Anterior fontanelle (bregma).

Reactive Muscles: Teres minor, infraspinatus, deltoids, supraspinatus.

Meridian: Heart.

Organ/Gland: Heart.

Nutrition: Vitamin E, vitamins B2, B3, vitamin C, carnitine.

Discussion: When exercise does not increase the heart rate as expected, subscapularis often tests weak. In this case, neurolymphatic stimulation will strengthen subscapularis and correct the heart's response to exercise. "Fluttering of the heart" contractions, breast and shoulder pains, and dizziness

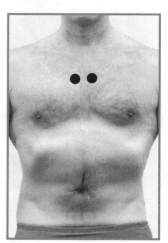

ANTERIOR NL

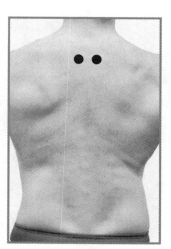

POSTERIOR NL

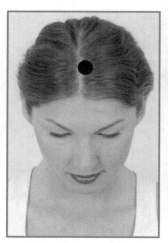

NEUROVASCULAR POINT

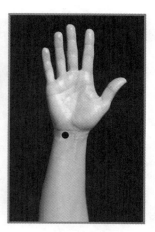

SEDATION POINT,
HEART 7

may be helped by strengthening the subscapularis. When the origin or proprioceptors of subscapularis require treatment, have the patient lift the hand up behind the back. This position lifts the medial edge of the scapula away from the back, allowing the examiner to reach under the scapula. For neuromuscular spindle cell manipulation, the examiner will have to reach under both edges of the scapula.

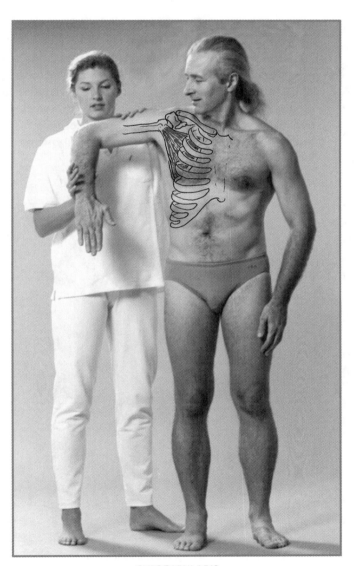

SUBSCAPULARIS

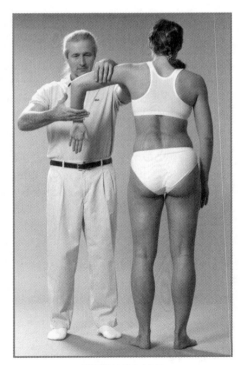

SUBSCAPULARIS

Supraspinatus

Origin: The inner two-thirds of the supraspinatus fossa, the part of the scapula above its "spine" ridge.

Insertion: Into the lateral surface of the head of the humerus at the level of the shoulder joint.

Action: Abducts the arm (directly to the side and slightly forward). Also holds the head of the humerus into the scapula (stabilizes the shoulder joint). Supraspinatus can never fully relax or the shoulder would dislocate.

Position: The patient brings the arm 15°-20° to the side and slightly forward. The palm is oriented toward the groin.

Stabilization: Upon the same or the opposite shoulder. Same side stabilization is preferred, allowing the examiner to feel the contraction of supraspinatus to make sure it is active during the test.

Muscle Test: The examiner pushes upon the arm proximal to the wrist in a direction caudal and medial to adduct the arm (down and in toward the groin).

Front Neurolymphatic: A line from just inside the shoulder joint down the anterior side of the shoulder in the depression between the anterior deltoid and pectoralis muscles, and slightly under the edge of the anterior deltoid.

Back Neurolymphatic: Under the edge of the occiput where it meets the neck, about 4 cm to the right and left of the atlas (posterior to the transverse processes of the atlas).

Neurovascular: Above the eyes on the little bony mounts of the forehead (frontal bone eminences).

Reactive Muscles: Rhomboids, pectoralis minor, teres major, teres minor, latissimus dorsi.

Meridian: Central (conception vessel).

Organ: Brain.

Nutrition: RNA, protein, amino acids, choline.

Discussion: Since the deltoid is active (synergistic) in this test, it is important to not allow the arm past 20° of elevation which is where the deltoid has a greater mechanical advantage and takes over most of the work of lifting the arm. Learning difficulties, especially in children, may be associated with a weakness of supraspinatus. Check for imbalances (such as reactive muscles) between supraspinatus, subscapularis and the deltoid muscles.

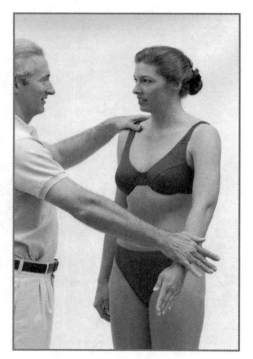

SUPRASPINATUS,
TESTED STANDING

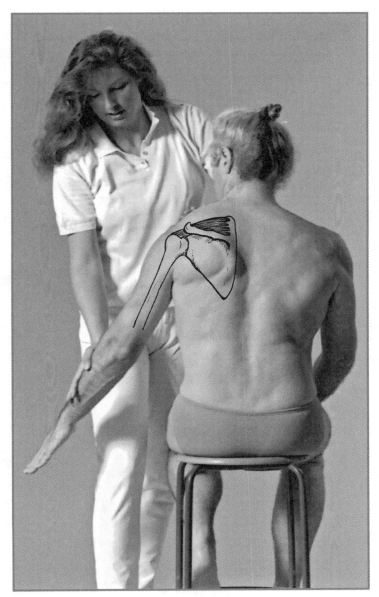

SUPRASPINATUS

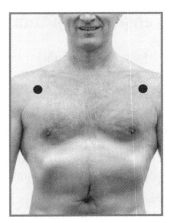

ANTERIOR NL

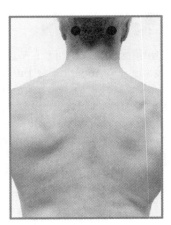

POSTERIOR NL

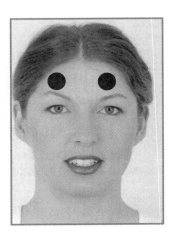

NEUROVASCULAR POINT

Tensor Fascia Lata

Origin: On the anterior lateral border of the ilium.

Insertion: Into the middle one-third of the iliotibial tract, the long tendinous ligament that connects the outer hip (iliac crest) with the tibia.

Action: Flexes, abducts and medially rotates the thigh. Pulls upon the iliotibial band, which stabilizes the knee against bending laterally.

Position: The patient lies supine with the knee completely extended. The leg to be tested is slightly abducted, medially rotated as much as possible and slightly flexed at the hip. The correct position for the test will cause the patient to feel strong contraction in the fascia lata.

Stabilization: With the patient lying on the back, the examiner can stabilize the opposite ankle. With the patient standing, the examiner should grasp around the patient's hips and clamp the hips to the examiner's chest. The patient should further place a hand upon the examiner's shoulder and/or the other hand upon a table for further stabilization.

Muscle Test: With contact proximal to the ankle, the examiner pushes the leg toward adduction and extension of the hip (toward the other leg).

Front Neurolymphatic: These are the largest neurolymphatic areas in the body, extending in a wide band on the sides of both legs from the hips to the knees.

Back Neurolymphatic: Two triangular areas from the hips up along the lumbar vertebrae. While stimulating these areas, the examiner must avoid pressing too firmly upon the kidneys.

Neurovascular: On the posterior portion of the parietal eminence.

Reactive Muscles: Adductors, peroneus tertius, gluteus maximus, hamstrings.

Meridian: Large intestine.

Organ/Gland: Large intestine.

Nutrition: Acidophilus, fenugreek, comfrey, folic acid, and vitamin D. If bilaterally weak, suspect iron deficiency.

Discussion: Fascia lata is often related to colon problems. When so, there is often severe lymph congestion. In such cases, stimulation of the neurolymphatic areas for the fascia lata and the colon can be helpful. Such stimulation may need to be continued by the patient as "homework."

The function of the large intestine can be stimulated by massage of the neurolymphatic areas for fascia lata on the sides of the thighs. The direction of muscular contraction and thus of the contents of the large intestine is ascending on the right abdomen, then transverse behind the stomach, and then descending on the left side of the abdomen. Following this direction with the corresponding neurolymphatic massage may be most effective in stimulating a lazy or constipated intestine. Notice that when one is standing, the reflexes on the thigh are located in the opposite direction to the movement of the colon, i.e., the ascending colon goes *down* (caudal along) the right thigh. If the knees are pulled up to the chest, the reflexes exactly follow the colon. To do so, use the fingers or knuckles to actively massage the neurolymphatic reflexes for fascia lata. Following the direction of the colon, begin on the side of the right leg just above the hip and massage vigorously down to below the knee. Then continue at the side of the left knee and massage up (in a direction cranial) to the left hip. Repeat this several times.

I visited a friend whose small dog had just had surgery for a blocked colon. She was worried that he might not survive because two days after the surgery he was listless and had not yet had a bowel movement. I moved his legs against his resistance to activate the fascia lata muscles. Then I massaged his neurolymphatic reflexes as described above. Finally, I moved his legs again against his resistance to activate the muscles. Within minutes he had a bowel movement. Later in the day he was back out in the garden digging vast holes, his favorite activity.

Bilaterally weak fascia lata muscles are often a sign of iron deficiency anemia. Goodheart postulates that if the lymph system is not draining properly, the pressure of the excess lymph can interfere with the production of red blood cells. Getting the excess lymph removed has first priority (see "Neurolymphatic Reflexes" on pages 100–106). Then such cases of anemia often respond well to homeopathic dosages of iron.

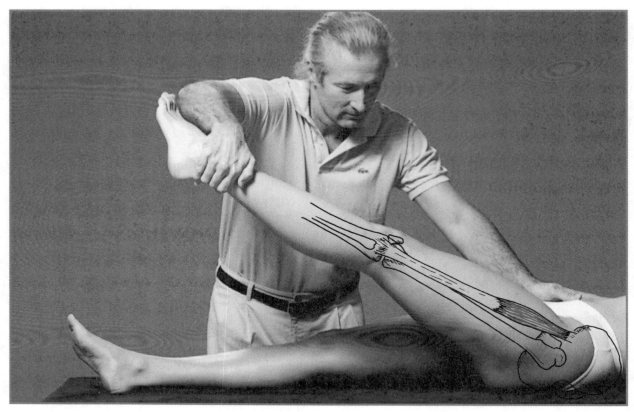

TENSOR FASCIA LATA

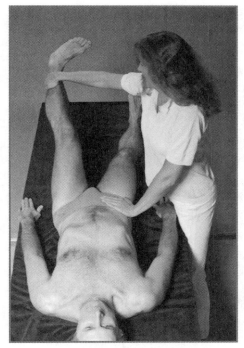

TENSOR FASCIA LATA

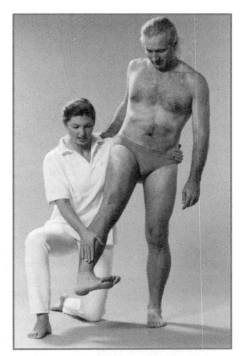

TENSOR FASCIA LATA,
TESTED STANDING

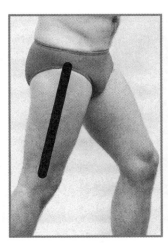

ANTERIOR NL

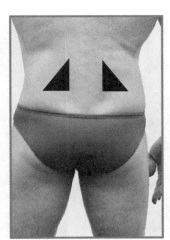

POSTERIOR NL

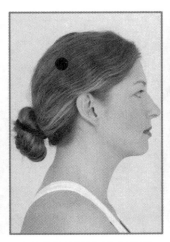

NEUROVASCULAR POINT

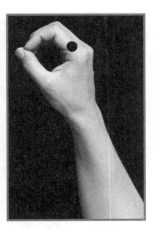

SEDATION POINT,
LARGE INTESTINE 2

Teres Major

Origin: From the lower one-third of the dorsal-axillary side of the scapula.

Insertion: Into the anterior surface of the humerus, just distal to the shoulder joint.

Action: Adducts and rotates the humerus inward (medially).

Position: The patient places the wrist upon the back of the hip with the arm bent 90°. The elbow is brought as far back (posterior) as possible.

Stabilization: With the patient prone, the posterior side of the opposite shoulder must be held down against the table. With the patient standing, the anterior side of the same shoulder must be stabilized. For bilateral testing (prone), no stabilization is required.

Muscle Test: The examiner presses the elbow in the direction of abduction and flexion (in an arc out and around the body). For bilateral testing, the examiner crosses his arms.

Front Neurolymphatic: Under the clavicle between ribs 2 and 3 about 7 cm from the midline of the sternum.

Back Neurolymphatic: In the intertransverse space between T2–3.

Neurovascular: Two finger-widths in front of the ear on a line just above where the top of the ear attaches to the head.

Reactive Muscles: Pectoralis major clavicular and sternal, anterior deltoid, teres minor, infraspinatus.

Meridian: Governing.

Organ: Spine.

Nutrition: When there is excessive sweating, organic iodine as found in kelp. Organic minerals. When the patient has difficulty tasting foods, zinc. Acid-alkaline balance may need evaluation.

Discussion: If the rhomboids or trapezius muscles are weak-testing, the scapula will move laterally during the test, making a strong teres major appear to test weak. To determine if teres major or teres minor is responsible for a "frozen shoulder," have the patient attempt to raise the arm with it rotated medially (teres major) or rotated laterally (teres minor). The rotation that produces the greatest difficulty in raising the arm defines which muscle is responsible. Often bilateral weakness indicates a vertebral fixation of the thoracic spine. If stretching and twisting do not help, this fixation may require chiropractic adjustment.

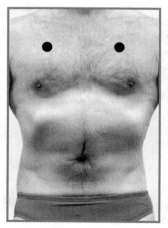

ANTERIOR NL

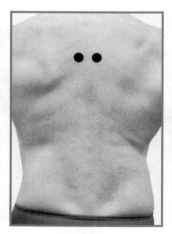

POSTERIOR NL

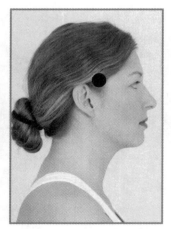

NEUROVASCULAR POINT

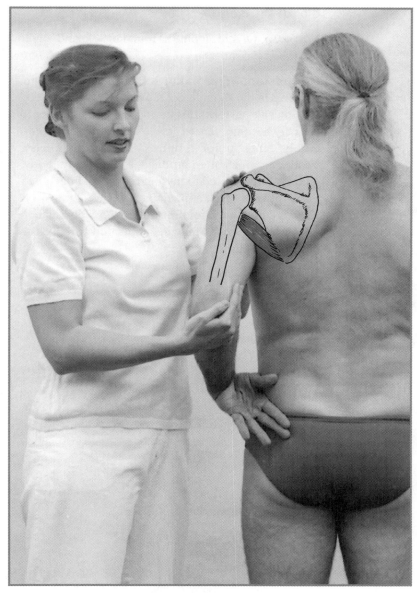

TERES MAJOR

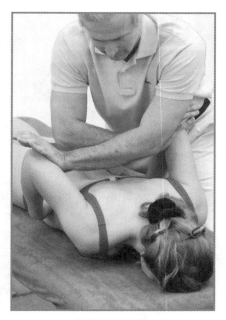

TERES MAJOR,
BILATERALLY TESTED

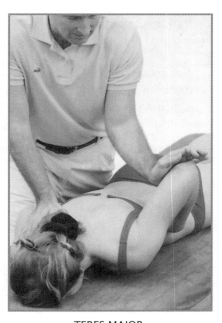

TERES MAJOR,
UNILATERAL, PRONE

Teres Minor

Origin: The middle one-third of the dorsal axillary border of the shoulder blade.

Insertion: Below the shoulder joint on the posterior surface of the humerus (distal to the insertion of teres major).

Action: Rotates the humerus laterally. Holds the head of the humerus into the glenoid cavity.

Position: With the elbow near the side, the arm is bent 90° at the elbow. The forearm is rotated laterally (away from the body to the side).

Stabilization: The examiner stabilizes the elbow to prevent any other motion besides rotation of the humerus. The patient's trapezius and rhomboids must be able to fix the scapula during the test.

Muscle Test: The examiner uses an open hand to press proximal to the wrist. The forearm is used as a lever to rotate the humerus inwardly.

Front Neurolymphatic: Between ribs 2 and 3 where they meet the sternum.

Back Neurolymphatic: T3 lamina.

Neurovascular: Two finger-widths in front of the ear on a line just above where the top of the ear attaches to the head. Also at the junction of the first rib, clavicle and sternum.

Reactive Muscles: Subscapularis, latissimus dorsi, deltoid, supraspinatus.

Meridian: Triple heater.

Gland: Thyroid.

Nutrition: Organic iodine as found in kelp and other seaweeds, tyrosine.

Discussion: Teres minor holds the head of the humerus in the shoulder joint when the arm is raised. If it doesn't perform this important task, the shoulder may become "frozen" (see "Teres major"). Commonly, teres minor requires the fascial release treatment, which often produces an increase of body temperature (related to thyroid function). Infections, problems with digestion, unexpected weight loss or gain, and crying without reason (all possibly related to thyroid function) may be associated with weakness in teres minor.

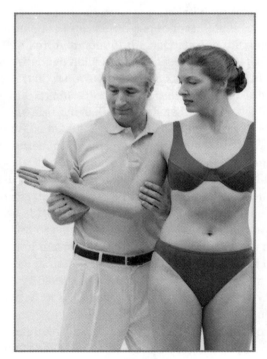

TERES MINOR

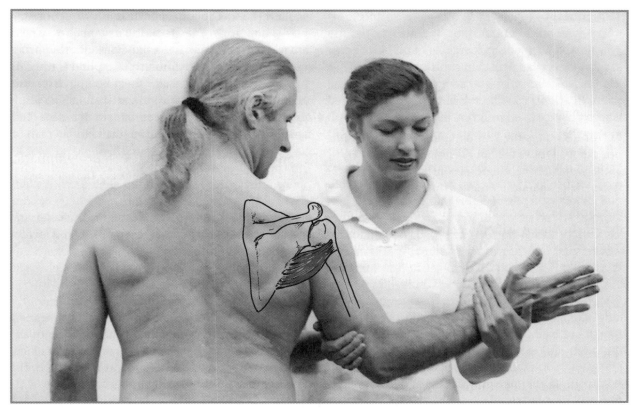

TERES MINOR

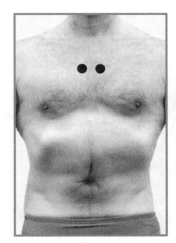

ANTERIOR NL

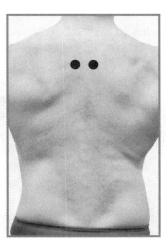

POSTERIOR NL

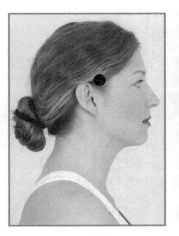

NEUROVASCULAR POINT

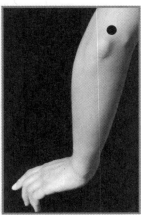

SEDATION POINT,
TRIPLE HEATER 10

Trapezius, Lower

Origin: Spinous processes from the thoracic vertebrae 6 to 12.

Insertion: Into the middle one-third of the spine of the scapula.

Action: Rotates the scapula and stabilizes its inferior aspect. Draws the lateral superior (acromial) tip of the scapula back. Bilateral contraction extends the spine (helps maintain erect posture).

Position: Prone or standing. The arm is elevated to the side to align it with the central fibers of the lower trapezius (about 150°). The arm is rotated externally so the thumb points posteriorly. The head is straight ahead or rotated toward the side of the test.

Stabilization: In the prone test, the examiner stabilizes the *opposite* hip to prevent rotation of the trunk. In the standing test, the examiner stabilizes the anterior side of the shoulder on the *same* side as the test. If the trunk is not stable in the standing test, the patient should stand with the back against a wall.

Muscle Test: The arm is pushed in a direction that brings it in front of the face. The examiner may push anywhere from the wrist to above the elbow, depending upon the desired amount of applied force. The posterior shoulder muscles must be able to fix the position of the humerus upon the scapula. The test is the fixation between the scapula and the spine. This must be observed or felt during the test.

Front Neurolymphatic, Back Neurolymphatic, Neurovascular: All reflex points are the same as for the middle trapezius.

Reactive Muscles: Pectoralis major clavicular and sternal, pectoralis minor, upper trapezius and levator scapula.

Meridian, Organ/Gland, Nutrition: Same as for middle trapezius.

Discussion: Bilateral weakness of the lower trapezius often indicates a fixation at the juncture of the thoracic and lumbar spine. This may require chiropractic correction. When the fixation is freed, the lower trapezius should test strong.

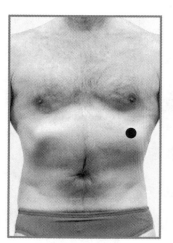

ANTERIOR NL

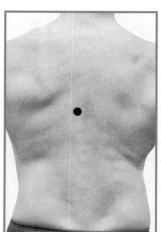

POSTERIOR NL

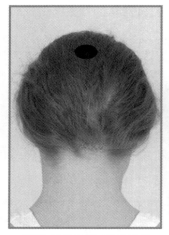

NEUROVASCULAR POINT

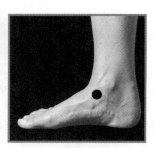

SEDATION POINT,
SPLEEN 5

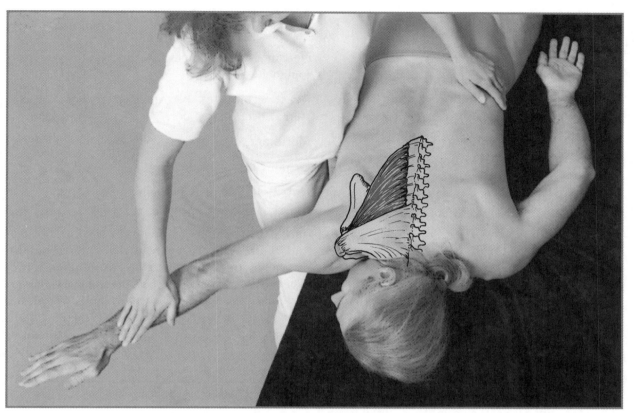

LOWER TRAPEZIUS

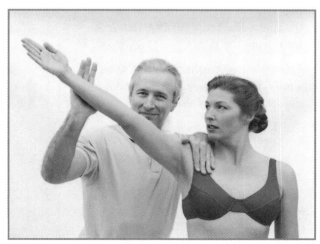

LOWER TRAPEZIUS

Trapezius, Middle

Origin: Spinous processes of thoracic vertebrae 1-5.

Insertion: Into the acromial process and the spine of the scapula.

Action: Adducts and slightly elevates the scapula, retracts the acromial process.

Position: Prone or standing. The patient lifts the arm laterally to 90° from the body. The arm is laterally rotated (thumb posterior) to place the synergistic rhomboids at a disadvantage. If the examiner presses proximal to the wrist, this angle of rotation also prevents bending at the elbow.

Stabilization: In the prone test, the examiner stabilizes the *opposite* shoulder to prevent rotation of the trunk. In the standing test, the examiner stabilizes the anterior side of the shoulder on the *same* side as the test. If the trunk is not stable in the standing test, the patient should stand with the back against a wall.

Muscle Test: The arm is pushed anteriorly. The examiner may push anywhere from the wrist to above the elbow, depending upon the desired amount of force. The posterior shoulder muscles must be able to fix the position of the humerus upon the scapula. The test is the fixation between the scapula and the spine. This must be observed or felt for during the test.

Front Neurolymphatic: Same as latissimus dorsi: between ribs 7 and 8 on the left side under the nipple.

Back Neurolymphatic: Between T7-8 near the laminae on the left.

Neurovascular: One inch superior to the posterior fontanelle (lambda).

Reactive Muscles: Pectoralis major clavicular and sternal, pectoralis minor.

Meridian: Spleen.

Organ-Gland: Spleen.

Nutrition: Vitamin C, calcium.

Discussion: Just because the arm comes forward during the test does not confirm a weakness of the middle trapezius. This may be due to the shoulder muscles not adequately fixing the shoulder joint. When middle trapezius is weak, the scapula will move away from the spine, and the vertebral edge of the scapula may flare up from the back. When the middle trapezius is weak on both sides, there is usually a vitamin C deficiency. To ascertain if this is the case, have the patient eat a slice of orange or other vitamin C-containing food and retest the middle trapezius. If now strong, a vitamin C deficiency is indicated.

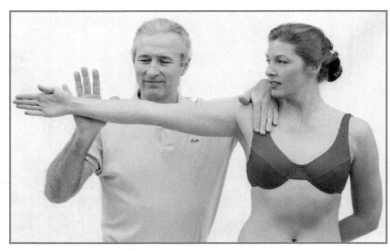

MIDDLE TRAPEZIUS, TESTED STANDING

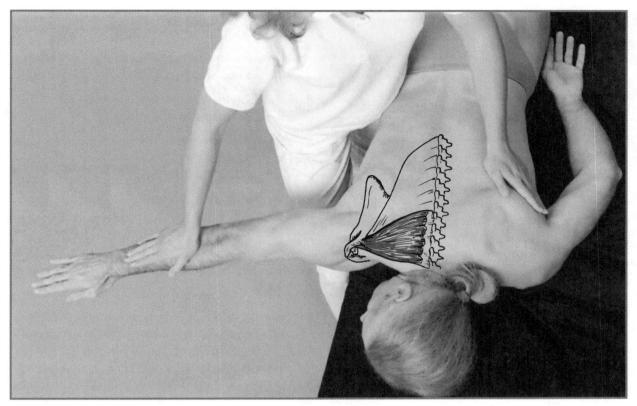

MIDDLE TRAPEZIUS

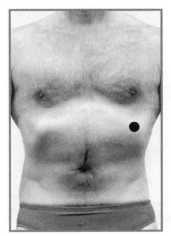

ANTERIOR NL

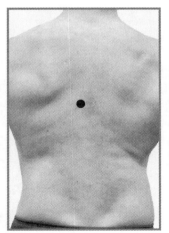

POSTERIOR NL

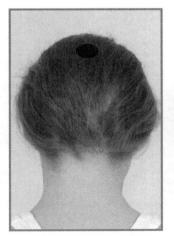

NEUROVASCULAR POINT

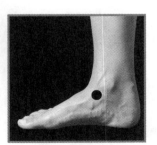

SEDATION POINT,
SPLEEN 5

Trapezius, Upper

Origin: From the base of the skull to the 7th cervical vertebra spinous process.

Insertion: Into the lateral one-third of the clavicle and the acromion process of the scapula.

Action: Rotates the scapula so the shoulder joint socket faces upward. When acting with the other portions of the trapezius, it pulls the scapula in medially. With reversed origin and insertion, it pulls the head forward and rotates the head away from the side of contraction. Bilateral contraction against resistance pulls the head back upon the neck.

Position: The patient raises one shoulder and leans the ear toward the shoulder. The head is slightly rotated away from the side tested. The shoulder should remain a few inches away from the ear to avoid over-shortening and thereby locking the muscle. Experience shows that if the patient is allowed to bring the shoulder and ear together, upper trapezius almost never tests weak.

Stabilization: Test pressure provides adequate stabilization.

Muscle Test: The examiner uses both hands to pull the shoulder and head apart.

Front Neurolymphatic: A 7 cm-long line between the anterior and middle deltoids.

Back Neurolymphatic: Under the base of the skull over the posterior arch of the atlas.

Neurovascular: Above the cheekbone, 2–3 cm behind the outside edge of the eye, where the temporal and sphenoid bones meet.

Reactive Muscles: Latissimus dorsi, biceps, subscapularis, contralateral upper trapezius, neck flexors.

Meridian: Kidney.

Organ: Eye and ear.

Nutrition: Vitamins A, B, F, G, calcium and water.

Discussion: The upper trapezius is often involved in certain eye problems, especially strabismus. Hearing loss can sometimes be corrected (though more in the lower ranges than the higher) by testing and correcting the upper trapezius. Neurolymphatic (and sometimes neurovascular) stimulation has the best effect upon related eye and ear problems. Dehydration can

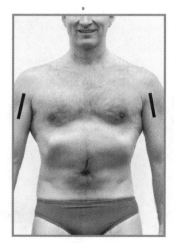

ANTERIOR NL

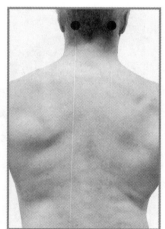

POSTERIOR NL

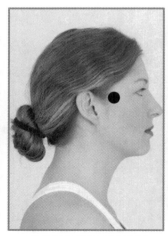

NEUROVASCULAR POINT

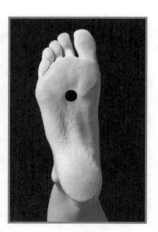

SEDATION POINT,
KIDNEY 1

cause pain and tension in the upper trapezius. It is a good first measure for excess tension in upper trapezius to drink two glasses of water and wait 20 minutes to assess the effect.

Excess upper trapezius tension is extremely common. It is often found to be a primary muscle, causing continued weakness in its antagonist, latissimus dorsi. In the "fright" response, the head is pulled back and the shoulders lifted, mainly by the upper trapezius muscles. This instinctual response protects the medulla (located at the lower posterior part of the cranium). Heartbeat and respiration are controlled from the medulla. As a direct blow to the medulla could cause death, instinctual protection of this area is important to survival. In patients with continual fear, tension in this area is more or less constant.

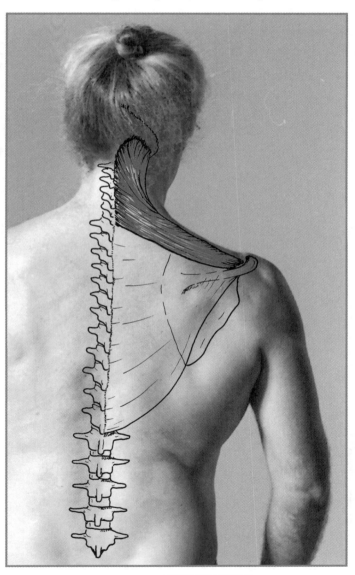

UPPER TRAPEZIUS

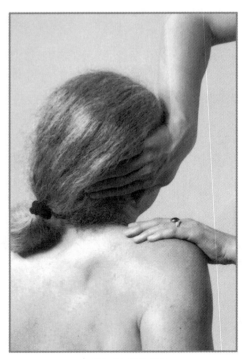

UPPER TRAPEZIUS

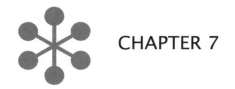

CHAPTER 7

Structure

This chapter teaches ICAK structural diagnostic and correction techniques, and a very effective stretching technique for extending the range of motion in shortened muscles. Topics include:

- Ligament Interlink: Contralateral joint correction. Treat your right wrist plus lateral pressure on the hyoid for your left ankle pain.
- Strain Counterstrain: Put the body into the position of no pain for awhile. Passively be moved back and the pain is gone.
- Gaits: Patterns of bilateral motion of arms and legs. Integrates the function of the two halves of the brain. Brings both coordination and clear thinking to the learning disturbed.
- Cloacal Synchronization: Integrating the upright reflexes of the head with the reproductive and excretory reflexes of the pelvis.
- Hyoid Bone: Balancing the gyroscope of the body.
- Injury Recall Technique: Getting rid of the aftereffects of old injuries.
- Ocular Lock, Eyes into Distortion, Eyes Out of Distortion, Body into Distortion: Looking into the direction of postural distortion stresses the system enough to bring up hidden positive reactions making subsequent treatments more complete.
- Proprioceptive Neuromuscular Facilitation: Tense the stretched muscle as you breathe out. Relax and stretch into a new range of motion as you breathe in.

Ligament Interlink

Goodheart had a patient with rheumatic fever that caused painful swelling in the knees. Interestingly, the pain was reduced when the patient bent his arms. The pain in the knee became worse when the patient extended his contralateral arm, straightening his elbow. Fascinated by this unusual finding, Goodheart looked for ways to apply it to help reduce pain in other patients. He found cases where a painful joint on a patient's arm would not therapy localize unless the corresponding joint on the other leg (contralateral upper and lower extremities) was simultaneously touched by the patient (two-handed therapy localization).

Goodheart found the two-handed therapy localization to function between the gait-related parts—the ones that move together in walking (shoulder and opposite hip, knee-elbow, wrist-ankle, fingers-toes). In four-legged (quadruped) animals with fingers, it is easy to see the simultaneous movement of the fingers with the toes of the opposite side. When humans freely and briskly walk, the swinging forward of the wrist can be observed to occur at the same time that the opposite ankle swings forward to take a step. There is a connection between the nerve signals (innervation) to one arm and the opposite leg. The correspondences found to function in two-handed therapy localization are given in the following chart:

Joint	Contralateral Joint
Fingers	Toes
Wrist	Ankle
Elbow	Knee
Shoulder	Hip
Sacroiliac (sacrum-hip)	Sternocostal (ICAK), Occiput (my own finding—not the standard ICAK relationship)
Coccyx	Xiphoid process (lower tip of breastbone)
Vertebra above T5–6	Opposite side of vertebra the same distance below the junction of the thoracic vertebrae 5 and 6 (Lovett Brother)
Any joint in the body	Temporomandibular (jaw) joint

Through experimentation, Goodheart found that holding the hyoid bone to one side eliminated the two-handed therapy localization to the joints. He proposed that stimulation to the nerves in the muscles attached to the hyoid somehow was affecting the nerve communication between the corresponding joints on the opposite sides of the body. Using this observation, he developed a technique to reduce joint pain. Here again we see Goodheart's genius for taking an unusual observation and developing it into a useful Applied Kinesiology technique.

First, the painful joint is therapy localized and an indicator muscle is tested. If the indicator muscle weakens, the usual Applied Kinesiology tests and corrections are performed until the positive therapy localization is eliminated. The corresponding joint on the other side of the body (see chart above) is similarly evaluated. Next, both the painful point in the joint (usually upon the ligaments) and the corresponding contralateral joint are therapy localized simultaneously. For example, in this test of both joints, the client may have her right hand on the hurting left elbow and at the same time her left hand on the contralateral right knee. Note that both of the hands of the patient are being used for this two-handed therapy localization. Because the arms are no longer available for muscle testing, a leg muscle may be used as the indicator muscle.

The client should not lean forward or otherwise change posture between the various tests (joint 1, joint 2, both joints). Changing position might inadvertently stimulate some other part of the body and change the results of the testing. Therefore, the body positioning used to test each individual joint should be chosen to be very near to the position required to test the two joints simultaneously.

The spots on the two extremities that therapy localize will be found to directly correspond. The inside of the ankle will correspond to the inside of the wrist. Caveat: Because the knee bends the lower leg backward and the elbow bends the forearm forward, the medial aspect of the left knee corresponds to the lateral aspect of the right elbow.

Next, the client holds her hyoid bone to one side and then the other while an indicator muscle is tested. If holding the hyoid toward either side causes the indicator muscle to test weak, the muscles attached to the hyoid must be evaluated and balanced before proceeding.

The examiner presses into both spots that therapy localized with equal pressure and asks which one is more painful. The *less*-painful joint is the one treated. During the treatment, the patient holds the hyoid bone toward the side treated (toward the side of the less-painful joint). The examiner presses upon the less-painful point with about 10 pounds of pressure for a few seconds and then releases the pressure. This cycle is continued for 30–40 seconds, or until pressure on the opposite joint no longer causes pain. During treatment, the examiner may lightly press upon the painful joint to determine if the pain is being reduced. This does not aid the therapy, but can be used to tell when to stop manipulation (when the pain is gone).

In rare cases, the corresponding joints may be on the same side of the body. Another unusual variation may be observed when both corresponding joints each therapy localize alone, cannot be individually balanced, but do not weaken the indicator muscle when therapy localized together. In both these unusual cases, the treatment remains the same: Hold the hyoid toward the less-painful side.

Ligament interlink is not a cure-all for joint problems. All of the other possible problems (subluxations, muscle weaknesses, and other imbalances of muscles such as muscle stretch reaction, repeated muscle failure, reactive muscles, strain counterstrain, etc.) need to be identified and eliminated. Ligament interlink can be effective in reducing arthritic pain. In the treatment of traumas such as sprains and other injuries, when the first "shock" reaction is over and initial healing has already begun, ligament interlink may be applied to swiftly reduce pain, inflammation, and swelling.

LIGAMENT INTERLINK TECHNIQUE

Assessment:

1. Patient assesses the level of pain in an articulation. TL the painful articulation. If active, perform standard AK techniques (muscle balancing, manipulation, etc.) to eliminate the positive TL.

2. Simultaneously TL the painful joint and its contralateral partner. If active, TL only the contralateral partner. If this single TL is active, balance the contralateral upper body-lower body partner joint first before continuing. If the double TL is now active, the ligament interlink technique is indicated.

3. Palpate the painful articulation to locate the area of greatest pain—usually upon a ligament.

4. Press simultaneously on the painful ligament and the corresponding contralateral upper body-lower body ligament, using the same amount of pressure on each side.

5. Ask the patient which side hurts more when you are pressing. The less-painful joint is the one to treat. This is usually, but not always, opposite the side where the patient's presenting pain is located.

Correction:

1. Press the hyoid bone to the left and muscle test. Press the hyoid bone to the right and test. If pressing the hyoid either right or left weakens the indicator muscle, evaluate and balance the muscles of the hyoid before continuing.

2. The patient holds her hyoid bone to the side to be treated.

3. The examiner presses firmly (about 10 pounds of pressure) upon the articulation/ligament to be treated for a few seconds and then releases his pressure. This is repeated for 30–40 seconds. Optional: The examiner may press lightly upon the opposite side and ask the patient to report any reduction of pain during the procedure.

Confirming the correction:

1. Simultaneously TL the painful joint and its contralateral partner. Muscle test. This should now no longer weaken the indicator muscle.

2. Have the patient move and assess the reduction in pain.

Strain Counterstrain

The Strain Counterstrain technique was developed by the osteopath Lawrence Jones in the 1950s as a method to treat neuromuscular and musculoskeletal disorders. Jones first published his method in an article entitled "Spontaneous Release by Positioning" in 1964. This article includes the specific positions and trigger points for all spinal and many other lesions.

The first patient Jones successfully treated with the Strain Counterstrain technique had bent over for an extended time while gardening. Upon standing up, he felt a sudden shooting pain in his low back (lumbago). Note that he had no pain while bending over. The pain started when he straightened up. This is a common occurrence that every examiner will likely hear from his patients.

Jones was able to help his patient relieve his pain by bringing him passively back into a position of strong flexion of the affected muscle(s), which was also the precise position he held for a long time while gardening. Jones hypothesized an explanation for this phenomenon: When a muscle is flexed for an extended period of time and then suddenly lengthened, the proprioceptors in the muscle have become accustomed to the shortened length and don't have time to adjust to the sudden lengthening. As a result, they send a volley of inappropriate impulses into the nervous system, which results in a disturbance of the function of the muscle, its synergists, and its antagonists. Passively holding the muscle in the shortened position, then passively and slowly lengthening it, allows the proprioceptors to reset and normalize the tone of the affected group of muscles.

Jones's technique is to hold the patient's body in the position that maximally reduces pain, ideally in the position of no pain, for at least three minutes. Then while the patient remains fully passive, the examiner slowly moves the patient's body so as to extend the shortened muscle.

The precise mechanisms of strain are not completely understood. It is now hypothesized that an injury to the muscles causes the spindle cells to fire inappropriately. This continued signaling initiates a neuromuscular reflex loop that inappropriately resets the tone in affected muscles, generates bodily pain, and is also believed to form what are called "tender points" in the tissues, often far removed from the directly affected muscles. These tender points are

exquisitely painful to the touch. These are the "trigger points" described by Travell and others. The location of trigger points can indicate the precise position of the lesion. The experienced examiner can palpate for tender trigger points to diagnose the position of the causative lesion. This is often far more effective in locating spinal lesions than direct palpation to the spine and tissues surrounding it.

The Strain Counterstrain technique is used to relieve the bodily pain in the tissues and in the tender points. The basic technique as taught today is quite simple: The examiner passively places the affected limb or the torso into a position that approximates the two ends of the affected muscle. The examiner experimentally moves the patient until a precise position is found in which all pain, including trigger point sensitivity, is absent. The examiner holds the patient's passive body in this position for 90 seconds. Then the examiner moves the patient's body back to a neutral position. For the technique to be successful, it is imperative that the patient does not attempt to move or tighten any muscles but rather remains completely passive throughout the procedure. This technique is often very successful in reducing the somatic pain and the sensitivity of the tender points.

Much research has revealed that for a specific lesion, the position that eliminates the pain is usually the same for all patients. This is likely because most lesions of a specific structure are nearly identical. There are, of course, exceptions but trying out the suggested positions first will save the examiner much time. These muscle-joint pain positions are well documented and provide a starting point for the examiner to utilize in treating his patients.

The specific positions to utilize for specific muscles are described in the literature and are also available to see as videos online. If the suggested position does not completely relieve the pain, the examiner varies the position until all pain is gone. In this position, the affected tight muscles can be felt to relax and the affected trigger points become pain-free to palpation. The examiner can also locate the treatment position by pressing on a related trigger point while moving the body to find the position that eliminates the pain in the trigger point.

If the patient moves his body out of this position, the muscles tighten up again—apparently in an attempt to splint up the affected joint to prevent further injury. Interestingly, the position that makes the lesion pain-free is usually the position where the lesion occurred. Actively moving away from the position of injury causes the muscles to tighten and the trigger points to become painful again.

Trigger points can be used diagnostically to determine the vertebral segment or other joint that has a lesion. A lesion between each two sequential vertebrae is correlated with specific active trigger points. Lesions can be easier to differentiate by using trigger points than by direct palpation of the subluxated area, which is often imprecise.

Note that the osteopathic "lesion" described above is called a "subluxation" in Applied Kinesiology.

Indications for the Strain Counterstrain technique include persistent pain in muscles and/or joints with tender trigger points.

STRAIN COUNTERSTRAIN TECHNIQUE: JONES

1. Ask the patient to describe precisely what occurred when he was injured. What was he doing? What position was he in when the pain began? Did something strike him? How did he fall? Deduce how the force of impact drove the body out of alignment. Palpate to confirm or correct your deduction.

2. Exaggerate the deformity found by your examination. Move the patient into the position that caused the subluxation. Vary the position until the position of maximal reduction of pain, maximal relaxation of the tightened muscles, and reduction of the trigger point pain is found.

3. The patient remains passively in this position for up to three minutes.

4. The patient remains passive while the examiner moves him back to a relaxed position.

Goodheart considered, further researched, and adapted the Strain Counterstrain technique for use in Applied Kinesiology. Its application not only resets muscle tone and relieves pain, it also improves neuromuscular function and patterns of movement throughout the body. He suggests that it be used whenever the patient complains of pain that is located away from the muscle needing treatment.

STRAIN COUNTERSTRAIN TECHNIQUE: GOODHEART

Assessment:

1. The muscle in question should test strong. If not, it should be initially strengthened with usual AK techniques.

2. The examiner assists the patient to maximally contract the muscle for 3 seconds and then to return to the relaxed position.

3. The muscle is again tested. If it now tests weak, the Strain Counterstrain technique is indicated.

Correction:

1. Palpate and locate the position in the belly of the muscle that is most painful to pressure. Hold the pressure as strongly as the patient can tolerate.

2. While the patient remains completely passive, the examiner moves the limb or other body part until the position of maximal reduction of the pain in the pressed point is located. In general, the farther the point is from the midline of the body, the more the limb or other body part must be not only flexed but also rotated.

3. The examiner holds the patient in this position. The patient refrains from tightening the muscle. If possible, the examiner lengthens the spindle cells under the pain point. This stretching apart of the spindle cell mechanism is illustrated on page 27. This stretching takes place during 5–7 cycles of respiration. If the treated muscle is on the anterior side of the body (psoas, rectus femoris, pectoralis, abdominals, etc.), the spindle cell stretching is performed during inspiration. If the treated muscle

is on the posterior side of the body (sacrospinalis, hamstrings, gluteus maximus, rhomboids, etc.), the spindle cell stretching is performed during expiration.

4. If spindle cell stretching is not performed, simply continue pressing upon the painful point while holding the patient in the position that reduces the pain to a minimum.

5. It is very important at the end of the treatment that the patient not tighten the treated muscle. He can return to a relaxed position in one of two ways. First, he can remain passive while the examiner very slowly moves his limb or other body part back to the beginning position. Or the patient can tighten the antagonist of the treated muscle against the slowly releasing resistance of the examiner.

Gaits

When a muscle is active, its synergists are facilitated and its antagonists are inhibited. This "reciprocal facilitation and inhibition" is described in length in the sections on neuromuscular spindle cells and Golgi tendon organs on pages 21–32. As discussed, this function occurs in the spinal segment and is active in very swift reactions such as the knee-jerk reflex.

More complex examples of reciprocal facilitation and inhibition can be seen in the organization of patterns of locomotion. Normal gait patterns involve contralateral movements of the upper and lower limbs. The word "gait" refers to the arm and leg coordination patterns that occur in walking and running. The different gait patterns are more easily seen in a horse than in humans. Horses use different gaits (walk, canter, trot, gallop ...) at different speeds. Although humans walk on two legs, in locomotion the arms swing contralateral to the legs in the same patterns of coordination that can be observed in four-legged animals. As the left leg swings forward, the right arm swings forward. At the same time, the right leg is stepping back and the left arm is swinging back.

When the right arm comes forward, contraction of the muscles of the left leg to bring it forward is facilitated. At the same time, muscles that bring the left arm forward and the right leg forward are inhibited. This reciprocal inhibition prevents the contraction of muscles that would interfere with the current muscular activity.

One does sometimes see people doing a "camel" gait, with same arm and leg, R-R and L-L. This indicates homolateral organization and is usually considered pathological. This homolateral gait indicates that the person is currently organized poorly and is using one hemisphere at a time to coordinate walking movements. A homolateral gait usually indicates neurologic disorganization. Neurologic disorganization can manifest as discoordination, as mental disabilities and incapacities, or as both. People with extreme cases of neurologic disorganization are categorized as "dyslexic." Dyslexia is considered a learning deficiency. However, some of the most creative and successful people (Cher, Tom Cruise, Steven Spielberg, Keanu Reeves, John Lennon, and many more) have had learning and/or coordination deficiencies to the extent that they were diagnosed as dyslexic.

When a person is walking, the head remains facing forward. This seemingly simple act requires sophisticated control. As the right foot steps forward, the pelvis and lower trunk rotate counterclockwise (as seen from above). As the left shoulder comes forward, the upper trunk rotates clockwise. To stop the head from following the motion of the upper trunk, the right sternocleidomastoid (neck flexor) and left upper trapezius (neck extensor) must contract while at the same time the left sternocleidomastoid and the right upper trapezius must relax. Rotation or inclination of the head while walking is evidence of a possible gait problem. The reciprocal facilitation and inhibition control of the many muscles of locomotion, including head position, requires more than spinal segment control. Control of the many muscles involved in locomotion also requires the activity of the cerebellum.

The muscles that work together (are facilitated) in walking should test strong when simultaneously tested. This is the basis of gait testing in Applied Kinesiology.

Gait testing is most easily performed with the patient supine. However, some gait problems can be detected only when the patient is in weight-bearing posture. When the walking gait is not well organized, but no gait imbalances are detected when testing supine, perform the gait tests with the patient standing.

GAIT TESTING TECHNIQUE

Assessment:

The patient lies supine. The examiner tests the contralateral gait postures. If any limb tests weak in the double test, the examiner tests it individually. If it tests strong individually, then the gait imbalance is confirmed. If it tests weak individually, the examiner strengthens it and repeats the double test.

1. Arm and hip flexors: The patient raises one arm and the contralateral leg up off the table about 20°. The examiner presses both down toward the table.

2. Arm and hip extensors: The patient pulls one arm and the contralateral leg down toward the table. The examiner pulls both upward from the table.

3. Arm and hip abductors: The patient holds one arm and the contralateral leg out to the sides. The examiner presses them back in toward the patient's sides.

4. Arm and hip adductors: The patient holds one arm and the contralateral leg in toward the midline. The examiner pulls both away from the midline.

5. Psoas and contralateral pectoralis major: The patient lifts one leg and rotates it outward. The contralateral arm is raised 45–90°. The examiner presses the leg and arm down and away from the body laterally. Note that this is a test of both pectoralis major clavicular and sternalis divisions simultaneously.

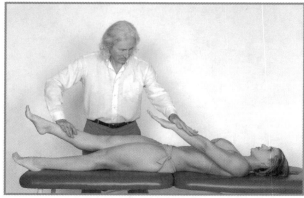

GAIT TEST: ARM AND HIP FLEXORS

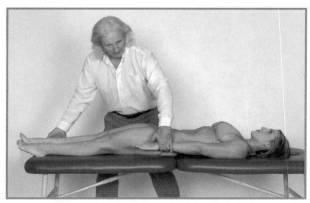

GAIT TEST: ARM AND HIP EXTENSORS

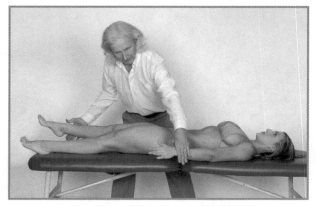

GAIT TEST: ARM AND HIP ADDUCTORS

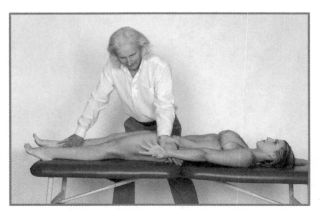

GAIT TEST: ARM AND HIP ABDUCTORS

6. Gluteus medius and contralateral abdominals: Supine, the patient lifts one shoulder and pulls it toward the opposite hip to contract the abdominals on that side. The patient also moves the contralateral leg out to the side. The examiner stabilizes the leg on the lifted shoulder side and presses the contralateral leg in toward the midline. Note that although the abdominals are contracted on one side, only the contralateral gluteus medius is tested for weakening.

7. The gluteus medius and contralateral abdominals can also be tested with the patient sitting. The patient sits and presses one leg out to the side against the examiner's legs. The patient rotates the upper body toward the examiner. The examiner presses the patient's shoulder in an attempt to reverse the rotation. Note that this tests only the abdominal part of the double test.

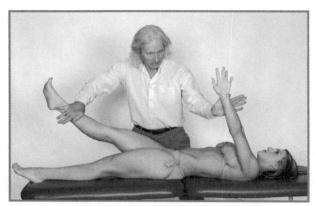

GAIT TEST: PSOAS AND PECTORALIS MAJOR

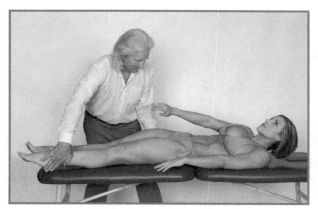

GAIT TEST: GLUTEUS MEDIUS AND
CONTRALATERAL ABDOMINALS—SUPINE

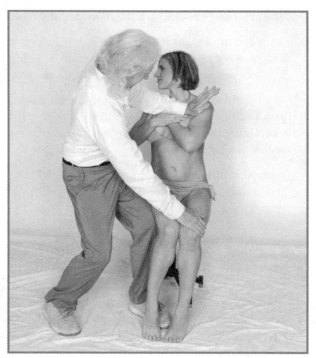

GAIT TEST: GLUTEUS MEDIUS AND
CONTRALATERAL ABDOMINALS—SITTING

Correction:

Firmly massage for about 15 seconds the acupressure points on the foot for the specific gait tests that tested weak.

There is a popular AK memory jogger for learning which acupressure points correct which gait imbalance. The first five letters of the city Palo Alto (PALOA) refer to the first five of the six gait positions beginning on the medial side of the big toe. These points are between the distal ends of the metatarsals of the foot. Massage between the root of the toes and up into the space between the metatarsals.

P—Posterior: The shoulder and hip extensors (that pull the limbs posterior)—Spleen 3

A—Anterior: The shoulder and hip flexors (that pull the limbs anterior)—Liver 2

L—Lateral: The shoulder and hip abductors (that move the limbs laterally)—Stomach 44

O—Oblique: The gluteus maximus and oblique abdominal test—Gall Bladder 42

A—Adductors: The shoulder and hip adductors—Bladder 65

The last point, the one for the psoas and pectoralis gait test, is Kidney meridian 1, located on the plantar (sole) side of the foot, proximal to the center of the ball of the foot.

Confirming the correction:

Retest the previously positive gait positions. They should now test strong.

FURTHER GAIT TESTING

As mentioned, the muscles that work together (are facilitated) in walking should test strong when simultaneously tested. This is the basis of gait testing in Applied Kinesiology. Conversely, when a gait position is taken (one leg and the opposite arm forward), all the muscles that are inhibited by this phase of the gait should test weak. More complete testing of these muscle circuits than the standard AK gait tests can be performed by having the patient stand in the gait position (one arm forward and the contralateral leg forward). In this gait stance, the synergists should be facilitated (test strong) and the antagonists should be inhibited (test weak). For a more complete test of muscle circuits involved in the gaits, have the patient take the gait stance and test all the muscles listed below. If any muscles fail to weaken as expected, one

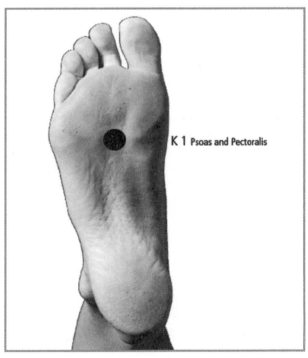

GAIT POINT ON BOTTOM OF FOOT

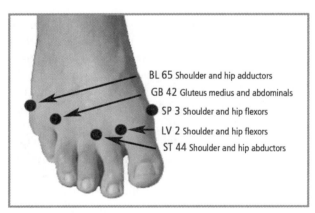

GAIT POINTS ON TOP OF FOOT

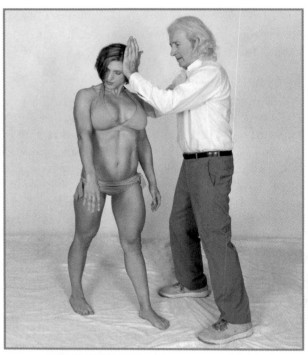

TESTING THE STERNOCLEIDOMASTOID IN
STANDING GAIT POSTURE. THE SCM SHOULD TEST
WEAK ON THE TRAILING LEG SIDE.

of the six gait positions listed above is likely at fault.
In *Applied Kinesiology Synopsis,* pages 163–164,
David Walther suggests that the muscles that failed
to appropriately weaken may have an active stress
receptor requiring treatment. Stress receptors are not
discussed in this book.

The right arm and left leg forward stance causes
the following muscles to be inhibited on the right side
and facilitated on the left side:

Latissimus dorsi
Sternocleidomastoid
Posterior deltoid
Triceps
Psoas
Rectus femoris
Tibialis anterior
Hand extensors
Foot flexors

The same right arm and left leg forward stance
causes the following muscles to be inhibited on the
left side and facilitated on the right side:

Upper trapezius
Anterior deltoid
Pectoralis
Biceps
Gluteus maximus
Piriformis
Hamstrings
Gastrocnemius
Hand flexors
Foot extensors

DISCUSSION

Shoes can improve or disorganize the gaits. The examiner should test the patient in weight bearing, both
barefoot and while wearing various pairs of shoes.
Inserts to correct leg length can improve or disorganize the gaits and should similarly be assessed.

A child with gait problems runs with discoordination and is often made fun of by the other kids. He
may then decide that sports are not for him and concentrate exclusively upon mental studies. This can disturb his self-image and lower the quality of his whole
life experience. Correcting the gaits can make a great
improvement in the quality of life.

Case history: A 45-year-old, extremely dyslexic
patient had both mental difficulties and physical discoordination. He wore special pants because he often
wet his pants uncontrollably. His wife made fun of
him and his personal image was *am Arsch* (German
for "on his butt"—really down). When he lifted an
arm, all leg muscles on both sides tested weak. When
he lifted a leg, all arm muscles tested weak on both
sides. He always wanted to learn to swim, but the
simultaneous coordination of arms and legs needed
was beyond his capacity.

With concentration, he was able to learn to do various contralateral gait (cross crawl) movements. He
went to the swimming pool, performed various cross
crawl movements corresponding to the various gait
motions and tests, rubbed the reflex points on his feet,

and again did cross crawls (self-correcting his gaits). He then got in the water and learned to swim in one hour. He returned to the examiner with a look of great pride in his eyes (like a child who says, "Look, Mommy, at what I can do!") and told of his success. The best part, he said, was that he had control of his prior problem and could now correct it "with my own hands."

The following paragraphs provide useful information that is not standard ICAK practice:

When the anterior gait tests weak, the patient has difficulty "stepping forward" out of current conditions toward desired conditions. Correcting the gaits may give the patient more ability to overcome inertia, fear, etc., and positively act so as to achieve desired goals. Testing the emotion involved with the dysfunctioning gait will give the examiner information that can be utilized for helping the patient to receive a psychological assist in parallel with the physical treatment of the gait.

Eliminating Gait Imbalances with Fluorite (Mineral) and Pink Ivory (Wood)

David Walther recommends that patients take off their watches and jewelry before being muscle tested, as these can "change the results of muscle testing." Fascinated by this observation, I tested gemstones and minerals to see if they indeed do change the results of muscle testing. The results are included in my doctorate thesis, *The Effect of Gemstones upon Human Neurological Functioning.*

I discovered that the mineral fluorite (CaF_2) and the South African wood pink ivory (*Berchemia zeyheri*) will eliminate any positive gait tests. This is not a correction of the gaits but is an effective antidote that works as long as the patient is within about 5 mm of the mineral or wood. Direct contact is not required, so the effect is not chemical. As the effect occurs at a distance, there must be a field effect at work. Because neither the wood nor the mineral have a measurable electromagnetic field, the field seems likely to be the human body.

Many such examples of gems, woods, herbs, and other substances eliminating imbalances detected by muscle testing have been discovered and confirmed. Carrying the tested substance can act as a "stress buster," giving the patient the ability to handle higher levels of stress without his typical energetic imbalances occurring. Although such substances do not correct imbalances, they do act as effective "crutches" to get the stress off a particular problem while healing is taking place. The use of energy-balancing substances has also proved valuable for athletes and others who seek high levels of performance.

Those interested in this fascinating and as yet unexplained phenomenon are invited to contact me for further details.

Cloacal Synchronization

Long before humans appeared on this earth, our ancestors went through a stage in which the excretory and reproductive function shared the same orifice. Snakes and chickens are examples of animals that still maintain this structure: one hole for both functions.

During prenatal development, the human fetus goes through what appears to be a recapitulation of the evolutionary process. At early stages, the human fetus has gills and a tail—and looks like a combination of a fish and a reptile. Although we no longer have a cloaca, primitive cloacal reflexes from these earlier stages of evolution still exist in humans and other animals.

The cloacal reflexes can be elicited by stroking a cat down its back to its tail. It is the cloacal reflex that causes the cat to lift its tail and straighten the back legs when so stroked. When a cow is touched on the outer side of its buttocks, it moves away from the stimulus. However, when a cow is touched on the inner side of its buttocks, the cloacal reflexes move the buttocks toward the stimulus. This reflex surely has one effect—that of assisting sexual intercourse to successfully occur. Evolutionary selection favors any factor that helps a species to successfully have offspring. It is likely for this reason that the primitive cloacal reflexes are still found in so many species.

In evolution, the cloacal reflexes developed long before language. It is perhaps for this reason that patients receiving cloacal synchronization often report an awareness of something ancient and may experience a kind of wordless wonder. It may be very difficult to verbalize the feelings that are generated by this correction. It involves "pre-verbal" parts of our consciousness.

The cloacal synchronization technique of Applied Kinesiology balances the energies of the cloacal reflexes (related to excretion and sex) with reflexes in the head and neck that are responsible for maintaining upright posture. So understood, it is a kind of cranial-sacral integration.

Many people have a rather dissociated relationship to their own sexuality. They live their lives more or less "in their head" until their drives take over and they live "from their pelvis" for a while. The cloacal synchronization technique can assist the patient to integrate sexual drives with intellectual self-awareness. A patient requiring cloacal synchronization may have a functional separation between the intellectual life and the sexual life. After successful cloacal synchronization, the patient may well be able to utilize the great powers of sex more consciously, integrating these two poles of human life into a functional unity. These are my own observations of the psychological aspects of cloacal synchronization.

The examiner often uses the cloacal synchronization technique to locate and correct causes of neurologic disorganization. It is believed that this technique examines the functional organization of the anterior and posterior cloacal reflexes with the visual righting reflexes, the tonic neck righting reflexes, and the equilibrium reflexes of the labyrinthine organs of the inner ear. There are many Applied Kinesiology techniques that seem to affect the function of these reflexes. What is known for certain is that when these reflexes are not functioning properly and not working together in harmony, homeostasis is disturbed and general integration of the body is negatively affected. Establishing cloacal synchronization can eliminate recurring problems of neurologic disorganization or "switching." Cloacal synchronization helps get the head upright and balanced upon the neck, spine, and pelvis below.

Like gait testing, cloacal synchronization tests an arm and a leg simultaneously. The examiner has two choices. He can first test the individual arm and leg that will be used in the cloacal synchronization tests, correcting any imbalances he finds with standard AK techniques. Or he may directly perform the cloacal synchronization double tests. In this case, should any of the double tests show weakness, he must test the individual limb that tested weak to make sure it is strong when tested alone. If not, he must correct it and repeat the double test. Otherwise, the examiner may falsely assume that the cloacal synchronization requires correction when the problem is actually only with a single limb. Both methods are described below.

Pretests: Testing the Individual Limbs First

1. The patient lies supine and lifts one arm up off the table and over his head. Test the arm in both directions: pushing it down and pulling it up. Repeat with the other arm.

2. The patient lifts one straightened leg about 30° up off the table. Test the leg, both pushing it down and lifting it up.

3. Any weakness on these single tests must be corrected before proceeding.

4. After all the single tests of pushing the arms and legs down and pulling them up test strong, the actual cloacal synchronization tests may begin.

Cloacal Synchronization Technique

Assessment:

1. The patient lifts the right leg about 30° from the table and the right arm up over the head, also about 30° from the table. Test both limbs by simultaneously pushing them down toward the table. Then test both arm and leg by pulling them up.

2. Repeat the same pushing down and pulling up tests with all four combinations of arms and legs (R-R, R-L, L-R, L-L), noting any weaknesses. Test all eight possible combinations. Pushing the arm

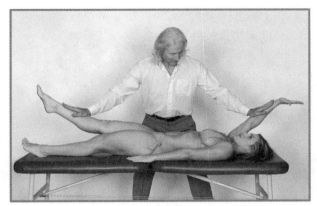

CLOACAL TEST: IPSILATERAL, PUSHING DOWN

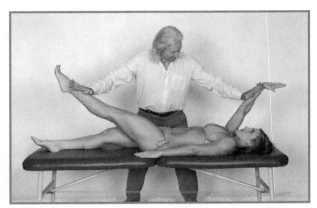

CLOACAL TEST: CONTRALATERAL, PUSHING DOWN

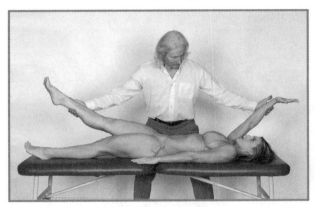

CLOACAL TEST: IPSILATERAL, PULLING UP

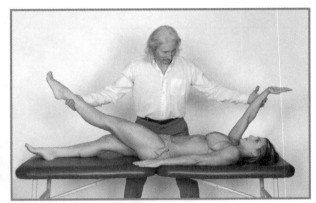

CLOACAL TEST: CONTRALATERAL, PULLING UP

and leg down tests the flexors. Pulling the arm and leg up tests the extensors.}

3. If a weakness is found on the pushing-flexor tests, use therapy localization to test each of the anterior cloacal reflex points located about one inch to the right and left of the center of the pubic bone. One of these points should be active. Then use therapy localization to locate the active visual righting reflex point located in the notch above the inner corner of each eye. One of these points should be active.

4. If a weakness is found on the pulling-extensor tests, use therapy localization to test each of two posterior cloacal reflex points, located on the right and left side of the junction of the coccyx and the sacrum. One of these lower points should be

active. Then test both the labyrinthine (at the mastoid process) and the neck righting reflex points (under the mastoid process between the occiput and the atlas, the atlas and the axis, and sometimes between the axis and the third cervical vertebra) right and left. One of these four upper points should be active. Note that therapy localization of all three positions of the neck righting reflex points can be performed simultaneously by touching along the side of the upper neck with three fingertips. If this TL is active, use a single point TL to determine the precise active point.

5. If active reflex points are not located where expected, test all the points, anterior and posterior. One will be found on the head and one on the pelvis.

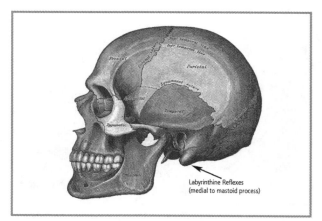

LABYRINTHINE REFLEX POINTS

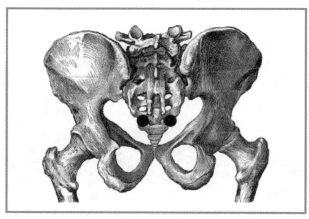

POSTERIOR CLOACAL REFLEX POINTS

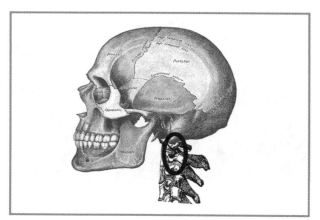

NECK RIGHTING REFLEX POINTS

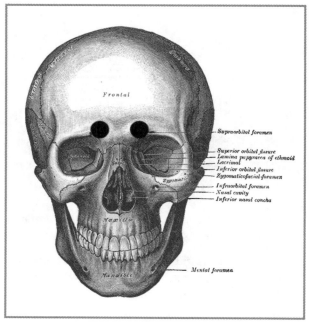

VISUAL RIGHTING REFLEX POINTS

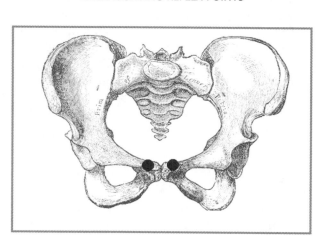

ANTERIOR CLOACAL REFLEX POINTS

Correction:

1. When cloacal synchronization is needed, there typically are powerful emotional issues involved. It is highly recommended that the examiner test the main issue related to the lack of cloacal syn-

chronization and discuss this with the patient before performing the correction. For a deeper look, the examiner can test the specific emotion corresponding to each of the two points (anterior or posterior cloacal points, visual righting, labyrinthine, and neck righting reflex points) involved in each cloacal synchronization correction. This is not a standard ICAK procedure.

2. Simultaneously hold the two active reflex points—one on the head and one on the pelvis. Contact is gentle and is held until synchronized pulsation in the two points is felt. This may take from 20 seconds to 2 minutes. Breathing in rhythm with the patient can assist the completion of the correction.

3. If the patient tested weak on both flexor and extensor tests, perform both the anterior and posterior corrections as needed.

Confirming the correction:

1. Retest the double cloacal synchronization tests that tested weak. They should now test strong.

2. If the related emotion(s) were tested before the correction, test now to see that they are no longer active (no longer weaken an indicator muscle). Double-check by stating the emotion(s) and repeating the previously weak cloacal synchronization tests.

Discussion

Walther says that if a phase of respiration (holding full inspiration or full expiration) eliminates the cloacal synchronization test weakness, the preferred correction to perform is treatment of the cranial-sacral primary respiratory system. This topic is out of the scope of this book.

Cloacal correction is indicated when switching recurs or when weaknesses reappear after walking or running. Correcting the cloacals usually does not require repetition unless there are problems with the cranial-sacral respiratory system. When walking, the sternocleidomastoid and upper trapezius muscles are alternately facilitated and inhibited. This produces a rhythmic set of pulls upon the cranium. If the gaits are out (imbalanced), these pulls can be altered, which can cause cranial faults. Correcting the gaits may be vital if cranial faults recur.

Hyoid Bone

The hyoid is the only bone in the body that is not attached to another bone through a joint. It is "free floating." The hyoid bone is shaped like a horseshoe and is located just above the thyroid cartilage of the larynx, to which it is attached by the thyrohyoid ligaments. The hyoid is attached to and serves as an anchor for the muscles of the floor of the mouth and the tongue.

The hyoid is held in place by ligaments and muscles that attach it to the jaw, skull, tongue, larynx, and even to the scapula. The hyoid is suspended by ligaments from the base of the skull (the styloid process of the temporal bone). Attached to the hyoid bone are muscles that move the tongue, larynx, pharynx, and the mandible. These muscles are involved with the processes of speaking, eating, and swallowing.

A little-known function of the hyoid is its effect as a kind of gyroscope. When any of the muscles attached to it have improper tone, the hyoid tilts. Here the gyroscope-like effect of the hyoid can be observed. When the hyoid tilts, the body segments (pelvis, shoulders, head) tend to reflect this tilt by tilting in the same direction.

Imbalances of the muscles of the hyoid can cause system-wide problems of organization. Suspect and test the hyoid whenever neurologic disorganization, gait problems, cranial faults, disorientation of body segments, or eyes into distortion are present or recur after correction.

The hyoid may cause other body segments to lose their proper orientation. Distortions of body segments will cause the hyoid muscles to adapt and thereby go out of balance. Whatever the cause, correcting the hyoid muscles may be needed for a lasting correction of the orientation of the head, shoulders, hips, and other body parts.

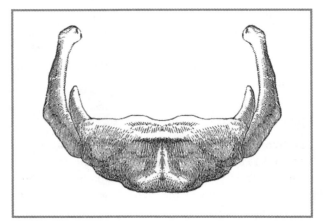

HYOID BONE

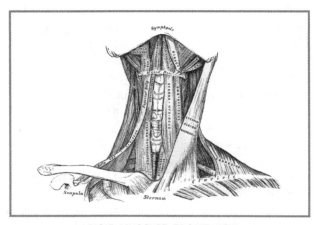

HYOID MUSCLES: FRONT VIEW

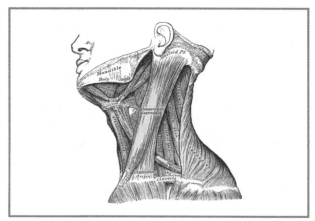

HYOID MUSCLES: SIDE VIEW

MUSCLES OF THE HYOID

The inferior hyoid muscles have their origins on the thyroid cartilage, the scapula, the clavicle, and the sternum. The inferior hyoid muscles are the thyrohyoid, omohyoid, and the sternohyoid.

The superior hyoid muscles are attached to the skull and the mandible. The superior hyoid muscles are the middle pharyngeal constrictor hyoglossus, digastric, stylohyoid, geniohyoid, and the mylohyoid.

The digastric muscle has the shape of a sling. At one end it is attached to the mastoid process. At the other end it is attached under the chin. In the middle, it has a fibrous loop of tendon that is attached to the lateral aspect of the hyoid bone.

Other hyoid muscles will not be individually discussed here. See the hyoid diagrams and the literature for the specific anatomy and function of these muscles.

HYOID TECHNIQUE

Assessment:

1. Lightly touch the hyoid with thumb on one side and first finger on the other.

2. Test an indicator muscle. If this touch weakens the indicator muscle, evaluate for injuries, skin irritations, or other pathology and correct as needed. The indicator muscle must test strong with TL to the hyoid before continuing.

3. For a group test of all the hyoid muscles, gently move the hyoid in all directions, including rotation and twisting.

4. Test an indicator muscle. If it tests weak, there is a dysfunction in one or more of the hyoid muscles.

5. Test each direction of moving the hyoid bone: up, down, right, left, rotate, tilt. For each direction that tests weak, consider which hyoid muscle was stretched. Moving the hyoid left stretches the muscles on the right. Pulling the hyoid forward and downward stretches the stylohyoid or the posterior belly of the digastric muscle.

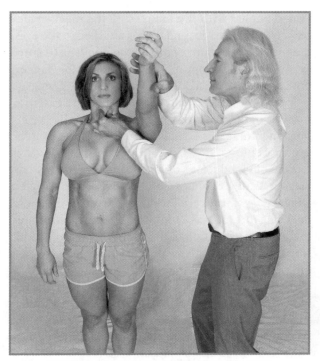

SUPERIOR CHALLENGE OF THE HYOID. THIS STRETCHES THE OMOHYOID, STERNOHYOID, THYROHYOID, AND STERNOTHYROID MUSCLES.

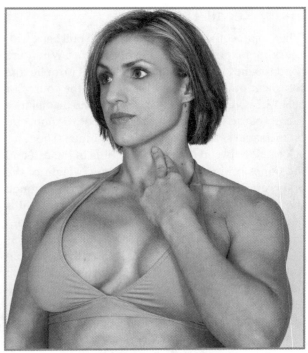

TL TO THE STERNOHYOID

6. Alternatively, stretch individual hyoid muscles by placing a finger into the muscle and pulling away from the hyoid. Immediately after stretching, test an indicator muscle for weakening. Note that some of the muscles are next to each other, partially overlapping, and difficult to fully isolate.

7. TL the belly of the suspect hyoid muscle and muscle test an indicator muscle. TL with just one fingertip and locate the position in the muscle belly that is active. Using two adjacent fingertips, one on top of the other, to make a small "test probe," eliminates any possible distortion of the test results by reason of differing fingertip polarity (this is not an ICAK technique).

Correction:

Spread the spindle cells in the belly of the muscle where the active TL was found. Use two fingertips to accomplish this. If the muscle can't be accurately contacted for this treatment, just do a general massage over the area.

Confirming the correction:

1. Repeat the previously active TL. It should now be inactive.

2. Shake the hyoid about in all directions and test the indicator muscle. If it now tests strong, the correction of the hyoid is confirmed.

Injury Recall Technique

When injured, the typical response is to pull back with a jerking response of the flexor muscles. When the hand touches something hot, the biceps (arm flexor) contracts, pulling the hand away from the source of heat. The podiatrist Robert P. Crotty found that injuries usually cause the talus bone of the foot to subluxate on the same side of the body as the injury. The talus is located between the fibula and tibia of the calf and the bones of the foot. Thus the whole weight of the body rests upon the talus and is transferred through the talus to the foot. It is possible that the talus becomes so subluxated because of the jerking contraction of the foot flexors when an injury occurs.

After an injury, until the talus is reset, the body continues to respond as if that injury is still in the acute phase. This means that even after the injured tissue has healed, stress hormones continue to be produced; and favoring of the limb, limping, and other compensations continue to occur. The increased signaling of the central nervous system caused by this perceived-to-be-current stress elevates the tone of many muscles, causing emotional disturbances (usually fear), and a body-wide stiffness and lack of flexibility.

The main exception to this rule of flexor contraction in response to injury is in the neck. When danger is imminent or an accident is occurring, the neck extensors contract, pulling the head back and elevating the shoulders. This instinctual response protects the medulla from injury. The medulla controls many bodily processes, including heartbeat and respiration. If the medulla receives a blow, heartbeat and respiration—and thus life—stops. This "startle reflex," which yanks the head back in situations of danger, can be lifesaving.

The joints and soft tissues (muscles, tendons, ligaments, facial tissues) of the neck contain more mechanoreceptors than the rest of the body combined. This concentration of proprioceptors allows the position of the head upon the neck and the neck upon the body to be carefully monitored by the central nervous system. Clearly, knowing the position of the head with relation to the body is highly impor-

tant. Coupled with the input from the mechanoreceptors in the muscles and tissues attached to the eyes, the mechanoreceptors of the neck allow us to accurately respond to capture prey and to escape danger, both vital to survival.

When the startle reflex is activated, the extensor muscles of the neck tend to remain overly tight. This tension inhibits the signaling from many of the neck proprioceptors.

One of Goodheart's original "dirty dozen" AK colleagues, Walter Schmidt Jr., DC, devised the Applied Kinesiology injury recall technique to deal with these lingering aftereffects of injuries. Schmidt postulates that normal activation of the flexors continually reinforces the old withdrawal reflex produced by past injuries. He gives the injury recall technique high priority and performs it with every new patient. He hands them a picture of a human body and asks them to mark everywhere they have had a past injury. Then he performs the injury recall technique as needed on each of these old injury sites.

The directions below are adapted from his method. Some authorities contend that the talus is the correction to perform for all injuries below the neck, and that the cervical vertebrae correction should be performed for all injuries in or above the neck. I recommend testing both talus and cervical injury reflexes for all previous injuries regardless of their location throughout the body.

INJURY RECALL TECHNIQUE: TALUS BONE

1. TL the talus bone of the foot. If the TL is active, clear it first so that it is inactive.

2. TL the area of an old injury. If the TL is active, clear it first so that it is inactive.

3. Simultaneously TL the old injury and the talus of the foot. If this double TL weakens the indicator muscle, the injury recall technique directed to the talus is indicated.

4. (alternate to step 3) Firmly tap on the heel of the foot. This gently jams the mortise joint between the talus and the tibia. The affected talus, if pres-

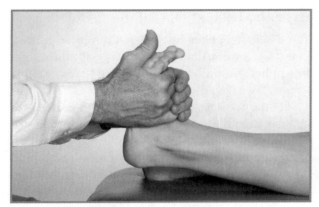

CHIROPRACTIC CORRECTION OF THE TALUS

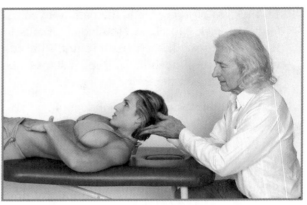

INJURY RECALL TECHNIQUE: FLEXING THE NECK

ent, is most often on the same side of the body as the injury. If the injury is medial, test both talus bones, left and right.

5. Immediately TL the old injury site and retest the indicator muscle. Weakness indicates the presence of the talus injury reflex pattern.

6. Test other injury sites in the same manner.

7. Measure the range of leg abduction by pulling the leg out to the side.

Chiropractic correction:

The chiropractic correction is as follows. The patient lies supine and TLs the injury site. The examiner stands at the patient's feet. The examiner fully flexes the patient's foot and holds it flexed with both his thumbs under the foot and his fingers crossed over on top of the foot. A corrective thrust is given by tugging the talus bone toward the bottom of the feet. The point of pressure is upon the talus bone with the little finger and ring finger of the examiner's hands.

Non-chiropractic correction:

Bruce Dewe, MD, et al. have devised a non-chiropractic correction for the talus. This is not an ICAK technique.

1. TL the injury site.

2. Take hold of, pull, and externally rotate the big toe on the side of the injury. Simultaneously pull and externally rotate the opposite thumb. The indicator muscle should now test weak.

3. Find the phase of respiration (usually full in or full out) that abolishes the indicator muscle weakness.

4. The patient holds this phase of respiration while the examiner pulls and rotates the thumb and big toe firmly several times.

Confirming the correction:

1. Again tap firmly on the heel.

2. TL the injury site and test the indicator muscle. If the TL is inactive, the correction is confirmed.

3. Retest the leg abduction. It should be greater now.

INJURY RECALL TECHNIQUE: CERVICAL VERTEBRAE

1. The patient hyperextends the neck by gently pulling it back as far as can be done without pain. Muscle test. If this weakens the indicator muscle, clear this before continuing.

2. TL the area of an old injury. If the TL is active, clear it first so that it is inactive.

3. TL the area of injury while the patient hyperextends the neck. Muscle test the indicator muscle. If it now tests weak, the patient requires the cervical injury recall technique. Repeat steps 2 and 3 for each of the other prior injury sites.

4. Test the possible range of leg abduction.

Correction:

While the patient TLs the site of injury, the examiner gently flexes the patient's head forward, nodding it several times. This is repeated for each active prior injury site.

Confirming the correction:

1. TL the injury site with hyperextension of the neck. The indicator muscle should now test strong, indicating that the correction is confirmed.

2. Test leg abduction and demonstrate the increased range of motion.

Input from the cervical mechanoreceptors forms a major part of our righting reflexes—of our awareness of our postural relationship to gravity. The cervical injury recall technique can alter our sense of balance. After performing the cervical injury recall technique, Dr. Dewe recommends "resetting the horizon" through simultaneously placing one hand on the navel, massaging the K 27s, and performing rotations with the eyes.

Ocular Lock, Eyes into Distortion, Eyes Out of Distortion

OCULAR LOCK: FURTHER CONSIDERATIONS

In Applied Kinesiology, much attention is given to cases where looking in a specific visual direction weakens most any indicator muscle. This has been discussed in the ocular lock section on pages 85–88. Ocular lock is usually connected with problems of integration between the two sides of the body and with cranial faults.

EYES INTO DISTORTION (EID)

There is another phenomenon that can cause muscles to test weak when the eyes look in specific directions. In Applied Kinesiology, this is called "eyes into distortion." When a postural distortion is present, such as a tilt of the pelvis, shoulders, or head, orienting the eyes in a direction that parallels the bodily distortion will weaken many muscles. Why is this? Any postural distortion of the body segments places imbalanced pulls upon the dura mater, which creates imbalanced tensions throughout the vertebral column and cranium.

In order to keep visual acuity, the eyes swiftly adapt to changes in body position. For example, one can read even while turning the head back and forth or tilting the head. Other righting reflexes (labyrinthine and head on neck reflexes) are not so responsive. The distortion caused by an upper cervical subluxation can cause the head on neck receptors to send incorrect information about the position of the head. Segments of the body will adjust their orientation to align with the incorrect signals from the head on neck receptors. Whatever the cause, when a segment of the body is in a distorted orientation, there are imbalanced pulls throughout the body, upsetting the delicate mechanisms of equilibrium. This can produce system-wide disorganization.

It is hypothesized that the muscles of the eyes compensate for such imbalances so as to maintain upright orientation. When the eyes are oriented into the same angle as the body distortion, this compensation is challenged or removed, resulting in a system-wide disturbance that weakens many muscles.

The direction of eyes into distortion can be determined by carefully inspecting the body language. There are eight main directions of eyes into distortion: up, down, right, left, up to the right, down to the right, up to the left, and down to the left. Up and down are active only if the distortion is only in the sagittal plane, such as hips tilted forward. If the shoulders are rotated to the right, the eyes into distortion direction will be level to the right. If the hips are tilted downward to the left, the eye direction will be down to the left. Many times, the body distortion is more complicated. For example, if the head is rotated to the left and tilted to the right, the patient can access eyes into distortion by looking down to the left and then slowly sweeping his downward oriented eye direction back to the right toward but not beyond the midline.

This phenomenon can be utilized to detect hidden problems. Visual inspection may reveal a gait problem, but testing the gaits (even in weight-bearing positions) may reveal no imbalance. In such cases, looking in the direction of distortion while retesting the gaits will cause the hidden gait problem to be revealed. Eyes into distortion will also cause hidden problems to therapy localize. Eyes into distortion produces "high-gain" therapy localization.

There is an unusual connection between eyes into distortion and the hyoid bone. This can be utilized to determine if an eye direction weakening of an indicator muscle is caused by eyes into distortion. When an eye direction weakens an indicator muscle, move the hyoid bone into the same orientation and hold it there. If this causes the eye direction to no longer weaken an indicator muscle and the other signals caused by the eye direction to disappear, the stressing eye direction is the direction of eyes into distortion.

Eyes into distortion is often secondary to hyoid imbalances. Correcting hyoid imbalances will often correct eyes into distortion and may be required for a lasting correction of eyes into distortion. For further information, see the section on the hyoid bone on pages 247–249.

Eyes Out of Distortion (EOD)

Schmitt discovered that when the eyes are oriented in the direction opposite to eyes into distortion, muscles that are weakened by the distortion become strong testing. This phenomenon is called eyes out of distortion (EOD). As discussed above, eyes into distortion is believed to remove the body's adaptation to postural imbalances and for this reason weakens muscles. Eyes out of distortion logically improves the eyes' adaptation to the imbalance and thus results in the related muscle strengthening effect.

Eyes out of distortion can be used to determine the precise orientation of the distortion of body segments, which is the eyes into distortion direction (opposite to EOD). In the unequal shoulder height example above, if looking upward to the right strengthens the weak-testing upper trapezius, then the eyes into distortion direction is downward to the left. Therefore, the left shoulder is low rather than the right shoulder being high.

Body into Distortion

The results of muscle testing are often different when the patient is standing than when sitting or lying. This may be due to the weight bearing of upright posture. Another factor to consider is the postural distortions present when the patient is standing. These may be absent when lying on the treatment table and thus be overlooked.

To find these kinds of problems, first carefully observe the patient's posture. If necessary, use eyes into distortion and eyes out of distortion to determine the precise postural deviation. Then orient the lying patient similarly and use pillows or blocks to imitate and exaggerate the postural deviations observed in standing. If the head is forward and leaning to the right while standing, have the patient lie supine. Place a pillow under her head to elevate it and lean her head over to the right. This added distortion will cause otherwise-strong-testing related muscles to test weak and thus be detected as requiring treatment.

Sometimes it is not easy to determine the parameters of body distortion. Is the shoulder high on the right or low on the left? When there is a postural distortion, there are weak-testing postural muscles associated with the distortion. If shoulder height is unequal, the muscles to suspect and test are the muscles that raise, stabilize, and lower the shoulder, including upper trapezius, serratus, subscapularis, rhomboids, levator scapulae, latissimus dorsi, pectoralis major sternal, and pectoralis minor. These should be tested to determine which one(s) test weak.

Use body into distortion:

1. whenever there are observed postural deviations, but no related imbalances can be located.

2. when patient progress slows or stops.

3. when after all tested corrections have been performed, there is still an obvious postural deviation or other symptoms.

Note also that the position of body into distortion can indicate the direction to perform chiropractic corrections of the vertebral column. A basic principle of chiropractic is to correct in the direction of the plumb line. So if body into distortion reveals a left leaning of the spine, then chiropractic corrections should be made toward the right. Vertebral challenge will reveal the ideal point of contact and vector of force to apply.

Proprioceptive Neuromuscular Facilitation

The range of motion of the joints should be equal on each side of the body. If one side is more flexible than the other, pain and dysfunctions will result. For example, daily movements such as walking with a longer stride on the more flexible side will produce an unequal pull upon the dura mater surrounding the spinal nerve. The dura mater is attached to the sacrum and to the inside of the skull. The constant unequal pull of one leg taking a longer step will cause cranial faults and system-wide problems. Stretching the side with less range of motion will reestablish bilateral symmetry and resolve many seemingly unrelated problems.

How does one stretch most effectively? Bouncing while stretching is to be avoided. Bouncing activates the proprioceptors, which cause the stretched muscle to tighten and resist the stretch. Passive, slow stretching is more effective. Prolonged passive stretches produce lasting changes in the fascia that allow a greater range of motion.

However, passively stretching has drawbacks. Passive stretching increases the range of motion of joints, but does not increase the strength of the muscles in this new range of motion. As a result, if the body suddenly slips or falls, stretching the joint into its new range of motion, the muscles may not be strong enough to protect the body from injury.

Whenever stretching a muscle, attention needs to be given to strengthen the muscle in its new full range of motion. The proprioceptive neuromuscular facilitation technique and its adaptation by Frank Mahoney in his Hyperton-X technique extend the range of motion and increase strength in this new range of motion. It is accomplished by alternating contraction of the muscle with relaxation and further extension of the muscle. By this method, the tissues are stretched and the proprioceptors are trained to allow more tension and length in the muscle before firing and causing the muscle to contract. With these techniques, more increase of range of motion can be acquired in one short session than through weeks of passive stretching.

PROPRIOCEPTIVE NEUROMUSCULAR FACILITATION TECHNIQUE

1. Place the body in a position that near maximally extends the chosen muscles and blocks the body in that position so the stretched muscles cannot shorten.

2. Contract the stretched muscles, using 80–90 percent of the available strength for 20–60 seconds until the muscles tremble.

3. Relax and further extend the chosen muscles.

4. Repeat steps 1–3 as desired.

FRANK MAHONEY'S HYPERTON-X TECHNIQUE

1. The examiner moves the patient's passive limb or other body part so as to gently bring the muscle into full extension.

2. Examiner isometrically provides resistance to keep the limb extended. Patient breathes in slowly.

3. Patient tightens the muscle being stretched to about 25 percent of maximal contraction while breathing out for about 5 seconds.

4. As patient relaxes and breathes in, examiner moves the limb to stretch the muscle farther.

5. Do this cycle of steps 3 and 4 three times.

6. After the third contraction, the patient relaxes the muscle and allows the examiner to stretch it a little farther. The patient continues to relax the muscle while the examiner passively brings it back to its resting position.

When used to correct shortness on one side of the body, give more attention to the shortened side. Apply PNF to the shortened side first. Then apply PNF more gently to the opposite side. Finish by treating the shortened side again.

Use caution with these techniques. Warm up before stretching. If the patient is not strong and in good condition, begin gently and use only a low percentage of the available strength in the muscles stretched. As the proprioceptor signaling is altered by these techniques, it is advised to avoid exercise or strenuous movement for a few hours. This gives the proprioceptors time to adjust to their new state and to be better able to respond to protect the body when needed.

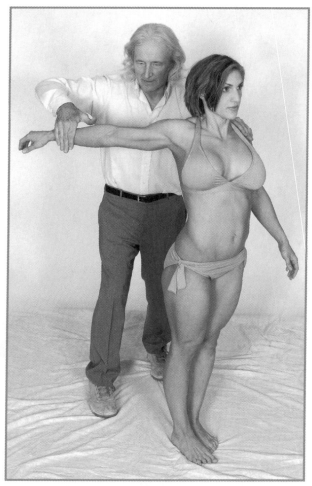

PNF/HYPERTON-X TECHNIQUE TO STRETCH
THE RIGHT PECTORAL MUSCLES

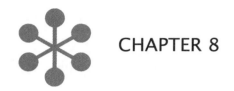

CHAPTER 8

Chemistry

The balance of chemicals in the body directly affects both the body's structure and the psyche. Using AK, the examiner can determine the nature of chemical imbalances and how to correct them. Chapter contents include:

- Substance Testing: Determine if a substance has a positive, neutral, or negative effect upon the body.
- Retrograde Lymphatic Technique: Check that the lymph system is properly draining.
- Hot or Cold?: Test whether hot or cold should be applied to a healing injury at a particular time.

Substance Testing

Substance testing is an important diagnostic tool of Applied Kinesiology. Common substances that often have a negative effect upon the body include chemicals, foods, metals, microbes, and pollens. Sources for test sets of such substances and for effective remedies are listed in Appendix X, "Contact Addresses."

When testing nutrients, supplements, medicines, and other chemicals, there are some basic Applied Kinesiology rules to follow:

Substances can be tested to determine if they have a negative, a neutral, or a positive effect upon the body.

In general, substances are tested in the way they are normally contacted. Substances consumed orally are tested in the mouth. Fragrances or air samples are inhaled. Topical creams are rubbed on the skin. This is standard ICAK protocol.

To test if a substance has a negative effect upon the body, use a normotonic indicator muscle and see if the substance weakens it or makes it hypertonic.

To test supplements and remedies that should have a positive effect upon a particular problem, the ideal indicator is a muscle that tests weak because of the problem.

If no muscle tests weak because of the problem, provoke the problem through TL or challenge in a way that makes an indicator muscle test weak or hypertonic. Use the resulting weakness or hypertonicity for testing possible remedies.

At the very minimum, any remedy to be taken should neither weaken an indicator muscle nor make it hypertonic.

Ideally, a substance to be taken (a remedy) should make a weak-testing or hypertonic muscle normotonic.

If the substance to be tested is a remedy for a particular organ dysfunction, test the muscles related to that organ. If a related muscle tests weak or hypertonic, that is an ideal test muscle to use for testing remedies.

If the intent is to determine what substances have a negative effect upon a particular organ, the ideal indicator muscle is a normotonic muscle associated with that organ. Substances that weaken the indicator muscle or make it hypertonic should be avoided.

When substances have been identified to have a negative effect upon the body, what should one do? The best plan is to avoid contact with and ingestion of those substances. Test possible remedies by placing them in the mouth with the problem substance and muscle test. Substances that, when in the mouth with the problem substance, make the indicator muscle normotonic can be used as remedies. Detoxification should be undertaken to remove metals, toxins, allergens, and other substances determined by muscle testing to have a negative effect upon the body. This may include taking remedies that counteract the tested negative effect.

If a particular organ is suspected or known to have dysfunction, but the related muscle(s) are neither weak-testing nor hypertonic, how can the examiner test for substances that have a positive effect upon that organ? Various techniques can be used to elicit hidden weakness.

Techniques to Elicit Hidden Dysfunctions and Muscle Weaknesses

1. TL over the organ, joint, or dysfunctional structure itself.

2. Eyes into distortion.

3. Body into distortion.

4. TL a treatment point for the muscle/organ and temporal tap.

5. TL two treatment points and temporal tap to detect nutritional needs.

6. TL to the organ neurolymphatic reflex points.

Organ Neurolymphatic Reflex Points

Kidneys: one inch above and to each side of the navel
Adrenals: one inch above the kidney points
Immune reflexes under the armpits
Thyroid: second intercostal space near the sternum
Heart and Lungs: third and fourth intercostal space
Pituitary: glabella
Hypothalamus: GV 21
Pineal: GV 20
Sinuses and Teeth: under the whole length of the clavicles

Stomach: six-inch-long space between ribs 5 and 6 on the left
Liver: approximately six-inch-long spaces between ribs 5–6, 6–7, 7–8
Spleen/Pancreas: 7–8 intercostal space on left, one and one-half inches lateral to the nipple
Bladder/Reproduction: pubic bone
Small Intestine: inferior to the lowest ribs, twelve inches long on each side
Large Intestine: lateral thigh from knee to hip

Michael Lebowitz, DC, discovered that TL/challenge can be made far more sensitive by performing it with the south pole of a small, strong magnet. Coloring the south pole red with paint or red duct tape will make the challenge even more effective and elicit even more hidden weaknesses. Using the red-colored south pole of a small strong magnet over an organ, the organ neurolymphatic reflex point, or any reflex point will elicit far more imbalances than TL alone. This is a good way to proceed. You can only treat what you can detect.

If a nutrient has synergists and antagonists, taking the nutrient alone may cause a deficiency in the synergist or antagonist.

Before prescribing a nutrient, consider any synergists and antagonists. Synergists and/or antagonists may also need to be taken, or the nutrient may cause a deficiency in the synergists. Some antagonists may need to be taken at a separate time of day. Learn the physiological ratios of synergists and antagonists. For example, the physiological ratio of zinc to copper is 7:1. If zinc tests well and it is to be prescribed, place copper in the patient's mouth simultaneously with zinc and retest. If the combination neither weakens the indicator muscle nor makes it hypertonic, prescribe both zinc and copper *en bloc*.

The patient may have a deficiency of magnesium because he is taking calcium. He may have a deficiency of copper because his levels of zinc are proportionally too high. In such cases, reducing the intake of a synergist or antagonist may normalize the levels of a deficient nutrient without the need for supplementation.

Although oral or nasal testing is standard ICAK protocol, direct presentation of a substance for testing may provoke an allergic reaction. Inhaling toxic solvents such as formaldehyde can cause mental confusion. Lebowitz has developed a method for substance testing that does not require direct contact. The results correlate very well with direct contact testing as reported by him and a great number of AK-using doctors. Although too new to be a standard ICAK technique, his protocol is recommended to all.

SUBSTANCE TESTING AND CONSEQUENCES

1. Find a normotonic indicator muscle. Find another muscle that tests weak (ideally one related to the organ system in question, but any weak-testing muscle will do).

2. Place the substance against the red-colored south pole of a strong magnet. Hold the substance between the magnet and GV 20. Muscle test the effect.

3. Substances that make a weak-testing or hypertonic muscle normotonic have a positive effect upon the body and ought to be prescribed.

4. Substances that weaken the indicator muscle or make it hypertonic have a negative effect upon the body and should be avoided.

5. If it is not possible or not desirable to completely avoid a substance that tests poorly, test it together with possible remedies. Locate a remedy that, when tested together with the poor-testing substance, makes the indicator muscle normotonic. Taking the remedy with the problem substance will reduce its negative effect upon the body.

6. Ideally, foods that tested poorly ought to be completely avoided for at least a few weeks. During that time, take measures to correct any dysbiosis and take any tested remedies that were found in step 5 to counteract the negative effect of the food. Then the food may be tested again. If it no longer tests poorly, it may be eaten again, sparingly at

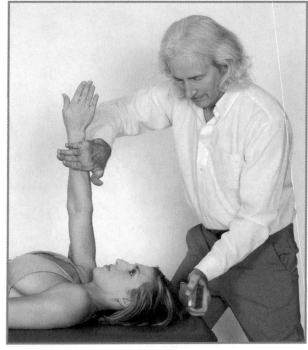

SUBSTANCE TESTING

first. Test regularly to be sure that sensitivity to the same food is not recurring.

7. To prevent recidivism, identify the sources of exposure to problematic substances and eliminate or avoid them.

Retrograde Lymphatic Technique

The lymphatic system drains toxins from the whole body. It is the slowest-moving fluid system in the body and is susceptible to partial blockage. Many times, poor posture or muscle imbalances partially close the right and/or left lymphatic ducts where the lymph from the whole body empties into the venous system under the clavicles. They have backpressure upon them from the semilunar valves that prevent blood from flowing back into the lymphatic vessels. For more detailed information, see the discussion of pectoralis minor on pages 178–179. Shortened, overly tense pec-

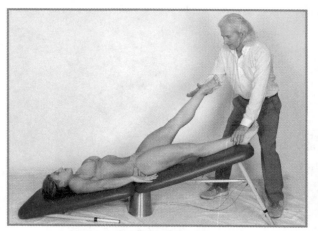

RETROGRADE LYMPHATIC TEST

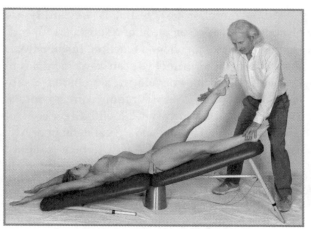

POSITIVE RETROGRADE LYMPHATIC TEST. IF
WEAKNESS IS ELIMINATED WITH HANDS OVER THE
HEAD, LYMPHATIC CONGESTION IS CONFIRMED.

toralis muscles are a common factor causing block-age of the lymphatic ducts.

Impaired lymphatic drainage is a common occur-rence. Because the lymph system removes waste prod-ucts from the body, any undue slowing of lymph drainage can increase toxicity and slow the process of healing and recovery. A variety of conditions can be caused or adversely affected by lymphatic conges-tion. Test for and correct lymphatic congestion when-ever these conditions are present or suspected: eye, ear, nose, and throat problems, upper and lower res-piratory infections such as bronchitis or pneumonia, colds, tonsillitis, problems in the extremities, joint problems, slow-healing joint traumas, grinding the teeth or shortness of breath while sleeping, edema, and frequent urination at night. Bed rest slows lym-phatic drainage. Symptoms that arise during sleep or prolonged bed rest may have lymphatic congestion as a cause.

In iridology, a "string of white beads" around the outer part of the iris of the eye indicates lymphatic congestion. Use a good hand lens and look for this telltale sign in the eyes of patients suspected to have lymphatic congestion. This is not an ICAK protocol.

The standard Applied Kinesiology test for poor lymphatic drainage through the lymphatic ducts is called the retrograde lymphatic technique. To per-form it, have the patient lie supine on a slant table with the head lower than the body. An adequate slant is 20°. In this position, the examiner tests a leg muscle for weakening. If it tests strong normally, but weak-ens when in the head-down slant position, lymphatic congestion is indicated.

The patient continues to lie on the slant table. If extending the arms over the head (which stretches the pectoralis muscles) causes the indicator muscle to strengthen, lymphatic congestion is confirmed. Alternately, while the patient is still on the slant table, an assistant can apply traction to the armpits, stretch-ing the pectoralis muscles and thereby relieving the pressure upon the lymphatic ducts. If this traction causes the indicator muscle to test strong, lymphatic congestion is similarly confirmed.

The slant table is considered to be the most accu-rate test for lymphatic congestion. Sometimes a slant table is not available. Although not as accurate as using a slant table, pillows can be placed under the hips of the supine patient as an alternative for this test.

While the patient is still lying in retrograde posi-tion, and before applying any correction procedure, test if low-potency vitamin A or nutritional iron in the mouth eliminates the retrograde lymphatic test weakness. If so, prescribe these and the tendency for retrograde lymphatic recurrence will be reduced. Similarly test herbs known to help lymphatic drainage such as *Vitex agnus-castus* (chasteberry), *Phytolacca decandra* (poke), *Iris versicolor, Galium aparine* (cleavers), *Baptisia tinctoria* (wild indigo), *Harpagophytum procumbens* (devil's claw), *Trifolium pratense* (red clover), *Taraxacum officinale* (dandelion), etc. Prescribe the ones that eliminate the retrograde lymphatic test weakness and test normotonic. These will assist the lymph system to drain more adequately.

Whenever this retrograde lymphatic test is positive, the pectoralis minor muscle is involved. The pectoralis minor muscles lie over the major lymphatic vessels: the thoracic duct and the right lymphatic duct. Lymph from most all of the body empties into the thoracic duct, which ends with a high arch before attaching to and emptying into the junction of the left subclavian vein and the left internal jugular. The pectoralis muscles are invested in the same fascia that surrounds the lymphatic vessels. When the pectoralis minor muscles are excessively tight, they pull the shoulders forward, round the back, and increase the pressure upon the lymphatic vessels. Usually the involved pectoralis muscles are found to be hypertonic, but they may test weak and require strengthening.

Most often, the pectoralis minor muscles test strong, but after a swift stretching they test weak. To stretch the pectoralis minor muscles, the examiner can pull the patient's shoulders up and back. Or the patient can accomplish the same stretch by pulling her shoulder blades together with a swift contraction of her rhomboids and upper trapezius muscles. Treatment of the muscle stretch response of the pectoralis minor muscle usually requires the fascial release technique. Also, test pectoralis major clavicular and sternalis for the muscle stretch response and treat as needed. Muscle stretch response and fascial release are described on pages 130–131.

When the antagonists to pectoralis minor, the lower trapezius muscles, test weak, their weakness will cause pectoralis minor to become too tight. A

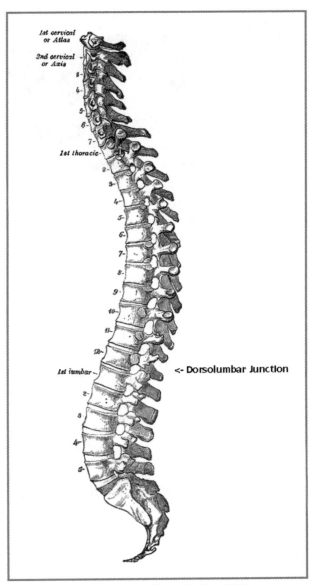

NATURAL CURVATURE OF THE SPINE

fixation of the vertebrae in the dorsolumbar junction (T10-L2) will cause the lower trapezius muscles to test weak. A lasting correction of hypertonic pectoralis minor muscles may require releasing this fixation through chiropractic or other methods.

Most acute injuries to the spine occur in the cervical spine and in the dorsolumbar junction. This is an unstable area of the spine. The thoracic portion

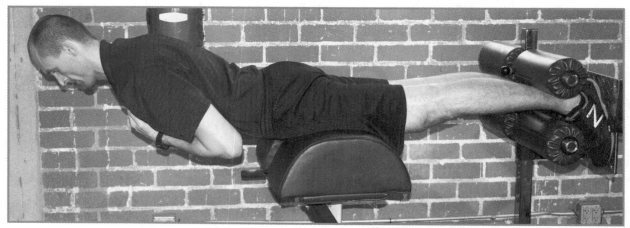

SPINAL EXTENSION. PHOTO BY SAM VISNIC.

(T10, 11, 12) has only floating ribs attached. Above T10, the ribs make the thoracic spine relatively stiff. Below, the lumbar spine is relatively flexible. This is also where the spinal curves reverse—where thoracic kyphosis meets the lumbar lordosis. Fixation in the dorsolumbar junction may be the body's attempt to protect itself where it is structurally weak. Lasting correction of this fixation may require strengthening the sacrospinalis muscles and other hip extensors, especially gluteus maximus. Sam Visnic of www.endyourbackpainnow.com reports that patients who build up adequate strength to hold the illustrated spinal extension pose for three minutes have a significantly reduced occurrence of back pain episodes as compared with individuals with poor spinal extensor endurance.

The anterior neurolymphatic reflex point for pectoralis minor (image on page 181) is located just above the xiphoid process at the base of the sternum. Firm massage (with care not to press upon the delicate xiphoid process) for about two minutes is recommended—both by the examiner and by the patient as "homework" to improve lymphatic circulation.

RETROGRADE LYMPHATIC TECHNIQUE

Assessment:

1. Patient lies supine on a 20° slant table, head down.

2. Examiner tests a leg muscle. If it tests strong in this position, the retrograde lymphatic test is negative. If the leg indicator muscle tests weak, continue to the next test.

3. Patient lifts extended arms above her head. Examiner retests the leg muscle. Alternately, an assistant pulls the patient's armpits to lift the shoulders and stretch the pectoralis muscles. If either of these causes the leg muscle to again test strong, the retrograde lymphatic test is positive.

4. Test if low-dosage vitamin A, nutritional iron, or herbs that assist lymphatic drainage strengthen the indicator muscle.

Correction:

1. Test the pectoralis minor muscle. If it tests weak, vibratory massage of the Golgi tendon organs located at the two ends of the muscle is usually effective.

2. If the pectoralis minor muscle tests strong, swiftly stretch it and immediately test it again. Note: Pectoralis minor is often so strong and tight that it is hard to elicit muscle-weakening in the muscle itself. If this is suspected, swiftly stretch the pectoralis minor muscle and then use an indicator muscle to test for weakening. If the muscle stretch of pectoralis minor elicits weakness directly or in an indicator muscle, use the fascial release technique upon pectoralis minor.

3. Check the pectoralis major clavicular and sternalis for the muscle stretch response and if present, treat it.

4. Muscle test the lower trapezius muscles. If weak, correct—preferably by releasing any fixation in the dorsolumbar junction. Demonstrate and recommend a program of strengthening the back extensors.

5. Prescribe the nutrients or herbs that tested positive in assessment step 4 above.

Hot or Cold?

A common treatment for injuries, strains, sprains, etc., is to apply cold or heat. The general rule is to apply cold first to reduce swelling. Then, after an unspecified amount of time, heat is applied instead of cold. How can one determine which will help with a specific condition, heat or cold?

TESTING WHETHER TO APPLY HEAT OR COLD

1. TL the injured area. Test an indictor muscle. It should test weak.

2. Apply cold to the area while continuing the TL, and muscle test.

3. Apply heat to the area while continuing the TL, and muscle test.

4. The cold or heat that made the muscle test normotonic is the one to apply at this time.

5. Test again often to see which to apply at that time.

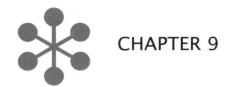

Psyche: Mind and Emotions

The psyche is the least explored of the three sides of the triad of health. In David Walther's approximately 600-page *Applied Kinesiology Synopsis,* only seventeen pages are dedicated to mental/emotional imbalances. Several further ICAK-accepted techniques are presented here to enable the examiner to identify and resolve mental and emotional imbalances:

- Emotional Neurovascular Reflex Points: Relieve stress with a hand on the forehead.
- Reversals and Conflicts: Identifying and disarming the saboteur.
- Temporal Tapping: Used to make suggestions more effective, reveal hidden problems, test nutritional supplementation, and perform certain chiropractic corrections without adjustment.
- Front Brain–Back Brain: What to do when eyes open or eyes closed changes the results of muscle testing.
- Phobias: AK adaptation of Callahan's Five Minute Phobia Cure.
- Homolateral Organization: Cross K 27 switching, hypersensitivity, and schizophrenia.

Emotional Neurovascular Reflex Points

What can an examiner using AK do for disturbances on the mental side of the triad of health? The first thing is to learn how to help the patient to reduce emotional stress. A simple technique for reducing stress is to place a hand (the examiner's or the patient's) upon the patient's forehead. This is done throughout the world by most everyone when under great stress. When highly stressed, we all put a hand upon the forehead, take a deep breath, and say something like, "Oh my God. What am I going to do?"

How does placing a hand upon the forehead reduce stress? The frontal parts of the brain deal with present-time awareness of what is. This prefrontal cortex is the area of our brain where conscious thinking and decision making take place. The functioning of the prefrontal cortex allows us to choose to act or not to act upon emotional impulses. Brain physiologists believe that the prefrontal cortex gives us the ability to decide how to act. It is here that we set goals and monitor if our activities are moving us toward them or not. It is the prefrontal cortex that gives us the ability to inhibit activities that are moving us away from our chosen goals. It exerts control over other parts of the brain to keep us moving toward our goals.

The mental functioning of the prefrontal cortex appears to be free of emotion. Motivation, planning,

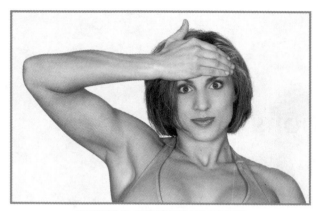

UNIVERSAL RESPONSE TO STRESS

organization, and focused attention are all functions of the frontal lobes of the brain.

When overwhelmed by emotion, we have no position of abstract isolation from which to observe. We lose the ability to function from the prefrontal cortex. We are, as it were, swallowed up by our feelings with little or no ability to see what is really going on. When our emotions dominate our mental processes, we mostly react in habitual ways. We react as we did in the past with the intention of avoiding pain. It is hypothesized that placing a hand upon the forehead brings energy, blood, and activity into the prefrontal cortex. This lifts us out of our feelings and allows us to see our situation with perspective. This gives us the ability to inhibit automatic reactions and to decide what we will do. It reduces stress and gives us the capacity to choose.

Here is a simple test of the efficacy of placing the hand upon the forehead to reduce stress:

HAND ON FOREHEAD TECHNIQUE

Assessment:

1. Locate a normotonic testing indicator muscle.

2. Have the patient recall a onetime situation that, when thought about, still produces a small amount of stress. For this simple example, avoid extremely stressful memories. It is not desirable for the patient to have a panic attack by recalling primal scream type situations. This simple technique is not adequate for that level of stress. Check that the memory is not a major stressor. For this simple example, avoid stressful situations that occur again and again (such as doing the ironing)!

3. Have the patient recall the stressful situation and tell you when she is mentally "in it."

4. While the patient is recalling the stress, retest the previously normotonic indicator muscle. If the stress chosen is adequate for this process, the muscle will now test weak. If it tests strong, touch the acupuncture sedation point for the meridian related to the chosen indicator muscle. If touching the sedation point fails to weaken the muscle, the thought of the stress has put the patient's indicator muscle into a hypertonic state. The experienced examiner may use this hypertonic response as the starting point for reducing stress.

Correction:

1. Have the patient place her hand upon the forehead.

2. Instruct the patient to breathe deeply (another well-known stress-reducing technique).

3. Have the patient look around in all directions. Have the patient look at your hand as you make slow circles. Observe closely the patient's eyes. If the eyes skip over a specific area, move your hand back and forth over this area. Tell the patient to really watch your hand. Watch closely to be sure that the patient does. For further information about using eye circles, see the section on ocular lock on page 85. For this simple example, this step may be optional.

4. Instruct the patient to recall the stressful situation in the following way: Begin before the event. Play the memory like a videotape in fast-forward until the situation is over. Without going backward, begin again from before the stressful situ-

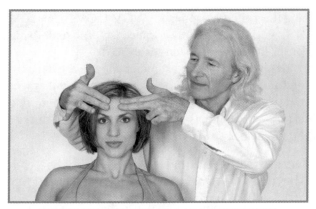

EMOTIONAL NEUROVASCULAR REFLEX POINTS

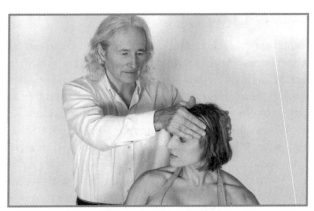

FRONTAL-OCCIPITAL HOLDING

ation and review the memory swiftly. Repeat this process until the memory has been reviewed swiftly ten times. This speeding through the memory doesn't give the patient time to "fall into" the negative emotions.

Confirming the correction:

Have the patient recall the chosen stressful situation while you retest the indicator muscle. If the correction was successful, the memory of the stress will no longer weaken the indicator muscle. If the indicator muscle was hypertonic while the stress was first elicited, it should now be normotonic.

FINE-TUNING THE EMOTIONAL NEUROVASCULAR REFLEX TREATMENT

The actual points on the forehead that are treated are the two frontal bone eminences. These are usually palpable as a bump located about two inches directly above the pupil of each eye. These were first described by Terrence Bennett and integrated into Applied Kinesiology by George Goodheart. Bennett called them "emotional points." In AK, they are referred to as the emotional neurovascular reflex points.

As with other neurovascular points, gently holding them can be effective. However, treatment of these and other neurovascular points is more effective when they are tugged gently in the direction that produces the greatest palpable pulsation under the examiner's fingertips.

As originally taught in AK, active TL to the frontal eminences can be used to indicate the need for emotional neurovascular reflex treatment. After holding the frontal eminences, TL to the frontal eminences is again performed. If the TL is no longer active, the treatment is considered to be finished. However, as Walther points out, it is considered to be more effective if the issue that is causing emotional distress is identified and considered while frontal eminence holding takes place.

FRONTAL-OCCIPITAL HOLDING

Placing one hand on the forehead and one on the back of the head helps to physically stabilize the patient, especially if performed while the patient is standing. The visual centers of the brain are located in the occiput. Placing a hand over the occiput while the other hand is on the forehead can help to release the stress stored in old visual memories. Present-time awareness occurs in the frontal lobes of the brain. Past-time memories are stored farther back in the brain. Frontal-occipital holding is a variation of emotional neurovascular reflex point holding and is recommended for relieving stress from events that occurred in the past. Frontal-occipital holding may be performed by either the examiner or the patient. This is not an ICAK technique.

Practical Applications

When experiencing emotional distress, hold the frontal eminences and breathe deeply! Before going into action, hold your emotional neurovascular reflex points, look around, breathe, consider how you would like to act, and allow the stress to diminish and subside.

When stressed, everyone tends to repeat habitual behavior. If it is your choice to act in a novel, creative way, reduce your stress first.

When you get into a heated discussion with someone, carefully watch her eyes. When white appears under one pupil, she is going into distress. When white appears under both pupils, she is so stressed that it makes no sense to continue the discussion. Nothing new will come of it. If you try to make a point, she will likely react like a cornered animal, lashing out. Instead, take a break, do something fun, and un-stress both of you!

If your partner also knows AK or is open to the idea, it is useful for each of you to hold your frontal eminences. Remember to relax and breathe deeply. Both holding the foreheads may seem so funny that you both laugh. Laughter is called the best medicine and it is an excellent way to reduce stress.

To test if an issue is emotionally stressful and could be helped with emotional neurovascular reflex point holding, ask the patient to imagine the issue while you muscle test. In this case, the patient's mental image is the challenge that is tested. If the indicator muscle tests weak, have the patient continue to imagine the issue. Hold the patient's emotional neurovascular reflex points, and retest the indicator muscle. If holding the emotional neurovascular reflex points eliminates the muscle weakness, holding the points can assist in relieving the stress. In order to most effectively relieve the stress with this simple technique, mentally imagine ways to resolve the issue while holding the points.

Holding the emotional neurovascular reflex points can reduce stress. For simple daily stresses, it works well. However useful this may be, trying to resolve more complex mental/emotional issues by holding the forehead is rather like clearing switching by rubbing the switching points K 27, GV 1, GV 27, and CV 24. It works but it is only a "quick fix." The underlying causes have not yet been resolved.

The more advanced examiner will use the hand on the forehead to determine if there is a mental aspect to any other imbalance and then proceed to muscle test other techniques to identify one that will resolve the imbalance.

Determining If There Is a Mental/Emotional Aspect to a Dysfunction

1. Examiner finds an imbalance that causes an indicator muscle to test either weak or hypertonic.

2. Patient (or examiner) places a hand on the patient's forehead.

3. Examiner retests the imbalance.

4. If the indicator muscle now tests normotonic, there is a mental/emotional aspect to the dysfunction.

Use this simple method as a screening test to determine if there is a mental/emotional aspect to a dysfunction. Then use further techniques from the mental side of the triad of health to identify and resolve such mental/emotional imbalances.

Reversals and Conflicts

This section is adapted from the practice of the psychologist Roger Callahan, founder of Thought Field Therapy and the Emotional Freedom Technique.

Callahan's original technique for psychological reversal uses only a single-arm pull-down muscle test and two possible treatment points: SI 3 and sometimes SI 1. This technique has been expanded below to include two types of sabotage programs (reversals and conflicts), bilateral testing of a reliable indicator muscle, and several further treatment points.

Concerning psychological reversal, the literature states that when a patient has a psychological reversal, his conscious mind wants one thing but his subconscious mind wants something different. The patient says, "I want to get well," but muscle testing reveals that some part of him does not want this at all. To say that this is a conflict between the patient's conscious and subconscious minds is a useful model, but it is probably too simplistic to be rigorously accurate.

CONFLICTS ELICIT SWITCHING

A conflict has two sides and both want what they want. You want to eat ice cream but you want to be healthy and thin. If you do too much of one, the other suffers. Either way, one side will be unhappy. This is not an optimal state of affairs! A typical response to a conflict is switching, usually in the right-left axis. In the switched state, the wrong thing feels right. One can eat the ice cream and feel good about it. One can do the wrong thing and it feels like the right thing to do. Neurologic disorganization is a typical reaction to unresolved conflicts.

Psychological problems can interfere with the healing process. It is well documented that when someone gives up the will to live, her prognosis is poor. Conversely, when someone really wants to live and fights to do so, her prognosis is much better.

When someone is in a state of psychological reversal, it is impossible to treat her effectively. According to Callahan, this is true for any kind of treatment. If a reversal is present, that complex will block any kind of treatment from being effective. If this is true, then therapists of all kinds, including medical doctors, ought to detect and correct reversals before attempting any kind of intervention or even prescribing a medicine.

Psychological reversals and conflicts are a kind of sabotage mechanism. Unless the saboteur is located and neutralized, good work done will later be lost. Foods and other substances that have a negative effect upon the body's energy will often, when consumed, cause prior energy balances to be lost. Such "energy allergies" often cause reversals.

When suffering from a psychological reversal, the conscious mind and the subconscious mind are in conflict. The conscious mind has one opinion, and the subconscious mind has an opposing opinion.

SABOTAGE PROGRAMS RUNNING

To test for reversals and conflicts, test with both arms simultaneously. State the goal or the desired state and muscle test. If both arms hold strong on the positive statement and go weak on the negative statement, all is well and you may proceed. If your results are the opposite (both arms go weak on the positive statement, and both arms hold strong on the positive), you have a reversal. If the positive statement causes only one arm to hold strong and the negative statement causes only the opposite arm to hold strong, you have a conflict (between the two sides of the brain/body).

Look for reversals or conflicts. Callahan claims that in one of eight cases they are present. Check for them whenever another correction doesn't hold. Better still, test for reversals and conflicts as a pretest. Caveat: Even if tested for and cleared at the beginning of a session, reversals or conflicts can arise around a specific issue during the session. Whenever the work is not progressing as expected or when a correction procedure does not have the desired effect, check for and correct any reversals or conflicts.

Diagnosing reversals and conflicts:

1. Define the goal of the session.

2. Have the patient say aloud, "It is true that I want to [achieve the desired goal]."

3. Muscle test bilaterally.

4. If both sides test strong, have the patient say, "It is not true that I want to [achieve the desired goal]."

5. Muscle test bilaterally.

6. If both sides now test weak, there are no reversals or conflicts present with respect to the stated goal.

7. If reversals or conflicts are still suspected, test other aspects of the goal or phrase the goal differently, repeating steps 1–5.

8. If both sides tested weak in step 3 and strong in step 5, there is a reversal present.

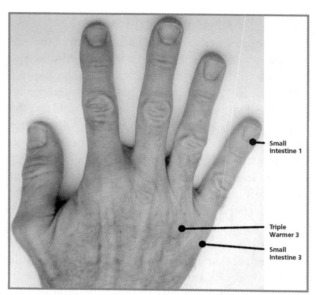

HAND CORRECTION POINTS FOR CONFLICTS
AND REVERSALS

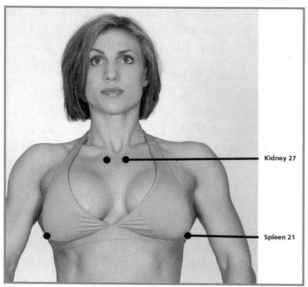

EXTRA REVERSAL POINTS

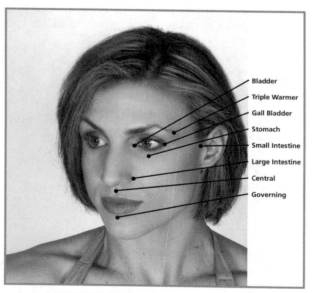

ACUPUNCTURE END POINTS ON THE HEAD

9. If one side tests strong and the other side tests weak in step 3 and/or step 5, there is a conflict present.

Correction for reversals and conflicts:

1. Repeat steps 2–5 while therapy localizing SI 3. This most often will cause strength on both sides in step 3 and weakness on both sides in step 5, indicating that there is neither a reversal nor a conflict present. If so, this is the point to use. If not, also try with TW 3, SI 1, K 27, Sp 21, or the beginning and end points of the meridians that begin or end on the face.

2. Tap the correcting acupuncture point bilaterally while

3. the patient makes full rotations with her eyes, preferably both with eyes open and with eyes closed, while

4. the patient says, "Although I have this reversal [or conflict] about [state goal or issue], I still fully accept, respect, and love myself." The patient says

this several times while making eye rotations and having the tested acupuncture points tapped.

5. All this happening at once may be a bit confusing or overwhelming to the patient. If the patient doesn't sound very convincing after a few attempts, ask the patient to pause, and explain to her, "This means something like, 'Although I am kind of crazy about my [goal or issue], I still totally love and accept myself.' Say it a few more times with a tone of voice that lets me know that you really mean it." While she does so, continue to tap the tested points and guide her to make rotations with her eyes.

Small Intestine 3 is the most common point needed for the correction of reversals and conflicts. Since SI 3 is on the side of the hand near the base of the little finger, Callahan suggests that the patient can repetitively "karate chop" the SI 3 points on each hand together (or against the edge of a table) during steps 3–5.

Confirming the correction:

1. Repeat diagnostic steps 1–5.

2. If you get the results listed in diagnostic step 6 above, the correction was successful.

3. Anchor the correction in by having the patient state, "It *is* true that I want to achieve [the desired goal]," and muscle test bilaterally. This statement should now test strong. Then test, "It is *not* true …" This statement should now test weak. Repeat the positive statement last, "It *is* true …," and test. This statement should test strong.

Temporal Tapping

Early practitioners of Applied Kinesiology often used palpation of the temporal sphenoidal line for diagnosis of muscular imbalances. Both sensitivity and persistence are required to master the use of the temporal sphenoidal line for diagnosis. However, this same line has several simple and effective therapeu-

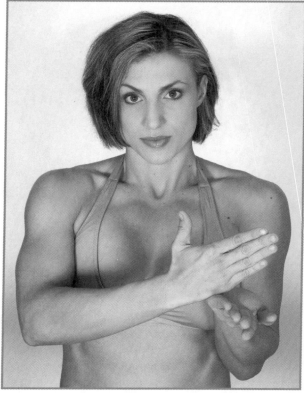

"KARATE CHOP" ACTIVATION OF SMALL INTESTINE 3

tic applications in the technique called temporal tapping. Temporal tapping can be used for extracting information from the client's subconscious mind. Its main use is in reprogramming the subconscious mind.

Temporal tapping may be used to:

1. reprogram the brain with suggestions,

2. test whether a particular muscle-meridian complex has been completely corrected,

3. test nutritional supplementation, and

4. perform certain limited structural corrections without the need for chiropractic adjustments.

Temporal tapping simplifies and increases the effectiveness of many other techniques. Mastery of its use is recommended to every practitioner of Applied Kinesiology.

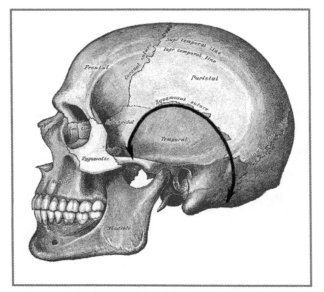

THE TEMPORAL SPHENOIDAL LINE

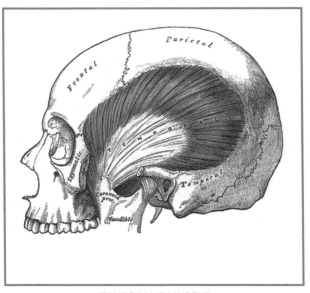

TEMPORALIS MUSCLE

Temporal tapping is performed by tapping smartly along the temporal sphenoidal diagnostic line beginning in front of the ear and continuing forward, up, and around the whole line. The tapping should be done with the palm surface of the fingertips. To perform the temporal tap upon yourself, tap the right TS line with the right fingertips and the left TS line with the left fingertips. When temporal tapping someone else, use your right fingertips (palmar surface) on their left TS line and your left fingertips on their right TS line. Tapping must be done firmly enough to penetrate curly hair or thick hairdos and to spring away from the skull after each light blow. Note that the temporal sphenoidal line begins between the temporal and sphenoid bones but continues farther around the temporal bone along the temporo-parietal and temporo-occipital sutures.

If the jaw is pulled back, or the posterior portion of the temporalis muscle (which lies over the TS line and has the action of pulling the jaw back) is overly tense (hypertonic), temporal tapping will not be effective. Therefore, observe that the patient does not pull the jaw back during temporal tapping. To test if the

posterior portion of the temporalis muscle is hypertonic, have the patient place two fingers into the belly of the muscle above and behind the ear. If this therapy localization weakens an indicator muscle, the touched portion of the temporalis muscle is hypertonic and requires spindle cell pinching to lower the tone. After such treatment, the therapy localization to the belly of the temporalis muscle will no longer weaken the indicator muscle, and temporal tapping should function normally.

A main effect of temporal tapping is to inactivate the brain's censoring mechanisms so that some chosen input may have a more powerful effect. Suggestions given while temporal tapping have a more profound effect. In a normally organized person, positive suggestions are given while tapping the left side. Negative suggestions ("There is *no* need for …") are given while tapping the right side.

Use of the following test will determine if temporal tapping can be effectively utilized and how it must be performed. Find a normotonic indicator muscle. Tap the left TS line with the palm surface of your right fingertips. While tapping, say aloud, "This muscle now tests weak," and retest. If the muscle does now test weak, the patient is normally organized and may be temporal tapped as described in this text.

Temporal tapping may be used to determine if all the factors directly affecting a muscle-meridian complex (the neurolymphatic and neurovascular reflex points, meridian alarm points, etc.) have been adequately treated. A muscle may test strong in the clear, yet test weak when one of its treatment points is touched. Because it tests strong in the clear yet can be made to reveal hidden problems, this condition is called a hidden muscle weakness. Using normal techniques, it would be necessary to test all of the possible treatment points to a specific muscle to be sure there are no hidden weaknesses. This technique may be simplified with temporal tapping. To do so, first see that the muscle tests strong while the patient touches any one of the related treatment points. Then while having the patient continue to touch the treatment point, the TS line on the left side is tapped.

If the muscle weakens after the tapping, there is a hidden weakness that can be located and treated. To do so, each of the treatment points is therapy localized, one at a time, and the muscle is tested. The ones that cause the muscle to test weak require further treatment. When all hidden factors have been correctly dealt with, touching a treatment point and tapping the left TS line will no longer weaken the muscle. Thus all direct influences affecting the muscle-meridian group may be detected in one test with temporal tapping.

Through experimentation, a way to use temporal tapping to determine the need for nutritional factors to correct muscle weakness has been found. To do so, first be sure that all neurolymphatic and neurovascular reflex points and meridian alarm points for the chosen muscle test strong. Next, have the patient touch two of these points simultaneously, temporal tap the left TS line, and retest the muscle. If the muscle now weakens, some sort of nutritional supplementation is required.

Check a list of possible nutritional supplements for the particular muscle. Nutritional supplements for specific muscles are given in this book and in Walther's *Applied Kinesiology Synopsis*. Have the patient chew

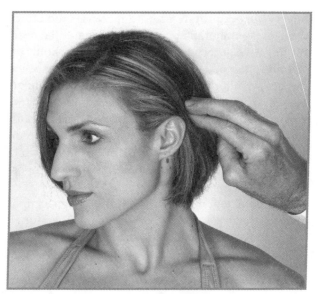

TAPPING THE TEMPORAL SPHENOIDAL LINE: LEFT SIDE

one supplement after another until a supplement is found that causes the muscle to return to strength (with the double therapy localization and the TS line tapping). This is the needed nutritional factor.

Temporal tapping is sometimes effective as an alternative to chiropractic corrections. After diagnosing a specific structural problem, the patient is put into the position proper for chiropractic correction (for example, with the pelvis correctly placed upon treatment blocks for the correction of pelvic faults). Then, instead of adjusting the fault by chiropractic manipulation, temporal tapping is provided upon the left side of the head. Often, without further treatment, the desired adjustment is accomplished automatically.

It appears that temporal tapping alerts the nervous system to the need for the correction indicated by the treatment position. The nervous system then corrects the structural problem without the need for chiropractic adjustment.

This use of temporal tapping has been developed and applied to various problems by Bruce Dewe, MD, in his Professional Kinesiology Provider program. This is not an ICAK technique. Dewe finds that the inclusion of the emotional finger mode (thumb to ring finger) plus eye rotations both increases the effectiveness of temporal tapping and eliminates the need for negative affirmations. To perform this, hold the thumb to the pad of the ring finger. Fold the other fingers together around the thumb and ring finger. Use all of the fingertips as a little hammer. Dewe reports success with his technique of tapping both sides simultaneously while the patient holds the emotional finger mode and performs eye rotations while the examiner stimulates the problem or gives a positive affirmation only.

Temporal tapping has so many useful applications that its practice and mastery is recommended for all Applied Kinesiology practitioners.

Front Brain–Back Brain

Many problems can only be accessed when the eyes are open or closed. When the eyes are open, the occipital and temporal cortices are accessed. When the eyes are closed, the frontal lobes and the temporal cortex are accessed.

Any imbalance that registers only when the eyes are open or closed, but not both, may be treated with this method. If eyes open causes the imbalance to be active, tap over the occiput. If eyes closed causes the imbalance to be active, tap over the top of the frontal bone. The tapping with eyes open or closed may need to be performed while the original correction is repeated.

It is advised after other corrections (that were performed with the eyes open) to test if closing the eyes makes the problem return. If so, use the front brain–back brain technique to clear this imbalance.

Phobias

Psychological dysfunctions are often the result of disturbed physiological function. Roger Callahan's popular treatment for phobias demonstrates this truth clearly.

Before treating any phobia, it is vitally important to check for and clear any psychological reversals or conflicts (see pages 268–271). Psychological reversals will sabotage other work.

Callahan discovered that phobias are energetic disturbances of specific meridians. The stomach meridian is usually the culprit. The kidney meridian is the next most popular one.

The treatment described here is David Walther's AK adaptation of Callahan's "Five Minute Phobia Cure." Extra techniques that bring up hidden problems are included to make the treatment more effective.

After treatment, have the patient confront the actual phobia as soon as possible. If possible, do it during the treatment session to stabilize and confirm the correction.

Phobia treatment:

1. Check for and clear any psychological reversals.

2. Use the pectoralis major clavicular as an indicator muscle.

3. Have the patient think of the phobia and test the PMC. It should weaken.

4. If it does not weaken, there is a psychological reversal or conflict about the phobia. Clear this by using the statements "I want to be free of my fear of [name the phobia]" and "I want to keep my fear of [name the phobia]." Perform this as described in the section on reversals and conflicts on pages 268–271.

5. When this reversal or conflict is cleared, thinking of the phobia should weaken the PMC.

6. While the patient thinks of his phobia, touch the stomach meridian alarm point, and retest. It the PMC now tests strong, the phobia is associated with the stomach meridian.

7. If thinking of the phobia plus touching the stomach meridian alarm point does not strengthen the PMC, test the other alarm points until the one that does is located. A graphic of the alarm points is in Appendix III on page 294.

8. Have the patient self-rate on a scale of 1–10 the level of discomfort he experiences when thinking of his phobia.

9. While the patient thinks of the phobia, tap the beginning and end points of the affected meridian. A graphic of the end points of the meridians is in Appendix III on page 295–296.

10. Repeat step 3. If the treatment was effective, the PMC should now test strong. If not, check for and correct any further reversals or conflicts.

11. Have the patient activate his right brain by humming an improvised tune. He should simultaneously hum and think of his phobia as you test the PMC. If this weakens the PMC, TL the affected alarm point again. If this tests strong, repeat the treatment while the patient hums.

12. Have the patient activate his left brain by doing mental mathematics out loud while thinking of his phobia. If this weakens the PMC, TL the affected alarm point again. If this tests strong, repeat the treatment while the patient thinks of his phobia and performs mental mathematics out loud.

13. Test the PMC while the patient thinks of his phobia while looking in the direction of eyes into distortion. Repeat this procedure with body into distortion. If either of these weaken the indicator muscle, repeat the same correction—this time with eyes into distortion (or body into distortion if that tested weak).

14. Have the patient again self-rate his level of discomfort while thinking of the phobia. If it is down to 1 or 0, confront the patient with the object or activity of his phobia to confirm the correction. If the phobia is still present (with a discomfort level of 2 or more), check for and correct any reversals or conflicts and repeat the treatment. Some reversals and conflicts may arise only during the treatment process. Sometimes the residual stress is in a different meridian. If so, test and treat the new meridian involved.

15. Instruct the patient on how to tap the affected end points. He can do this later if the phobia should again arise. He can also do this later if the phobia requires an activity (like flying on an airplane) that can't be elicited by the examiner during the session.

Homolateral Organization

Cross crawl movements (gait motions with arm and contralateral leg) generally improve functioning. They are often helpful for those who have neurologic disorganization. Practicing cross crawl movements requires that both sides of the brain function at the same time in a coordinated manner. Performing the contralateral physical movements usually helps to integrate the function of the two halves of the brain.

Goodheart noticed that some patients are weakened by performing normal gait movements (cross crawl) with one arm and the contralateral leg. In these same patients, making homolateral movements (arm and same leg) causes weak-testing muscles to strengthen.

These homolaterally organized individuals have an active TL to the Kidney 27 points, but only if the hands are crossed over so the left hand touches the right K 27 and the right hand touches the left K 27. Care must be taken so the right and left hands do not touch each other and "short-circuit" the signal. Care must also be taken that K 27 is precisely touched. K 27 lies immediately caudal to the sternoclavicular joint at the point where the sternum, first rib, and clavicle meet.

All AK tested schizophrenics have been found to be homolaterally organized and have an active cross K 27 therapy localization. However, not all homolaterally organized individuals are schizophrenics.

The simplest and most accurate diagnostic technique for schizophrenia is the Hoffer-Osmond Diagnostic Test (HOD). The short form of the test has been found to be more accurate than the long form in the diagnosis of schizophrenia. Patients with a high perceptual score may have difficulty understanding explanations. A high paranoid score indicates poor interpersonal relationships and a tendency to misunderstanding. A high score on depression may indicate the need for psychiatric care. The ratio between the

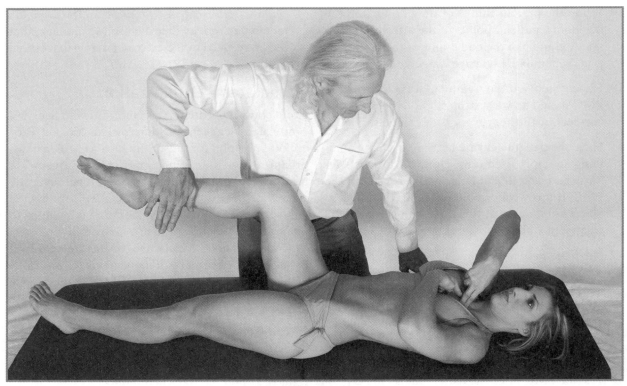

CROSSOVER K 27 TEST

total score and the depression score is the most accurate factor for diagnosing schizophrenia.

Homolaterally organized people are hypersensitive to all types of stimuli. They are easily overwhelmed.

The original AK treatment for homolateral organization (and schizophrenia) was orthomolecular supplementation with niacin or niacinamide, vitamin B6, and other substances as tested. Performing homolateral movements was also prescribed, as these are the homolaterally organized person's forte—that which strengthens them.

After performing homolateral movements for some time, the patient may switch over so that homolateral movements test weak and contralateral movements test strong. When this occurs, the crossover K 27 test will no longer be active, and symptoms of hypersensitivity (and schizophrenia if present) will be absent. It is important at this stage to cease making homolateral patterning movements as these can

bring back the former imbalances and symptoms.

As the patient is not always aware of when the switch to normal organization occurs, other methods of correcting crossover K 27 and shifting homolateral to contralateral organization were sought. Techniques for correcting neurologic disorganization can work for crossover K 27 as well. The technique found to correct most cases of crossover K 27 is cloacal synchronization. Cranial and pelvic corrections that correct cloacal synchronization are the most effective and lasting corrections for crossover K 27. Other factors to check include gait, foot, and dural tension. Many patients shift to normalization with such structural corrections. Others need to chew niacin or niacinamide, or vitamin B6. Some need both.

After eliminating crossover K 27, the usual tests for neurologic disorganization should be made, and any imbalances found should be corrected using the standard methods.

CHAPTER 10

Diagnostic Protocol

Standard Applied Kinesiology Diagnostic Protocol

How does the AK examiner know where to start with a patient? Should the examiner check for structural dysfunctions first? Does the patient need specific nutrients? Are there mental/emotional issues to clear?

There are many approaches to answering the question of how to test and treat a patient with Applied Kinesiology.

George Goodheart advised examiners to "fix what you find."

The standard AK protocol is to first gather information from anamnesis, laboratory tests, and body language observations. Then make educated guesses, and use muscle tests, challenges, and TL to find what there is to do. Then do it. This protocol is very general. Some examiners may still find it difficult to decide where to start and how to proceed.

Let's say the patient's presenting problem is painful tension in his right upper trapezius with the shoulder elevated on the side of pain.

Body language gives possible points of entry. One high shoulder may indicate an ipsilateral hypertonic upper trapezius, an ipsilateral hypertonic levator scapulae, an ipsilateral hypotonic latissimus dorsi, or a contralateral hypotonic upper trapezius. There may be excess tension pulling the hyoid out of balance, causing the body segments to slant parallel to the imbalanced hyoid. There may be a short leg on one side, which is slanting the pelvis. Dural tension and other tensions from the slanted pelvis may be pulling one shoulder down. The tight upper trapezius could be a reactor muscle, turning off its ipsilateral antagonist, the latissimus dorsi, and then tightening up to take up the slack.

Even when the high shoulder has been diagnosed as a hypertonic upper trapezius, is this primary or secondary to a hypotonic latissimus dorsi? Is the hypertonic upper trapezius caused by an old injury? Is toxicity or nutrient deficiency causing the excess tension? Is the signaling from muscle proprioceptors overstretched in a past accident causing the excess tension? Is the phenomenon of muscle memory creating the patient's excess tension in an effort to "be ready" in case a similar accident happens again? Is a lack of hydration causing the upper trapezius, which is associated with the kidney meridian and water handling, to painfully tighten? Is the patient protecting himself from danger, real or imagined? Are several of these causes at work simultaneously?

With experience in interpreting body language, the examiner learns to judge the likely cause for the observed postural imbalances and uses this knowledge to guide his approach.

Doing most any correction will make a weak-testing muscle test normotonic, at least temporarily. Spindle cell pinching will often relax a hypertonic muscle and make it normotonic. But is the cause correctly treated or will the tension return there or elsewhere? How does the examiner find further work that needs doing if the muscle is now normotonic?

These are questions facing the examiner as he begins to correct the imbalances he finds.

A wise approach is to use temporal tapping after any correction to reveal hidden, subclinical weaknesses in the muscle. Eyes into distortion and body into distortion will also bring hidden weaknesses to light. Clearing all the hidden weaknesses will go far toward correctly treating the causes.

Screening techniques can help the examiner to determine what needs to be done.

STRUCTURAL SCREENING

Structural screening is accomplished by observing body language. Muscle testing with TL and challenge will reveal what to do.

If a particular body part has a dysfunction, test and correct all muscles directly connected to or affecting that body part. Have the patient then stand and move. Then test all the muscles that were in an imbalanced state again. Retest all these muscles during the next session as well. Those that again test weak (or hypertonic) after motion or again during the next session indicate a need for further diagnostic work to locate the cause.

Consider any hypertonic testing or tight/painful-feeling muscle to be a reactor muscle. Locate the reactive muscles it is turning off, and correct this reactor-reactive relationship as explained in the section on reactive muscles on pages 131–138. This is a very effective technique for painful muscles and joints with a limited range of motion.

Check for bilateral symmetry in the range of motion of the same muscle and related joint(s) on each side of the body. If the range of motion is not identical on the right and left sides of the body, use the proprioceptive neuromuscular facilitation technique to increase the range of motion on the side with more limited range of motion. Also train the patient to continue using this technique as homework. This will equalize the tension that the muscle exerts on the two sides of the body and will thereby eliminate many pains and problems.

MENTAL/EMOTIONAL SCREENING

Begin with a weak-testing muscle. The muscle may be one that tests weak in the clear. Alternately, weaken an indictor muscle through TL or challenge.

If placing a hand on the forehead strengthens the muscle, mental/emotional work is needed.

HIDDEN WEAKNESS SCREENING

Nearly any muscle-strengthening technique can make a weak-testing muscle test normotonic. How can the examiner determine if there is more to do to fully treat all imbalances that may be affecting that muscle?

The standard method to test for hidden weaknesses is to TL and muscle test every treatment point for the muscle. This process can be awkward and time-consuming. Through the use of temporal tapping, all direct influences affecting the muscle and its associated meridian can be detected in one step.

Even when there is obvious dysfunction in an organ or gland, the related muscle may test normotonic. Hidden problems can be detected in a muscle that tests normotonic in the clear. Temporal tapping can be used to reveal any subclinical weakness or weaknesses hidden by compensations. This method can be used anytime a muscle tests normotonic, whether corrections have been applied or not.

Use this method to locate hidden weakness for any normotonic muscle. If testing an organ or gland, use the related muscle. Touch one of the main treatment points for the muscle (neurolymphatic, neurovascular, or origin-insertion) and test. The muscle must test normotonic with the TL. Then continue the TL, tap the left TS line, and retest. If this does not weaken the indicator muscle, there are no hidden weaknesses. If the muscle now tests weak, there is a hidden problem. To determine which one is active, individually TL each treatment point, including the neurolymphatics, neurovasculars, neuro-emotional points, origin and insertion, spindle cells, Golgi tendon organs, acupressure points, associated points, etc., and retest the muscle as each one is TL'd. The ones that test weak require treatment.

When all the hidden factors have been treated, TL with left-side temporal tapping will no longer weaken the muscle.

Should the muscle weaken or other related problems return after treatment, possible indirect causes such as reactive muscles, cranial faults, neurologic disorganization, or imbalances from any of the three sides of the triad of health must also be evaluated and treated for lasting results.

CHEMISTRY SCREENING

Start with a normotonic muscle or perform minimal corrective procedures (such as spindle cell stretching) so the weak-testing muscle tests strong. TL the related neurolymphatic reflex point, neurovascular reflex point, and alarm point one at a time and test to be sure they are not active. TL two of these three points, temporal tap the left side of the head, and retest the muscle. If it now tests weak, chemistry work (nutritional support) is needed. The substance that, when chewed, makes the test with double TL and left-side temporal tapping normotonic is the nutrition that is needed.

Use the standard AK protocol and the screening techniques to determine what to do. After each completed step, use the hidden weakness technique to locate and correct further imbalances that do not appear in the clear.

As George Goodheart wrote in the foreword,

The name of the game, to quote a phrase, is to get people better. The body heals itself in a sure, sensible, practical, reasonable, and observable manner.... Man possesses a potential for recovery through the innate intelligence or the physiological homeostasis of the human structure. The recovery potential with which he is endowed merely waits for the hand and the heart and the mind of a trained individual to bring it into manifestation, allowing health to come forth....

This benefit can be performed with knowledge, with physiological facts, with predictable certainty. It should be done, it can be done, and this book offers a means and a measure of how it can be done.

APPENDICES

I. Glossary of Anatomical Terminology

In defining the origin and insertion of muscles upon bones, I have not always used the correct anatomical nomenclature. In order to do so, extensive definitions of the topography of bones would have been necessary. Instead of this, I have described their physical location upon bones and the relation to known structures. For the correct scientific nomenclature of the origins and insertions of muscles, the reader is referred to anatomical texts (Walther, 1981, 1988; Leaf, 1995; Platzer, 1991).

I also attempted to describe the positions and motions for the muscle tests with everyday vocabulary such as "to the front, to the side, rotate inwardly, pull the arm back," etc. This proved to require excess verbiage and could still be unclear. For example, "up" can mean different directions, depending on the position of the body. I was able to be more clear and use fewer words by mostly using the correct anatomical terminology. For those unfamiliar with anatomical terms, a brief list of definitions is given here:

ANATOMICAL POSITIONS AND DIRECTIONS

Lateral—Of or pertaining to the side. Notice that the lateral side of the hand is the little finger side, even though the hand can invert. A lateral rotation of the arm rotates the thumb over the little finger to a position with the thumb pointing away from the body. A lateral rotation is also referred to as an external rotation.

Medial—Toward the middle. A medial rotation is the same as an internal rotation.

Internal—An internal (or medial) rotation of the leg brings the toes inward toward the medial line of the body.

External—An external (or lateral) rotation of the leg brings the toes outward away from the medial line of the body.

Anterior—Situated on the front side (in human anatomy).

Posterior—Situated on the back side (in human anatomy).

Cephalic (Cranial)—Situated or directed toward the head.

Caudal—In the direction of the tail end of the trunk or torso.

Superior—Situated on the upper aspect (toward the head).

Inferior—Situated on the lower aspect (toward the feet).

Dorsal—The vertebral side.

Ventral—The belly side.

Axillary—Toward the armpit.

Proximal—Near to, toward the middle.

Distal—Away from the center, toward the extremities. Thus the distal joint of a finger is the one with the fingernail.

Prone—Lying upon the belly. In standing posture, the pronated hand has the palm posterior.

Supine—Lying upon the back.

Flexes—Closes the joint, pulls the attached bones together.

Extends—Opens the joint, pulls the attached bones apart.

Adduct—Pull or push in medially.

Abduct—Pull or push out laterally.

Eversion—To turn outward. Used here to describe the abduction of the straightened foot and ankle caused by the contraction of peroneus longus and brevis.

Inversion—To turn inward. Inversion is only used in this book to describe the direction of the pressure applied to test peroneus longus and brevis—in the direction of adduction of the straightened foot and ankle.

THE RIB CAGE, SHOULDER, ARM, AND HAND

Sternum—The breast bone.

Intercostal—Between the ribs.

Mammillary line—A vertical line intersecting the nipple.

Xiphoid process—The small delicate bone situated caudal to the sternum.

Scapula—Shoulder blade.

Coracoid process—The anterior wing of the scapula felt on the anterior superior side of the shoulder.

Acromion—The posterior wing of the shoulder blade that is palpable as the bone on the posterior side of the shoulder. The acromion extends into a long ridge (called the spine) in a direction slightly caudal across the posterior of the scapula toward the vertebral column.

Glenoid cavity—The shoulder socket in the scapula between the acromion and the coracoid process.

Clavicle—The collar bone. The clavicle lies between the acromion and the sternum.

Humerus—The upper arm bone.

Radius—The forearm bone on the thumb side.

Ulna—The forearm bone on the little finger side.

Carpals—The bones that form the base of the hand at the wrist.

Metacarpals—The bones that form the body of the hand.

Digits—The bones of the fingers (and toes).

THE HEAD

Cranium—The skull.

Frontal bone—The bone that forms the forehead and extends one-third of the distance over the forehead toward the back of the head.

Zygomatic bone—The cheek bone.

Temporal bone—The bone under and around the ear.

Sphenoid bone—The bone between the eye and the ear.

Parietal bone—The bone above and behind the sphenoid. The left and right parietal bones meet at the sagittal suture on the top of the head.

Parietal eminence—The ridge on the superior, posterior, lateral aspect of the cranium (on the side of the top of the head, above and behind the ear).

Sagittal suture—The junction of the parietal bones running from the apex (top-center) to the top of the back of the head.

Squamosal suture—The junction of the temporal and the parietal bones.

Bregma—The anterior fontanelle (the soft spot on a baby's skull) where the frontal bone meets both parietal bones. This is found by placing the base of one's own hand between the eyes at the root of the nose. Then where the middle finger reaches upon the top of the head is the location of the bregma.

Lambda—The posterior fontanelle where the occiput and both parietal bones meet.

Lambda suture—The junction of the occiput and each parietal bone.

Mastoid process—The portion of the occipital bone directly behind the ear lobe.

Occiput—The bone in the back and underside of the back of the head.

Occipital condyles—The two knobs on the inferior occiput that sit into the two depressions (facies articularis superior) in the atlas (the first vertebra).

Vertical auricular line—An imaginary line arising vertically from the hole in the ear to the top of the head.

The Vertebrae, Pelvis, and Legs

Atlas—The first vertebra upon which the head sits. The condyles of the occiput rest in two depressions on the superior aspect of the atlas. The movement of the cranium upon the atlas is a tiny rocking movement, forward and backward, sometimes called "the atlas rock."

Axis—The second vertebra. The atlas rotates upon the axis.

Cervical—The seven vertebrae of the neck.

Thoracic—The twelve vertebrae with ribs attached.

Lumbar—The five lowest and most massive vertebrae.

Sacrum—The "keystone of the pelvic arch." The vertebral column rests upon the sacrum, which hangs on strong short ligaments between the two Ilia, the two pelvic or hip bones.

Coccyx—The tail bone at the caudal end of the sacrum.

Ilia—Plural for ilium, the pelvic bones.

Iliac crest—The edge of the "pelvic bowl," palpable as the top and front edges of the pelvis.

Iliac spine—Four small, pointed, raised areas of the pelvis.

PSIS—The posterior superior iliac spine. The top edge of the pelvis across the back from the side to where it meets the sacrum and fifth lumbar vertebra.

Ischial tuberosity—The "sit bones" at the base of the pelvis.

Symphysis pubis—The area in the front center of the pelvis where the two pelvic bones meet caudal to the navel.

Pubic crest—The superior ridge on each side of the symphysis pubis.

Tuberculum pubicum—The two protuberances 2–3 cm to the right and left of the center of the pubic bone.

Acetabulum—The hip socket into which the head of the femur inserts.

Femur—The thigh bone.

The greater trochanter—The knob at the superior lateral side of the femur, which can be felt on the side of the leg at the height of the pubic bone.

The lessor trochanter—The small knob on the medial side of the femur just below the hip socket, upon which the iliopsoas muscles attach.

Patella—The flat bone of the knee—the "knee cap."

Meniscus—The cartilage discs within the medial and lateral sides of the knee joint.

Tibia—The shin bone in the lower leg.

Fibula—The smaller, more lateral, lower leg bone.

Malleoli—The lower heads of the tibia and fibula, the ankle bones.

Achilles tendon—The large tendon connecting the calf muscles to the posterior aspect of the heel.

Calcaneus—The heel bone.

Tarsals—The bones of the mid-foot.

Metatarsals—The last bones of the foot to which the toes are attached.

Digits—The bones of the toes (and hands).

THE STRUCTURES OF A VERTEBRA

Spinous process—The most posterior part of a vertebra. The spinous process is the part that can be seen and felt sticking out of the back from the vertebral column.

Transverse process—The two side "wings" of the vertebrae.

Vertebral lamina—The area on the posterior curve of the vertebrae between the spinous process and the transverse process. They are located in the groove about 2.5 cm directly to the side of the spinous process.

Vertebral bodies—The weight-bearing portion of the vertebrae.

Intervertebral discs—The gel-filled cartilage cushion between the vertebral bodies of two adjacent vertebrae.

Vocabulary

A

Actin—Actin and myosin filaments are chemicals in muscle fibers that slide together under the stimulus from motor nerves. This is the basis of muscular contraction.

Active—An active reflex point, acupuncture point or other area upon the body is one that will therapy-localize (will change the results of muscle testing).

Acupressure—Acupuncture with only pressure applied to the surface of the skin, without needles or penetration of the skin by any object.

Acupuncture—An oriental technique of placing needles in chosen meridian points to move the Chi energy.

Adjustment—A rearranging of the structures of the body. Adjustment usually refers to chiropractic realigning of bones that are out of alignment.

Aerobic—Requiring oxygen.

Afferent nerve—Transmits nerve impulses from structures of the body to the spinal cord.

Agonist—The prime mover, which is the main muscle involved in a movement.

Anaerobic—Taking place in an absence of oxygen.

Anatomy—The study of the structures of living beings.

Antagonist—The opponent of the agonist. A muscle that works against the main muscle involved in a movement.

Applied Kinesiology (AK)—A system for evaluating and correcting bodily function that uses muscle testing as its main tool of evaluation.

Arteriole—The smallest arteries.

Artery—Blood vessels that distribute blood from the heart to the body.

Avulsion—A tearing away. Used in this book to describe the partial tearing away of a tendon from the periosteum of the bone to which the tendon is attached.

B

BB—A spherical ball about 3 mm in diameter.

Bennett's reflexes—Points used to stimulate vascular circulation in chosen body areas. Called in AK "neurovascular reflex points."

Bilateral muscle weakness—A muscle that tests weak on both sides of the body. When possible, the muscles on both sides of the body are tested simultaneously to determine if bilateral muscle weakness exists.

Biological medicine—A new movement in medicine and biology that integrates the insights of quantum and chaos theories to view and treat the patient as a whole, including his nutrition, posture, social situation and all the various areas of his life that affect his health. In biological medicine, not the cell but rather the relationship of the ground substance, nerves and cells is seen as the basic building block of the body.

Biology—The scientific study of life and living matter, including all of its forms and processes.

Biomechanics—The mechanics involved in the posture and movement of living beings.

C

Calibration—The adjusting of a device so that accurate measurements can be made. The initial muscle tests and pre-tests often performed by examiners can be considered an act of calibrating the muscle test reactions of the patient's body. Subsequent to such calibration, the results of further tests will be more accurate.

Capillaries—The smallest blood vessels, located between the arterioles and the venules.

Central meridian—The meridian that flows directly up the anterior midline of the body. Also called the conception vessel.

Central nervous system—The brain and spinal cord.

Cerebrospinal fluid—The fluid that circulates through the spinal column and around the brain, providing shock cushioning and delivering various chemicals to the brain.

Challenge—The Applied Kinesiology technique of measuring the response of an indicator muscle to some external stimulus.

Challenging a correction—The Applied Kinesiology technique utilized after a successful correction to check if the correction is complete. Usually this challenge consists of reapplying the stimulus that previously made the normotonic muscle weak, or the weak-testing muscle strong, after the correction has been made. If the stimulus can no longer change the strength of the indicator muscle, the correction was performed adequately.

Chapman's reflexes—The neurolymphatic reflex points that, when massaged, activate the drainage of lymphatic fluids from specific organs and body areas (and strengthen the associated weak-testing muscles).

Chemical challenge—Applying nutrition, medicine or other chemicals to the patient and observing the effect upon the results of muscle testing.

Chi—The Chinese name for life energy. The energy that flows through the meridians.

Chiropractic—A technique of improving health and overall functioning by improving the structural alignment of the body.

Circulation-sex—A meridian without an organ name. The function of this meridian is the circulation of bodily fluids. The circulation-sex meridian is associated with the adrenal glands and with all the reproductive organs and glands.

Compensation—The body's reaction of adjustment to a chronic problem. This may mask and effectively hide the original problem, which will no longer show up in muscle testing without special techniques (see "Hidden Problems").

Conception vessel—Another name for the central meridian.

Condyle—The rounded end of a bone that makes up part of a joint.

Connective tissue—The unstretchable tissues that give the body structural stability. This includes ligaments, tendons, blood vessels, and all types of fascia in the body. Every organ contains connective tissue that gives the organ its internal and external structure.

Cranial fault—A misalignment of the bones of the cranium.

Cranium—The skull. All the various bones that make up the head except for the jaw.

D

Dehydration—A state in which the body does not have adequate water for optimal functioning.

Double therapy localization—An accepted Applied Kinesiology technique for locating the cause of a problem. If therapy localization of a problem area makes an indicator muscle test weak, any other point therapy-localized simultaneously that makes the weakened muscle then test strong is considered to be involved as a cause (and to indicate a possible correction) of the problem.

Dysfunction—Not functioning correctly.

E

Edema—Excess fluid in the tissues.

Efferent nerve—A nerve that transmits nerve impulses from the spinal cord to other structures of the body. In this text, the efferent nerves described transmit nerve impulses from the spinal cord to the muscles.

Endocrine—A gland that produces hormones and releases them into the bloodstream.

Exocrine—A gland that produces and releases chemicals onto the internal or external surfaces of the body.

F

Facilitation—Literally "aiding." When a muscle contracts, its synergists and stabilizers are automatically contracted (facilitated) at the same time.

Fascial release—A technique to stretch and smooth fascial tissues.

Fast fibers—The white anaerobic "twitch" phasic muscle fibers that enzymatically split glucose for energy. They contract very rapidly and tire quickly.

Five-element theory—The Chinese principle of the five phases of life (active growth, maximal activity, balance, decline, rest) used in Chinese philosophy to order and understand all growth processes. Understanding and use of this principle reveals the functional unity within all phenomena.

Fixation—The locking together of two or more vertebrae maintained by unnaturally high tension in the little intervertebral muscles. Fixations may also occur between other structures of the body.

Fixation, patient—In many muscle tests, the patient must be able to hold (fix) certain body parts motionless as a platform for the testing of specific muscles.

Flaccid—Used here to describe a muscle lacking in most or all tone, usually as a result of not receiving adequate motor impulses to contract.

Flexor digitorum longus—The muscle on the anterior side of the lower leg that pulls back the toes superiorly, flexing the foot.

Fluoroscope—An x-ray machine used in the early part of this century.

Foramen—An opening, a hole through a bone such as the sacrum.

G

Gland—An organ that produces fluids which are delivered inside or upon the surface of the body.

Glucose—The form of sugar that the body uses as a source of energy. As the available glucose is used up, glycogen is transformed into glucose to replace it.

Glycogen—The body's storage form of sugar.

Golgi tendon organ—Proprioceptors in the junction where muscle becomes tendon (before connecting to bone). Golgi tendon organs measure the tension in a muscle. When the tension increases too rapidly or becomes too intense, they signal for the muscle to relax which protects the muscle (and other attached structures) from possible injury.

Governing vessel—The meridian that runs up the spine, over the head and down to the area between the nose and upper lip. It is the partner to the central meridian (conception vessel).

Ground substance—The viscous fluid-gel and the connective tissue that surrounds and interconnects all cells. The ground substance forms a network for information transfer throughout the body and determines which chemicals enter and exit the cells.

H

Hidden problem—A problem that (when therapy-localized or challenged) does not weaken a normotonic indicator muscle. This may be a muscle that tests strong in the clear because of compensation. The hidden muscle problem will only be revealed if some other particular stimulus (such as touching a reflex point, performing an activity with only one side of the brain, etc.) is presented while the muscle is tested.

Hormone—Information-carrying chemicals produced in endocrine glands and distributed through the blood. Even in very dilute concentrations, hormones in the blood influence the metabolism of specific tissues in characteristic ways.

Hypertonic—Refers to a muscle that will not test weak, even when weakened with techniques such as spindle cell pinching or TL to its sedation point. *See also* Palpatory hypertonic.

Hypotonic—Refers to a muscle that has less than normal tone. *See* Palpatory hypotonic.

I

ICAK—The International College of Applied Kinesiology, founded by Dr. George Goodheart and his colleagues in 1974.

ICAK-D—The German branch of the ICAK.

IMAK—The International Medical Society for Applied Kinesiology (Austria/Germany).

In the clear—Without the application of any extra stimulus.

In the clear muscle testing—Testing muscles in and of themselves with neither therapy localization nor challenge.

Indicator muscle testing—Using a muscle that tests strong in the clear as an indicator for some other applied stimulus.

Inhibition—The blocking or holding back of one physiological process by another. In muscle function, when a muscle is active, it lowers the tone of (inhibits) its antagonists.

Insertion—The attachment of a muscle to the bone that moves when the muscle contracts.

Intercostal—Between the ribs.

Interstitial—Between the cells.

J

Joint—The moveable articulation between two neighboring bones.

K

Kinesiology, traditional—The science of human and animal posture and movement—also referred to as biomechanics.

L

Lacteals—The small intestine's four million small, finger-like protrusions that extend into and greatly increase its inner surface area. In each lacteal are capillaries and lymph vessels that absorb digested nutritional substances.

Ligament—A strong connective tissue band providing structural stability between bones.

Ligament stretch reaction—The pathological condition revealed by an indicator muscle testing weak after the gentle stretching of a ligament.

Locking—When a muscle tests strong, one can feel it holding the joint motionless (locking the joint).

Lymph—The fluid that gathers between the cells consisting of the blood plasma that was exuded from the capillaries and waste products from the cells. The lymph also transports fats from the lacteals of the small intestine. There is about twice as much lymph in the body as blood.

Lymphatic drainage—The natural job of the lymph system is to drain lymph from between the cells and return it to the bloodstream. When the lymph system isn't doing its job well enough, techniques that assist the lymph to better drain may be applied.

M

Mechanoreceptors—Nerve receptors that measure changes that occur inside (proprioceptors) and outside the body.

Mental challenge—Applying a thought or an emotion as a challenge in muscle testing.

Meridian—Energy channels just under the skin that guide the Chi through the body.

Metabolism—All of the chemical and physical processes within an organism that make energy available and produce, maintain or destroy substance.

Modality—A mode, a method, a technique.

Motor nerve—An afferent nerve that conducts the signals from the central nervous system to the muscles, stimulating the muscles to contract.

Muscle—The meaty parts of the body that contain tissues that contract, making human posture and movement possible.

Muscle fibers—The strand-like structures that contain the chemicals actin and myosin that pull together (contract) in a muscle under the influence of a signal from a motor nerve.

Muscle proprioceptors—Neuromuscular spindle cells and Golgi tendon organs.

Muscle stretch response—The reaction when a normotonic muscle tests temporarily weak after it is extended and then stretched a bit more. In such a case, it requires fascial release or the chill and stretch technique.

Muscle tone—The continual, gentle, unconscious contraction of a muscle active in maintaining the posture of the body.

Myosin—Partner of actin, the two chemicals that make up the contracting fibers of a muscle.

N

Nervous system—The brain, spinal cord, motor and sensory nerves, and nerve receptors.

Neurologic disorganization—A state of confusion in the nervous system and body in which observed elements of body language, including the results of muscle testing, are confused and yield conflicting results.

Neurology—The study of nerves and the structures and functions of the whole nervous system.

Neurolymphatic reflex—Massage points that activate lymphatic drainage in specific organs and body areas. They are also used to make weak-testing muscles test strong.

Neuromuscular spindle cell—Nerve receptors concentrated in the belly of all muscles that measure the length of the muscle fibers. When quickly stretched (as in the knee-jerk reflex), neuromuscular spindle cells signal for the muscle to contract swiftly. Slow stretching of the neuromuscular spindle cells (as happens in muscle testing) causes a slow increase in the contraction of the muscle to oppose the lengthening produced by the patient's and the examiner's increasing pressure during the muscle test.

Neuron—A single nerve cell.

Neurophysiology—The function of nerves.

Neurovascular reflex points—Points, mostly on the head, that when gently held and tugged stimulate local and remote increase of vascular circulation. They are also used to make weak-testing muscles test strong.

Normotonic—A muscle that tests strong and can be weakened by standard means such as TL to its sedation point.

O

Ocular lock—A test for neurological disorganization in which looking in a specific direction or making a specific movement of the eyes makes a normotonic indicator muscle test weak.

Organ—A single structure of the body consisting of connective tissue covering and containing groups of cells that have specific functions.

Origin—The end of a muscle that is attached to the bone that does not move during contraction of the muscle.

Origin-insertion technique—Heavy massage of the two extreme ends of the tendons of a muscle down upon the bone where they are attached. This was Goodheart's first method to strengthen weak-testing muscles.

Osmosis—Diffusion through a semi-permeable membrane.

Osmotic pressure—The pressure produced when one substance is in higher concentration on one side of a semi-permeable membrane. If the holes in the membrane are large enough, the substance passes through in the direction of lesser concentration.

Osteopathy—A medical therapeutic system with emphasis upon the manipulation of bones and muscles to produce structural balance and resultant improvement of organic function.

P

Palpation—Examination by touch, used especially to diagnose disease and the state of tissues in general.

Palpatory hypertonic—The state of a muscle (or other tissue) that has too much tone, feels hard, and may be painful to the touch.

Palpatory hypotonic—The state of a muscle (or other tissue) that has too little tone, and feels soft and mushy to the touch.

Palpatory normotonic—The state of a muscle (or other tissue) that has optimal tone and feels firm but not hard to the touch.

Periosteum—The skin-like tissue that surrounds all bones.

pH—A measure of the hydrogen ion concentration and thus of the acidity of a solution.

Phagocyte—White blood cells that digest foreign particles, cell remnants and microorganisms.

Phasic muscles—Muscles that make only quick bursts of activity, have a high ratio of fast fibers, and many neuromuscular spindle cells, exhibit high coordination, and tire quickly.

Physiology—The study of the function of the structures of the body.

Postural analysis—The assessment of the structural alignment of the human body. This is usually done with the subject standing and compared to a "plumb bob" (a weight on a string) and to horizontal lines.

Primary muscle—A muscle that, because of excess tone, inappropriately inhibits other muscles.

Prime mover—The agonist, the main muscle involved in an action.

Proprioceptors—Nerve receptors that measure stimuli within the body.

Protein—A large family of organic chemicals constructed from amino acids that make up the bulk of the substance of the body.

Purulent—Pus-containing.

R

Reactive muscles—Muscles that test weak after activation of other "primary muscles" (often the antagonists), which have too much tone.

Rebound challenge—An Applied Kinesiology technique of pressing a vertebra, pelvic or cranial bone, releasing it, and then testing the effect with an indicator muscle. A rebound challenge in the direction needed for correction will temporarily weaken an indicator muscle.

Reciprocal facilitation and inhibition—This occurs naturally due to the action of the muscle proprioceptors. When the agonist acts, its synergists and stabilizers are automatically facilitated while its antagonists are inhibited.

Recruiting—In AK muscle testing, when a muscle tests weak, the patient will often (consciously or unconsciously) change the parameters of the test to bring in (recruit) other muscles to take over the job of contraction.

Regulating System—See System of ground regulation.

Repeated muscle testing—The testing of a muscle several times in rapid succession. This tests the endurance of the muscle—the capacity for sustained muscle use.

S

Sedation point—An acupuncture point upon a meridian that, when touched, should cause all muscles associated with the same meridian to test weak.

Sensory nerves—Nerves that connect nerve receptors with the central nervous system, bringing in information about what is going on in or upon the body.

Slow fibers—Red postural aerobic muscle fibers that contract comparatively slowly and are capable of long or repeated contractions without tiring.

Spindle cell—See Neuromuscular spindle cell.

Stabilize—To fix in place. In muscle testing, it is often necessary for the examiner to stabilize parts of the patient's body so they cannot move.

Stabilizer—A muscle that holds parts of the body motionless, fixing them in place as a platform for other muscles to work.

Strabismus—The condition in which the two eyes do not look in the same direction.

Strong-testing—In early Applied Kinesiology, a strong-testing muscle was defined as one that can resist the pressure applied in muscle testing. In modern AK, this is often further differentiated into normotonic or hypertonic.

Structural balance—The proper alignment of the bones and tissues of the body. The goal of chiropractic and osteopathy.

Structural challenge—A stimulus (consisting of some body movement such as walking or pressing upon an area of the body) whose effect is examined by muscle-testing an indicator muscle.

Sub-clinical—Too small or too weak to have a observable effect.

Subluxation—The misalignment of a bone.

Switching—See Neurologic disorganization.

Synergist—A muscle that assists the agonist and is automatically facilitated by the action of the agonist.

System of ground regulation—The interconnected system of nerve endings, ground substance and cells responsible for the control of most bodily processes.

T

Temporomandibular joint—The jaw hinge.

Tendon—A strong connective tissue band connecting muscle to bone.

Therapy localization—The effect of touch (usually provided by the patient) upon a body area whose effect may be measured with muscle testing. A "touch localization challenge."

Tonic muscles—Postural muscles that make long steady contractions, have a high ratio of slow fibers and few neuromuscular spindle cells, exhibit low coordination, and can work for long periods of time without tiring.

Triad of health—The basic principle of chiropractic. Structural, chemical and mental factors form the three sides of the triad, affecting each other in health and disease.

Triple heater—The yang partner of the yin circulation-sex meridian. The triple heater has a connection with the thyroid and thymus glands and has the function of the distribution of bodily warmth. When a patient has cold hands or feet, meridian therapy to the triple heater is often indicated.

V

Vascular system—The system of arteries, capillaries and veins that the blood flows through.

Vein—Blood vessels that return blood from the body to the heart.

Venules—The smallest blood veins.

W

Weak-testing—In Applied Kinesiology, a weak-testing muscle is one that cannot resist the pressure applied in muscle testing.

II. Correspondences Of Meridians, Muscles, And Organs/Glands

Meridian	Muscle	Organ/Gland
Central	Supraspinatus	Brain
Governing	Teres major	Spine
Stomach	Pectoralis major clavicular	Stomach
	Pectoralis minor (Dewe)	Stomach
	Sternocleidomastoideus	Stomach
Spleen	Latissimus dorsi	Pancreas
	Trapezius (middle & lower)	Spleen
Heart	Subscapularis	Heart
	Subclavius (Dewe)	Heart
Small Intestine	Rectus femoris	Small Intestine
	Rectus abdominis	Small Intestine
Bladder	Peroneus tertius	Urinary Bladder
	Peroneus longus and brevis	Urinary Bladder
	Sacrospinalis	Urinary Bladder
Kidney	Iliopsoas	Kidney
	Trapezius (upper)	Eye and Ear
Circulation-Sex	Gluteus medius	(Ovaries) Reproductive Organs and Glands
	Adductors	Reproductive Organs and Glands
	Gluteus maximus	Reproductive Organs and Glands
	Piriformis	(Prostate) Reproductive Organs and Glands
	Sartorius (& Triple heater)	Adrenals (esp. the medulla portion)
Triple heater	Teres minor	Thyroid
	Infraspinatus	Thymus
Gall Bladder	Popliteus	Gall Bladder
Liver	Pectoralis major sternal	Liver
	Rhomboid major and minor	Liver/Stomach
Lung	Serratus anticus	Lung
	Deltoids (ant., med., & posterior)	Lung
Large Intestine	Tensor fascia lata	Large Intestine
	Hamstrings	Rectum

III. Charts

Sedation Points

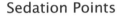

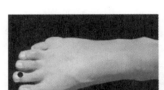

Stomach 45 - St45
Pectoralis major clavicularis
Sternocleidomastoideus
Pectoralis minor

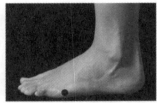

Bladder 65 - B65
Peroneus tertius
Peroneus longis and brevis
Sacrospinalis

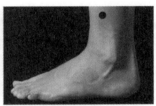

Gall Bladder 38 - GB38
Popliteus
anterior Deltoid

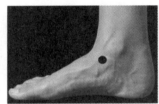

Spleen 5 - Sp5
Latissimus dorsi
middle and lower Trapezius

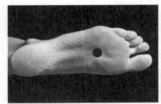

Kidney 1 - K1
Iliopsoas
upper Trapezius

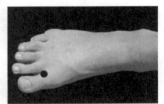

Liver 2 - Lv2
Pectoralis major sternalis
Rhomboids

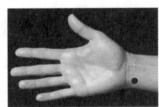

Heart 7 - H7
Subscapularis
Subclavius

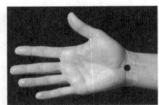

Circulation-Sex 7 - Cx7
Gluteus maximus & medius
Piriformis, Sartorius
Adductors

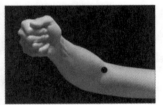

Lung 5 - Lu5
Serratus anticus
middle & posterior Deltoids

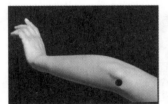

Small Intestine 8 - SI8
Rectus femoris (Quadriceps)
Rectus abdominis

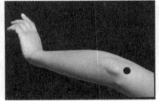

Triple Heater 10 - TH10
Teres minor
Infraspinatus

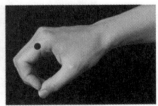

Large Intestine 2 - LI2
Tensor Fascia lata
Hamstrings

Alarm Points

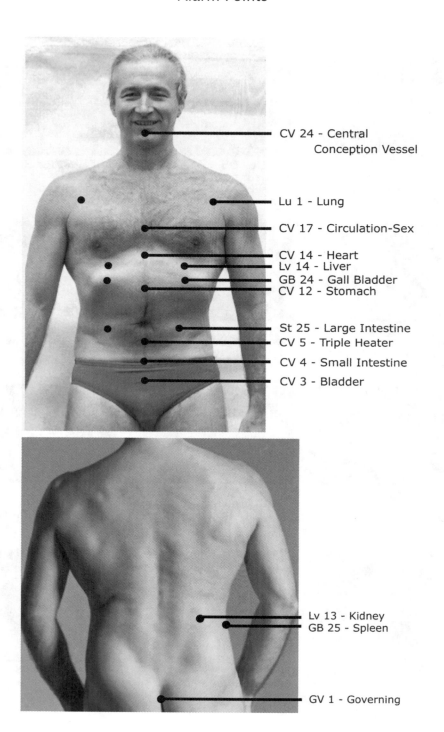

CV 24 - Central
        Conception Vessel

Lu 1 - Lung

CV 17 - Circulation-Sex

CV 14 - Heart
Lv 14 - Liver
GB 24 - Gall Bladder
CV 12 - Stomach

St 25 - Large Intestine
CV 5 - Triple Heater

CV 4 - Small Intestine

CV 3 - Bladder

Lv 13 - Kidney
GB 25 - Spleen

GV 1 - Governing

End Points

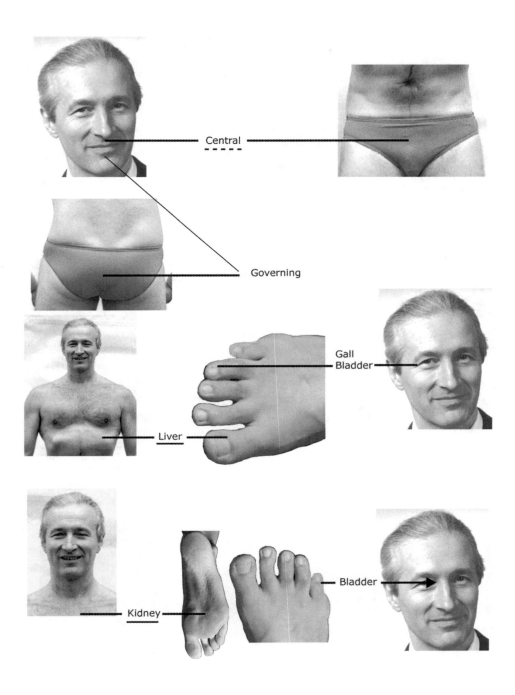

Central

Governing

Gall
Bladder

Liver

Kidney

Bladder

End Points (Continued)

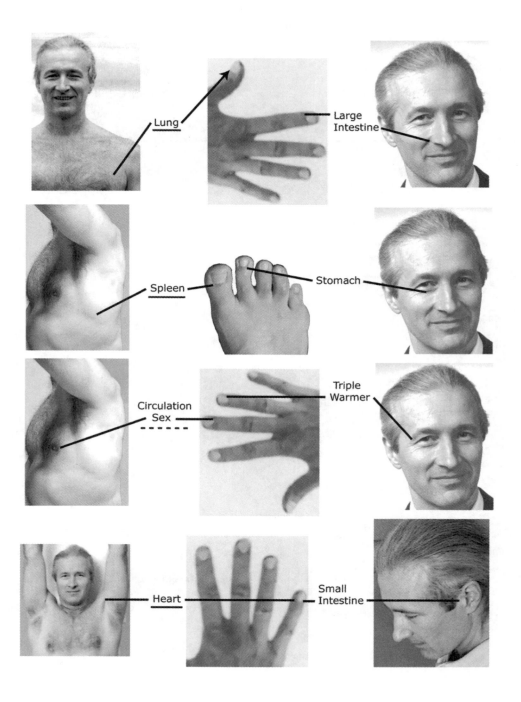

Muscle Test Circle

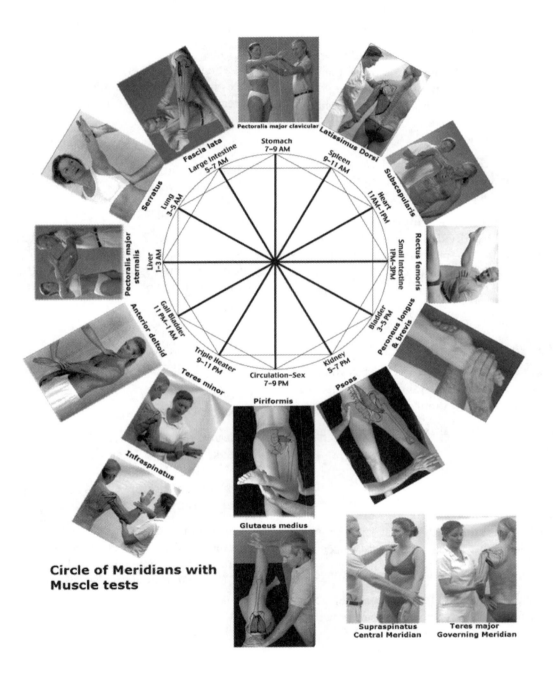

Circle of Meridians with Muscle tests

IV. Step-By-Step Plan for Conducting a Session with AK Techniques

(using the techniques described in this book)

Obviously, an AK session could include a vastly greater range of techniques and a more complex methodology than are found in the following directions for conducting a session. I designed this simplified treatment plan to include only the techniques described in this book.

1. (If qualified to do so) take a case history. Consider the results of lab tests. Inquire about the presenting problem. Observe the body language.

2. Perform the pretests and any pretest corrections necessary. The individual page numbers given below indicate where to find more complete descriptions of the pretests:

   A. *Dehydration* (p. 79)

   Examiner and patient both drink a glass of water.

   B. *Does the Muscle Test Strong?* (page 79)

   Ask, explain, show, "Press as hard as you can," provide isometric resistance to maximal contraction. Increase examiner pressure 2–5%.

   If strong, ok. If weak, strengthen it or choose and test another muscle.

   C. *Can the Muscle Be Weakened?* (page 82)

   Pinch the neuromuscular spindle cells, TL or tap the sedation point, stroke the meridian backward or place the north pole of a magnet upon the belly of the muscle and retest (weak).

   D. *Is the Individual Muscle Hypertonic?* (page 83)

   Spindle cell or Golgi tendon organ correction to the muscle itself, "Be here with me now, relax, breathe and be testable,"

   Or: Contract the muscle in the opposite direction while it is in a position of extreme contraction and extreme extension.

   Or: Drink water.

   If you find a case of bilateral hypertonic muscles or general hypertonicity, and you wish to treat it now, see the section on "General Hypertonicity," page 93.

   E. *Ocular Lock* (page 85)

   Test eye rotation clockwise, counterclockwise. Locate the weak-testing direction.

   F. *Kidney 27s?* (page 86)

   TL each Kidney 27 plus navel, both K 27s, cross K 27s and muscle test each. If any pair of points test weak, massage them both for 20 seconds. Check that any positive TL and ocular lock has been eliminated.

   G. *Auxiliary K 27s* (page 89)

   TL lateral to the transverse processes of T11 (or L1–2). If weak, massage point plus navel.

   H. *Conception Vessel 24, Governing Vessel 27* (page 89)

   TL and test CV 24 and GV 27. If either test weak, press CV 24 and CV 2 (top of pubic bone). Then hold navel and GV 1 (tip of coccyx). Or massage the CV 24 and/or GV 27 that had a positive TL.

3. Identify all muscles that may have a connection with the problem. This connection may be due to location of the problem (e.g., all leg and hip muscles for problems with the knee), or by the organ/gland associations (e.g., muscles associated with the bladder meridian for urinary bladder problems).

4. Identify, if possible, the priority muscle to work with first.

Therapy localization to the problem will usually cause any normotonic muscle to test weak. Continue this therapy localization (touch) to the problem and simultaneously touch the belly of muscles believed to be associated with the problem, one at a time. If the double therapy localization of the problem and the chosen muscle reverses the result of single therapy localization to the problem, the chosen muscle is the priority muscle to work with for the correction. Do all you can to balance the function of this priority muscle, including testing for hypertonicity and using the techniques for locating hidden weaknesses. This involves touching the corresponding treatment points for the priority muscle, one at a time, while retesting the muscle for each point touched. If a muscle tests strong in the clear, but weak when one of its treatment points is touched, it has a hidden weakness. Treat that point and retest for hidden weakness. Repeat this process until all hidden weaknesses are cleared.

For a palpatory hypertonic muscle, begin by strengthening all the antagonists. Then check if the hypertonic muscle itself is a "primary" muscle. To do so, contract the hypertonic muscle and immediately test its antagonists. Any that now test weak are reactive muscles. If so, clear this condition with the reactive muscle technique.

Note: A "primary" muscle refers to the topic of reactive muscles. Excess tension in a primary muscle causes reactive muscles. "Reactive" muscles are muscles that test strong in the clear but test weak immediately after contraction of the corresponding primary muscle. There are exceptions, but the reactive muscles are most often the antagonists to the primary muscle.

For a dysfunction in an organ (or gland), use double therapy localization of the organ and the muscles associated with the organ to locate the priority muscle to investigate and correct. If no muscle can be found that (when touched) eliminates the first TL to the organ, double therapy-localize the organ and another organ. If TL to the second organ eliminates the TL of the first, the presenting problem is a secondary result of a problem in the second organ. In this case, therapy localization to the second organ will likely weaken an indicator muscle. If so, again use double therapy localization to find the priority muscle that eliminates an active TL to the second organ.

5. If the muscle tests weak, have the patient taste a tiny amount of each of the various nutrients associated with the muscle/organ and retest the muscle. If any of them make the muscle test strong, advise the patient to eat them at a later time. Have the patient wash out her mouth with water after each nutrient is tested. The muscle should again test weak for further testing.

6. If the muscle tests weak, next TL the O/I (origin and insertion), the belly of the muscle for neuromuscular spindle cells, the junction of the muscle and its tendons for Golgi tendon organs, the NL (neurolymphatic reflex points), and the NV (neurovascular reflex points), and apply corrective techniques to the one(s) that made the muscle test strong.

7. After correcting, TL the same point again and retest the muscle. If it is again weak, repeat the treatment.

8. If (or when) the muscle tests strong, TL any points (I/O, spindles, Golgis, NL or NV) not yet treated and test the muscle again. If any make the muscle test weak, treat them until they cease to do so.

9. If the muscle does not test weak initially and no points can be found that make it test weak (or if you suspect that there is more to do with this muscle), use the activation of the right and left halves of the brain (page 122) to locate what needs to be done and do it.

10. Perform repeated muscle testing. If this weakens the muscle, check the related nutrition. Then check whether TL of the NL or NV points eliminates the repeated muscle test weakness. Massage the neurolymphatic reflex points for 2–5 minutes or hold and tug the neurovascular points for about 1 minute as required. Retest to confirm that repeated muscle testing no longer weakens the muscle.

11. Completely extend and then further stretch the muscle. If this weakens the muscle, extend and pluck it like a string instrument. If the muscle has pain when extending it, twitches when plucked (and has extremely tender "trigger" points), it needs the chill and stretch technique (page 131). This is more often the case with structural problems. If there is no twitch reaction, employ the fascial release technique (page 130). This is most often needed for problems of dysfunction in the related organs. After application of the chosen corrective technique, confirm that stretching no longer weakens the muscle.

12. Consider which muscles could be primary muscles to the muscle tested above (hereafter referred to as the "main muscle". The first suspect primary muscles to test are the antagonists to the main muscle. Further suspects can be found in the chart of reactive muscles on pages 137138. Test one suspect primary muscle andimmediately test the main muscle. If the main muscle tests weak after testing a suspect primary muscle, weaken the primary muscle by pinching its neuromuscular spindle cells (together in the belly of the muscle, parallel to the muscle fibers). Then immediately and strongly test the formerly reactive main muscle to reset it. Repeat this procedure with each of the primary muscle suspects. Then test if the main muscle is a primary muscle to other (reactive) muscles. If so, correct this condition with the reactive muscle technique here briefly described. Refer to the text on pages 131–138 for a more detailed description of the treatment of reactive muscles.

13. For structural problems, test for and correct the next priority muscle. If no further muscle shows as a priority, and the problem still exists, test and correct all the muscles in the area of, or related to, the problem.

For organic problems, therapy-localize the organ. If it still therapy-localizes, repeat the process (with the next priority muscle). If the problem no longer therapy-localizes, but the problem still exists, continue as above with the other muscles associated with the organ.

V. Applied Kinesiology Techniques of Examination and Diagnosis

This section describes AK techniques used in a session by the doctor, chiropractor or other therapist with a license to diagnose. As many of these techniques are not otherwise mentioned in this book, this will give the reader a foretaste of methods that go beyond the scope of this introductory book.

When examining a patient to determine the probable causes of his health problem, a professional examiner using AK investigates the interaction of all three sides of the triad of health (structural, chemical, mental). The primary assumption is that the body and all of its systems and functions form an integrated, interacting whole. Based upon this assumption, and assuming that the primary cause of the problem is not readily detected, the examination procedure is to first analyze and correct possible secondary problems and compensations in order to reveal the primary cause of the health problem.

The work is a combination of various tasks beginning with the search for bodily malfunctions. Then the therapeutic options are tested to determine the optimal treatment for the problem(s) found. When this is found, it is carried out. Finally the correction is challenged to see if it was performed successfully. If the health problem is not eliminated, or if it recurs (during the examination or later), the process is continued and the area of search is expanded. When the primary causes have been located and suitably treated, the health problem should be permanently corrected.

An AK examination does not depend only upon the symptoms reported by the patient. The observations and tests made by the examiner often reveal potential health disturbances before symptoms of illness emerge. Corrective measures may then be implemented before tissue pathology and illness develop. This is true preventive health care.

AK techniques of examination do not replace more standard diagnostic procedures. Moreover, the examiner should be familiar with traditional diagnostic procedures such as feeling the tissues (palpation) and laboratory tests such as blood and urine analysis. When a patient needs such tests, the examiner should perform them or refer the patient to the appropriate specialist or lab. The results of AK testing should in general concur with the results of other diagnostic procedures. When a patient has a health problem that has not progressed far enough for him to notice, or far enough to produce identifying symptoms, his doctor cannot be faulted for failing to perform the specific diagnostic tests that could reveal the problem. On the other hand, muscle testing has turned up problems that neither the patient, his examiner using AK nor his doctor suspected. For example, heart problems have been revealed by muscle testing before symptoms become extreme enough for the patient to notice. Once muscle testing results indicate the possibility of the existence of heart problems, the nature and extent of the problems can be confirmed by standard medical diagnostic tests (Omura, 1979).

Sometimes lab testing will locate problems missed by muscle testing. Conversely, muscle testing may find subclinical problems missed by lab tests. Since each may locate problems missed by the other, it is wise (whenever practical) to perform both kinesiologic muscle testing and standard laboratory tests and compare the results.

To diagnose, the examiner will ask about the patient's symptoms and also observe characteristics of the patient's body including color, odor, skin and hair quality, etc. In fact, to really master his trade, he needs to be able to recognize and interpret more subtle factors of "body language" such as tone of voice, posture, movements, breathing, coloration, etc. The examiner should give careful consideration to all factors of body language that can be either observed, or revealed by testing. For such examination of body language, the examiner may touch the patient or otherwise present a stimulus (challenge) and observe the effect this has upon manual muscle testing. The examiner may ask the patient to touch herself upon specific spots (therapy localization) and check the effect with muscle testing.

Originally in AK, the three most important techniques for evaluating the state of health of patients during the first examination were postural analysis, palpation of the temporal sphenoidal line, and evaluation of the meridian system. In AK, the muscles, organs and all bodily functions are grouped into fourteen "regulating systems" related to the fourteen main meridians of oriental medicine. Examiners originally used all three of these diagnostic methods early in an examination because they evaluate the body function as a whole and often provide direct indicators of the bodily areas involved in health problems. While postural analysis and evaluation of the meridian system are still commonly used, the palpation of the temporal-sphenoidal line is seldom employed in AK today.

VI. Additional Tips for Correcting Weak-Testing Muscles

Test, Treat, Test

For a correction technique such as massage of the neurolymphatic points to be effective in strengthening a weak-testing muscle, the muscle must be activated immediately before and after application of the strengthening technique (i.e., by testing or otherwise contracting it). If simply massaging the neurolymphatic points would strengthen the associated muscles, a whole-body massage would make all muscles test strong. Experience shows that this is not the case. Many muscles have the same neurolymphatic points. And yet, even though one of these muscles has been strengthened by massaging its neurolymphatic points, another muscle that shares the same points may still test weak. When the other muscle is tested and then the same neurolymphatic points are rubbed again, the effect of this treatment is connected with this muscle and usually it too will subsequently test strong.

It appears necessary to activate a specific muscle's neural circuits before Applied Kinesiology correction techniques will have the desired effect upon the function of the muscle. It appears that the corrective effort will only strengthen a muscle if that muscle's circuit has been freshly awakened by contracting the muscle. The energy freed by the correction seems to become coupled with the muscle and its circuit by again testing the muscle after the correction is applied. This second muscle test after the corrective effort "locks in" (and confirms) the correction. The effective formula is: "Test, treat, test."

LOCATING ACTIVE REFLEX POINTS

The position of many reflex points (and other treatment points such as the origin and insertion of muscles) is often difficult to determine from the description in words, drawings or pictures in a book. How can one determine the exact position of the various treatment points used in Applied Kinesiology?

When a muscle tests weak, reflex points that (when properly stimulated) will make it test strong are said to be "active." This means that they will therapy-localize. Similarly, a muscle that tests strong but has hidden (subclinical) problems will often test weak when the points needing treatment are touched. This phenomenon may be used to locate the precise position of an active reflex point. To do so, the patient (or the examiner) may use the whole palm of the hand to therapy-localize the area. The results are more dependable when the patient touches the area to be tested. But if the point lies where the patient cannot reach (like between the shoulder blades), or if the examiner wants to save time by not having to explain and demonstrate where the patient should touch, TL (actually a challenge) by the examiner will usually give the same results. If this touch causes the weak-testing muscle to restrengthen (or the normotonic muscle to weaken), touch with the fingertips to locate the precise area that therapy-localizes. Voila! That is the exact location of the treatment point. This technique will give the examiner the needed "hands-on" experience. With practice and attention, finding the exact location of treatment points will become second nature.

CHALLENGE ALL CORRECTIONS

Whenever a weak-testing muscle has been strengthened, challenge the correction by therapy localizing the point that was used to strengthen the muscle. If this causes the muscle to again test weak, repeat the correction.

Challenge all the work done in a session as well. After a complete session, have the patient get up and move. If any activity caused problems before (such as climbing stairs), have the patient perform that activity. Do whatever is necessary to attempt to cause the problems to return. Then retest all the muscles that were found to test weak during the session. Any weaknesses that have returned need to be more deeply explored and treated. Reactive muscles are often the cause of these recurring weaknesses. If so, find and correct them. Provoke the recurrence of problems while the patient is still in the office and correct them so they cannot return later.

"Unsolvable" Problems

Some weak-testing muscles will not restrengthen with the techniques given in this book. A muscle may test weak because of a subluxation in a joint, a fixation in the vertebral column, a cranial fault, a damaged nerve, a brain tumor or many other causes not discussed in this text. If none of the techniques described here succeed in strengthening a weak-testing muscle, advise the patient to seek the assistance of an examiner qualified in AK techniques, a medical doctor or other qualified health professional.

VII. How to Improve and Maintain Optimal Health

GENERAL HEALTH TIPS FOR THE THERAPIST
TO TELL TO HIS PATIENTS

Health depends upon regular repeating cycles of biochemical activity in your body. You can assist the process by living on a regular schedule. Make a regular daily time schedule for sleep and meals.

Eat approximately the same amount of similar kinds of food at the same time each day. This helps your body to prepare the proper amount and type of digestive enzymes to digest your food well.

Eat a big nourishing breakfast, a good solid lunch, and a small dinner. Oriental medicine states that the stomach meridian has its highest energy at 8 AM and its lowest energy at 8 PM. This means that your stomach is most capable of digesting food in the morning and least capable in the evening.

Eat the highest-quality, freshest, untreated foods possible. If vegetables are cooked, steam or stir-fry them rather than boil. Otherwise their minerals are lost in the boiling water. Do not overcook vegetables. They should be crisp and crunch when you bite them. Avoid prepared and refined foods such as white flour and sugar, pasta, fast food, etc. Butter is more healthy than margarine, which is made from hardened oils. Avoid all hardened oils. Do not overheat oils. Some research indicates that overheated oils stick to the lining of blood vessels. Buy good quality oils in small quantities and store them closed, cool and in the dark. Virgin olive oil is excellent, but be sure the quality is good. Eat at least a tablespoon of flax seed oil daily. Buy it fresh and keep it refrigerated!

Do not eat raw foods or excess amounts of food for dinner. Otherwise, these will ferment in the gut during the night. Separate proteins and carbohydrates whenever possible. Proteins travel through the intestines very slowly. Carbohydrates move through intestines very rapidly. When eaten together (meat with potatoes, cheese with bread), the carbohydrates are forced to move slowly with the protein and therefore have time to ferment. Fermentation of carbohydrates in the intestines produces gas, alcohol, ketones, and other toxic chemicals.

Vary your diet. Each food has its own mixture of vitamins, minerals and trace elements that your body needs. Learn to enjoy various grains (buckwheat, millet, oats, quinoa, amaranth, etc.) instead of only eating rice and wheat products.

Many people muscle-test as sensitive to wheat and milk products. If you do, avoid these. Avoid all foods (and other substances) that have a negative effect upon your body as revealed by muscle testing.

Do not make a habit of repeatedly grabbing something and throwing it in your mouth between other activities. However, if your blood sugar falls (hypoglycemia), take one nourishing snack between each meal. The hypoglycemic person eats too much sugar, her blood sugar rises quickly, her pancreas overreacts and produces more than enough insulin to bring the blood sugar down, the blood sugar falls too low, craving for sweets occurs, she eats sweets again and the cycle repeats. Other symptoms of hypoglycemia include hunger that suddenly arises and cannot be controlled, bad moods, lack of concentration, dizziness, attacks of hunger soon after eating and possible coffee addiction. If this cycle of eating sugar, which produces high and then low blood sugar is not broken, there may come a time when the pancreas gets exhausted and cannot make the needed insulin anymore. Then the blood sugar will rise and not come down. The result is that excess blood sugar is excreted in the urine, which draws a great amount of water and minerals out of the body, producing excessive thirst. This illness is called diabetes. Do not snack on sweets. These make the hypoglycemic problem worse. A hearty vegetable soup makes an excellent snack. A mixture of various whole grains cooked in water makes an excellent breakfast for the hypoglycemic person. Each type of grain digests and turns to sugar at a different rate, keeping the blood sugar level relatively constant for several hours.

Eat consciously. Taste the foods and chew them very well before swallowing. Do not read, watch TV, discuss or mentally involve yourself with any stress while eating. Pay attention to your food and invite it, with gratitude, to become you.

Replace nutritional factors missing in your diet. Chew at least a small amount of each supplement you take. This alerts your body, via taste, to prepare for assimilating and utilizing the nutrients.

Whenever possible, when taking nutritional supplements, take them with natural foods that contain the same nutrients. The natural factors that make the nutrients more biologically active are in the natural sources of the same nutrients. For example, when taking extra vitamin C, eat an orange or drink some fresh-squeezed diluted lemon juice. Eat some of the white inside peel the citrus as well. The bioflavonoids that help make veins, skin and other tissues elastic are concentrated there. In a study, rats were fed a diet lacking vitamin C until their bones got soft. Then one half received powdered chemical vitamin C. The other half received dried orange juice with a known amount of vitamin C content. Both vitamin C sources eliminated the symptoms of vitamin C deficiency. But to have the same clinical effect, the amount of chemical vitamin C had to be twenty times as great as the vitamin C in the orange juice powder. This demonstrates how much more effective vitamin C is when administered with the various other chemicals with which it is found in nature. According to Helmut Heine, vitamin C is the most important vitamin for furthering the health and proper functioning of the ground substance.

Maintain a good acid-base balance. Buy pH paper with a range of 5.5–8 from a pharmacy. Before drinking or brushing your teeth, test the pH value of your morning saliva. The color of the pH paper wet with saliva compared to a scale provided with the paper reveals the pH value. 7.0 is neutral. Lower numbers are acidic. Higher numbers are basic. Ideally the morning pH of the saliva should be between 6.6 and 7.2. Typically, most people are too acidic. Degenerative diseases (rheumatism, arthritis, tumors, etc.) typically begin only in a body that is too acidic. If you are too acidic, you may use an alkali powder (also from the pharmacy). Check the formulation of the powder. Some companies use aluminum, nickel or other toxic substances in their alkali powder. Do not take such poisons! If you have difficulties with milk products, avoid mixtures that contain lactose or milk powder. If your pharmacy doesn't have a good formulation, have them make up the following recipe:

Sodium bicarbonate	15.0
Potassium bicarbonate	2.5
Calcium phosphate	3.5
Calcium citrate	3.5
Magnesium citrate	0.5

When you find a good product, take a spoonful in water before sleeping until your morning pH is in the desired range. Do not take it near mealtime as it will neutralize the hydrochloric acid that the stomach releases for digesting food. Also, do not depend upon such an alkali powder. Use it for a limited time to break out of the excess acid condition. Then keep your pH in the desired range by changing your diet. In general, fruits and vegetables make the system more alkaline. Grains, sugars, and meats make the system more acidic. The only grains that are not acid-producing are quinoa and millet. Potatoes, as long as you have no allergies to the nightshade family of plants, are one of the most alkaline-producing of foods. Get a good book that lists the acid or alkaline reactions of foods and experiment with your diet until you know how to eat to preserve a good pH balance.

Drink lots of pure water with minimal mineral content. Mineral waters with a high content of mineral salts are only recommended for the treatment of specific ailments. Drunk regularly, such mineral water can leave mineral salts in your joints like they do in pipes. Get your minerals in organic form from foods.

A reverse osmosis and/or carbon block water filter is recommended.

Breathe lots of fresh air. Take a run in the woods. At least regularly open the windows and breathe deeply several times. When you exercise, you naturally breathe more deeply. In the morning, there are less pollutants and less ozone in the air. For this reason, it is advised to exercise early in the morning.

Get sunlight on your skin (before 10 AM and after 3 PM to avoid excess UV radiation). In sunlight, vitamin D is produced in the oils excreted by your skin. To be of use to the body, these oils need to be reabsorbed by the skin. For this reason, do not shower for at least 20–30 minutes after sunning.

Wear sunglasses when the sun shines. Ultraviolet light can permanently damage the lenses of your eyes.

Eliminate the foci (of infections or prior infections in the teeth, tonsils, appendix, sinuses, gall bladder, intestines, or anywhere else in the body). Use muscle testing to determine effective methods of purification for your individual case (homeopathic remedies, nosodes, nutrition, colonics, etc.). If the infection cannot be cleared with less aggressive methods, the affected organ or structure may need to be removed surgically. But let this always be a last choice after natural remedies and methods have all been tried.

Correct the energy blockages that are caused by scars. Use neural therapy, application of the light of a laser, Bach Rescue Cream®, APM Cream®, or Ionen Salbe Forte® as muscle testing reveals best for your individual case.

Clear out candida overgrowths and fetid matter from the intestines. Excess candida depresses the function of the immune system. It is important not to fast or go on a candida diet without taking an antifungal substance. If starved, candida may change into an invasive form, penetrate the intestinal wall, and via the bloodstream invade other tissues. Use muscle testing to determine which antifungal substance such as lapacho (pau d'arco), cat's claw (unicaria tormentosa), grapefruit seed extract, nystatin, or a systemic anti-fungal drug works best for you (makes the hyper-

tonic rectus femoris normotonic). See pages 95–96.

Candida feeds mainly upon sugars, all carbohydrates (pasta, grains, bread, fruits, etc.), and milk products. Fermented products (vinegars, sourdough, soy sauce, etc.) should also be avoided. For an anti-candida diet, eat only non-starchy vegetables, nuts, seeds (sunflower, poppy, sesame, etc.), and meats. While on this diet, eat high quantities of the natural intestinal flora Lactobacillus acidophilus and bifidis. After the diet, continue to eat less of the foods that feed candida. Antibiotics destroy the natural intestinal flora thereby allowing the candida to proliferate freely. If antibiotics must be taken, take an antifungal substance simultaneously. Replace the natural intestinal flora for at least a few weeks beginning on the last few days of taking the antibiotics.

Get adequate sleep (7–8 hours). The hours before midnight are important so go to sleep no later than 11 PM. Twenty-minute naps can refresh and increase alertness and energy. When you take naps, you need fewer total hours of sleep per day.

Keep the body warm and the head cool. Thermal chilling or overheating is a major stress factor for the body.

Do warm-ups, stretching, aerobic and anaerobic exercises.

Get rid of excess fat. You can do so by either eating less or exercising more. If you eat less, be sure you are getting adequate quantities of the nutrients your body needs daily. A good multi-vitamin, mineral, trace element supplement is recommended.

Do not do things that poison your body (smoking, drinking excess alcohol, drugs, breathing poisonous vapors, using hair dyes that contain lead, etc.).

Use natural herbs, vitamins, minerals, trace elements, enzymes, homeopathic remedies, nosodes, essences, etc., as determined by muscle testing for correcting various imbalances.

Reduce stress. Balance mental stress with physical stress such as exercise. Balance intellectual stress with creative stress (such as playing music). Practice forgiveness and gratitude. Perform good deeds. Praise yourself for the things you do right. Carefully choose what you expect as this will tend to come true. Be joyful and laugh lots. Laughter is biochemically health-promoting.

When you do get ill, allow your body to fight against the illness in its natural way. Your body needs to fight against infectious agents to strengthen the immune system. People who get and naturally overcome infections a few times each year have a reduced rate of cancer. Use no medications that when taken over a long period of time can cause damage and other diseases. Use allopathic chemical medicines for short periods of time only, and only as a last resort for severe or life-threatening illnesses.

VIII. Case Histories

The following cases were treated successfully using only the techniques described in this book:

1. A secretary complained of pain in the low back. The low back pain typically occurred while sitting at her desk. Palpation of the low back revealed hypertonic sacrospinalis muscles. Following Goodheart's "swing-door" model, the hypertonic muscles were not treated. Their opponents, the rectus abdominis, were tested and found weak. Strengthening the rectus abdominis caused the back pain to cease. The patient was asked to stand, walk, arch her back, etc. This caused the pain to return and the rectus abdominis to again test weak.

The return of the pain in the low back and weakness in the rectus abdominis after various motions implied the existence of a primary-reactive muscle relationship. Rectus abdominis was again strengthened. After arching her back (contracting the sacrospinalis), rectus abdominis again tested weak. This confirmed the primary-sacrospinalis to reactive-rectus abdominis muscle relationship.

The patient lay upon the side. Her sacrospinalis muscles (from about T8 to L5) were neuromuscular spindle cell weakened. Since such a large area of the back was involved, the neuromuscular spindle cell weakening took a few minutes to complete. Efforts were concentrated upon the areas of the sacrospinalis that felt especially tight. Since the weakening effect only lasts a short time, the patient was instructed to tighten her abdominal muscles about every ten to fifteen seconds during the treatment. (This technique with these two muscles is described in detail and illustrated in the section on reactive muscles, page 135). After this treatment, rectus abdominis could no longer be weakened by tightening of the sacrospinalis, and the pain did not recur during the treatment session. Postural training in how to sit and work at a desk correctly (Alexander Technique) was given to prevent recurrences of the problem.

2. A patient had a long history of repeatedly spraining her ankle and of having recurring bladder infections. During one sprain of the ankle, the peroneus tertius suffered partial separation of tendon from its insertion upon the dorsal surface of the base of the 5th metatarsal. Since peroneus is associated with the bladder meridian and the urinary bladder, a possible connection between the ankle sprains and the bladder infections was suspected. The patient had experience with kinesiology through Touch for Health and other non-AK kinesiology courses. Peroneus, when tested as described in Touch for Health, always tested strong over a period of one year. Touch for Health testing of the alarm points revealed no excess of energy in the bladder meridian. And no reactive conditions with peroneus were detected. Using Touch for Health techniques, there seemed to be nothing to do for this organic problem.

The recurring bladder infection began again. Testing peroneus tertius without the toes being pulled back (which is allowed in Touch for Health and which recruits assistance from the flexor digitorum longum) revealed no weakness. However, repeated muscle testing with the toes flexed quickly produced weakness in peroneus tertius. When the lower margin of the pubic bone (the anterior neurolymphatic point for peroneus) was therapy-localized, peroneus tertius remained strong even after repeated testing. The patient was asked for permission to massage this sensitive and personal area. Contact was made at the upper inner thigh. Excursion of the skin allowed contact with the underside of the pubic bone without pressing upon the labia. The area was then massaged, which was painful to the patient. This was repeated on the other side. The two points on the underside of the pubic bone that were massaged (the inferior surface of the tuberculum pubicum) lie about 4–8 cm apart. No attempt was made to massage under the center of the pubic bone. Prolonged massage of the anterior neurolymphatic reflex points on both sides (and the posterior reflexes) eliminated the repeated muscle weakness. This had to be performed three times at an interval of two days each before the repeated muscle testing weakness ceased to recur.

Therapy localization to both the origin and insertion of peroneus tertius was positive. Deep, heavy massage was painful and eliminated the TL to the origin and insertion. As the ankle had not been sprained for several months, it was decided that the peroneus could be stretched without danger of further damaging injured tissues. Muscle stretch reactions were present in peroneus tertius. Stretching and plucking peroneus tertius produced no jump sign. Application of the fascial release technique was exquisitely painful to the patient. After this treatment, stretching the peroneus tertius no longer caused weakness. This single treatment did not have to be repeated. Peroneus tertius remained free of muscle stretch reactions during subsequent sessions. No primary muscles were found to weaken peroneus tertius. After this treatment, none of the various types of tests (single, hidden, repeated, muscle stretch, reactive) caused weakness of peroneus tertius.

Peroneus longus and brevis tested strong. Careful observation revealed that the patient was not performing the test properly. It required several attempts for the patient to achieve the proper test position without pulling the toes back or flexing the foot on the ankle. When the proper test position was achieved (foot extension and eversion), peroneus longus and brevis tested extremely weak.

Therapy localization of the underside of the pubic bone (the anterior neurolymphatic reflex point for peroneus) caused peroneus longus and brevis to test strong. After massage of the anterior and posterior neurolymphatic points (the same ones as for peroneus tertius), peroneus longus and brevis tested strong.

Repeated testing again weakened peroneus longus and brevis. Prolonged stimulation of the neurolymphatic reflex points allowed repeated testing to be performed without weakening.

TL of the neurovascular points and of the origins and insertions caused no weakening of the peroneus longus and brevis.

Peroneus tertius was found to be a primary muscle to reactive peroneus longus and brevis. Neuromuscular spindle cell pinching of the belly of peroneus tertius was exquisitely painful to the patient. Immediately after this treatment, peroneus longus and brevis were reset by testing them strongly. After this, contraction of peroneus tertius caused no subsequent weakening of peroneus longus and brevis.

After this work with peroneus tertius, longus and brevis, the bladder infection ceased without any other sort of treatment. This was surprising as the patient usually had to take strong antibiotics to stop her bladder infections. In the one and one-half years since this treatment, the bladder infection has not occurred again.

3. A professional tennis player stated that he felt that he couldn't hit the ball as hard as he believed he should be able to do. Further questioning revealed that he couldn't perform a single chin-up. He was able to make the chin-up motion with great weights when pushing with his elbows upon an exercise machine. But when grasping the bar above his head, he had not the strength to lift himself.

Latissimus dorsi (the main muscle involved in the chin-up motion) tested strong but became extremely weak when he grasped anything with his hand. Specific testing revealed that when he pulled his thumb across his palm (activating opponens pollicis, the muscle that connects the entire radial side of the first metacarpal bone of the thumb to the wrist), latissimus dorsi and pectoralis major sternal became subsequently weak. This confirmed the primary-opponens pollicis to reactive-latissimus dorsi and pectoralis major sternal muscle relationships.

Opponens pollicis was weakened by pinching its neuromuscular spindle cells. Latissimus dorsi and pectoralis major sternal were reset immediately by testing them strongly. This was performed on both sides of the body. After this treatment, the client could perform chin-ups for the first time in his life and could hit the tennis ball more strongly.

4. A young mother had a weak-testing pectoralis major sternal. The muscle strengthening techniques in this book including manipulation of the neuromuscular spindle cells and Golgi tendon organs plus various meridian balancing techniques (acupressure, etc.) all failed to strengthen the muscle. Pectoralis major sternal is associated with the liver meridian. The main nutrition for this muscle and meridian is vitamin A. A source of vitamin A (some parsley, which was growing in the window box) was placed in her mouth and she was instructed to chew it and keep it in her mouth. Immediately, the weak-testing pectoralis major sternal tested fully strong. During the next session, testing revealed that cod liver oil made the pectoralis major sternal muscle normotonic. She was advised to include a spoonful of cod liver oil in her diet daily. She did so and her pectoralis major sternal was no longer found to test weak during subsequent sessions.

5. A patient had painful menstrual cramps. Therapy localization of the uterus weakened an indicator muscle. Double-handed therapy localization of the uterus and the gluteus medius muscle restrengthened the indicator muscle. Double TL of the uterus and of the other circulation-sex meridian muscles (associated with the reproductive organs and glands) did not have the restrengthening effect. Therefore, corrective efforts were confined to the gluteus medius muscle.

The gluteus medius muscle tested weak. A small quantity of vitamin E oil placed in her mouth returned gluteus medius to testing strong. She was advised to include vitamin E in her daily diet. After rinsing her mouth, gluteus medius again tested weak.

Therapy localization of the pubic bone (the anterior neurolymphatic reflex point for gluteus medius) made gluteus medius test strong. Neurolymphatic reflex point massage of this anterior point and the posterior point was performed. Gluteus medius then tested strong. Subsequent therapy localization of the neurolymphatic reflex point did not weaken gluteus medius.

Therapy localization of the neurovascular point for gluteus medius caused it to again test weak. Neurovascular point-holding was performed. TL of the neurovascular point again weakened the gluteus medius. Neurovascular point holding was again performed with great care to find the exact direction of tugging that caused the greatest pulsation. After this, TL of the neurovascular point no longer weakened the gluteus medius.

Therapy localization of the origin and insertion of gluteus medius both weakened the gluteus medius. Heavy massage of these areas removed this positive therapy localization.

Repeated testing of gluteus medius caused weakness. Prolonged stimulation of the neurolymphatic reflexes removed this finding.

Stretching of the gluteus medius caused weakness. Extending and plucking it caused no jump sign nor were there active trigger points. Therefore the fascial release technique was employed. This caused the patient great pain. Afterwards, stretching the muscle had no further weakening effect.

No primary muscle could be found to weaken the gluteus medius. No muscles were found to be reactive to gluteus medius.

After this extensive work on gluteus medius, the menstrual cramping ceased and did not return during this menstrual cycle.

6. When babies begin to eat solid food, many suffer from colic. The gas, diarrhea, and obvious suffering with crying and sleeplessness are common symptoms. When the family doctor is asked about these symptoms, many mothers receive the answer, "Ah, this is colic. It is normal. It will go away in about six months to one year."

The examiner visited the mother with a baby suffering from colic. All the foods that the baby had been eating were placed upon the table. The mother was muscle-tested and an easily testable normotonic muscle was located. With the baby in her lap and skin contact between the mother and child, a bite of one kind of food was placed in the baby's mouth. The mother was again muscle-tested. This was repeated with all of the foods. When a food in the baby's mouth caused the mother's muscle to test weak, the baby was given a drink of water and the mother's indicator muscle-tested to ensure that it again tested strong before proceeding.

After the testing, the mother was advised to not give her baby the foods that had tested weak. She did so and the colic disappeared and did not reappear.

7. During a holiday in France, one of the group brushed her bare leg against a bush of stinging nettles. Touching the spot provided an active TL. Leaves from plants growing nearby were gathered and placed one at a time upon the spot. The active TL was abolished by contact with plantain. A mash of plantain leaves rubbed upon the area soothed the itch and reduced the swelling.

IX. Bibliography

Athenstaedt, H., *Pyroelectric and piezoelectric properties of vertebrates,* Annals of the New York Academy of Science 238, 1974, pp. 221–242.

Bergsmann, O., *Bioelektrische Phänomene und Regulation in der Komplementärmedizin,* Wien, Austria, Facultas Universitätsverlag, 1994.

Bergsmann, O., *Grundsystem, Regulation und Regulationsstörung in der Praxis der Rehabilitation,* in A. Pischinger, *Das System der Grundregulation,* eighth edition, Heidelberg, Germany, Haug Verlag, 1990, pp. 89–139.

Bergsmann, O., and R. Bergsmann, *Projektionssymptome,* Wien, Facultas Universitätsverlag, 1988.

Chaldni, Ernst, *Entdeckungen über die Theorie des Klanges,* Leipzig, 1787.

Dewe, Bruce M.D. and Dewe, Joan, *Professional Kinesiology Practice 1,* Queensland, Australia, International College of Specialized Kinesiology and Natural Therapies, 1989.

Frost, Robert, Ph.D. , Grundlagen der Applied Kinesiology, Freiburg, Germany, VAK, 1998.

Gerz, Wolfgang, M.D., *Bio-logische Präparate für Diagnose und Therapie in der naturheilkundlichen Praxis,* München, AKSE Verlag, 1997.

Gerz, Wolfgang, M.D., *Hilfe durch Naturheilweisen, Ein Ratgeber für den Sport und das tägliche Leben,* Oberhaching, Germany, Sportinform Verlag, 1989.

Gerz, Wolfgang, M.D., *Lehrbuch der Applied Kinesiology (AK) in der naturheilkundlichen Praxis,* München, AKSE Verlag, 1996.

Gleditsch, J.M., *Mundakupunktur,* second edition, Schorndorfr, WBV Biologische-Medizinische Verlag, 1981.

Goodheart, George J., Jr., D.C., *Applied Kinesiology,* thirteenth edition, Detroit, Self-published, 1977.

Goodheart, George J., Jr., D.C., "The interosseous vertebral holographic subluxation, Part II," Chiro Econ, Vol 29, No 2 (Sept/Oct 1986).

Goodheart, George J., Jr., D.C., *You'll Be Better, The Story of Applied Kinesiology,* Geneva, Ohio, USA 44041, AK Printing, year not given.

Hauss, W. H.: *Die unspezifische Mesenchymreaktion (UMR.) Das essentielle Erignis der in den Industriestaaten häufigsten Erkrankungen,* in: Perfusion 9 (1994), pp. 312–322.

Heine, Hartmut, *Lehrbuch der biologischen Medizin,* Stuttgart, Hippokrates Verlag, 1991, 1997.

Heine, Hartmut, *Neurogene Entzündung als Basis chronischer Schmerzen,* New York, Plenum Publishing Company, 1990: pp. 127–159.

Horrigan, Joseph, and Robinson, Jerry, *The 7-Minute Rotator Cuff Solution,* Los Angeles, Health for Life, 1991.

Jenny, Hans, *Cymatics,* Vol. II, Switzerland, Basilus, 1974.

Kellner, G., "Wundheilung-Mikrowunde (Nadelstich) – chirurgischer Laser – Laser-Regulationstherapie," in: *Deutsche Zeitschrift für Akupunktur,* 22, 1979, pp. 86–95.

Kendall, H.O. / Kendall, F.P. / McCreary, E.K., *Muscles – Testing and Function,* Baltimore: Williams & Wilkins, first edition 1949; third edition 1983.

Klinghardt, Dietrich: *Lehrbuch der Psycho-Kinesiologie,* Freiburg: Bauer, 1996.

Leaf, David W., D.C., *Applied Kinesiology Flowchart Manual,* Published privately and available from the author: David D. Leaf, 159 Samoset St., Plymouth, MA, USA 02360, 1995.

Leaf, David W. D.C., "Nutrient testing evaluation," in: *Proceedings of Summer meeting,* Santa Monica, California, ICAK, 1985.

Lebowitz, Michael, and Steele, Mark, *Correcting chronic health problems. A doctor's manual,* Reprint: München, AKSE, 1989.

Lippert, Herbert, *Lehrbuch Anatomie,* München-Wien-Baltimore, Urban & Schwarzenberg Verlag, 1990.

Mandelbrot, Benoit B., *The Fractal Geometry of Nature,* W. H. Freeman, 1982.

Mann, Felix, *Acupuncture. Ancient Chinese art of healing,* London: Heinemann Medical Books.

Maturana, Huberto, and Varela, Franzisco: *Der Baum der Erkienntnis,* München, Goldmann, 1987.

Omura, Yoshiaki, "Acupuncture and Related Unorthodox Methods of Diagnosis and Treatment: ... Applied Kinesiology," *ACUPUNCTURE & ELECTRO-THERAPEUT. RES., INT. J.,* 1979, 4: pp. 69–89.

Pischinger, A., *Das System der Grundregulation. Grundlagen für eine ganzheitsbiologische Theorie der Medizin,* Heidelberg, Haug, fourth edition 1975.

Platzer, Werner, *Taschenatlas der Anatomie für Studium und Praxis, Band 1: Bewegungsapparat,* Stuttgart/New York, Thieme, 1991.

Popp, A., *Neue Horizonte in der Medizin,* Heidelberg, Haug, second edition 1987.

Prigogine, I., *Vom Sein zum Werden,* München and Zürich, Piper, 1979.

Schäffler, Arne, M.D., and Schmidt, Sabine, M.D. (Hrsg.), *Mensch, Körper, Krankheit; Anatomie, Physiologie, Krankheitsbilder; Lehrbuch und Atlas für die Berufe im Gesundheitswesen,* Neckarsulm, Germany, Jungjohann Verlag, 1993.

Schmidt, Walter, D.C., *Common Glandular Dysfunctions in the General Practice,* Applied Kinesiology Study Program, Chapel Hill, North Carolina, 1981.

Schnering, H.G., "Die Krümmung chemischer Strukturen," in: *Nova acta Leopoldina NF,* 65, 1991, pp. 89–103.

Schumann, W.O., "Über die strahlungslosen Eigenschwingungen einer leitenden Kugel, die von einer Luftschicht und einer Ionosphärenhülle umgeben ist," in: *Zeitschrift für Naturforschung* 7a, 1954, pp. 149–154.

Selye, Hans, *Einführung in die Lehre vom Adaptionssyndrom,* Stuttgart, Thieme, 1952.

Selye, Hans, *Stress Without Distress,* New York, Signet, 1974.

Stecco, L., *La manipolazione neuroconnettivale,* Roma, Marrapese, 1996.

Travell, Janet, "Myofascial trigger points—clinical view," in: *Advances in pain research and therapy,* Vol. I, editors Bonica, J.J., and Albe-Fessard, D., New York, Raven, 1976.

Travell, Janet, und Rinzler, S.H., "The myofascial genesis of pain," in: *Post-graduate medicine,* Vol. II, Number 5, May 1952.

Virchow, R., *Die Cellularpathologie in ihrer Bedeutung auf physische und pathologische Gewebslehre,* Berlin, Hirschwald, 1858.

Voll, R., *Topographische Lage der Meßpunkte der Elektroakupunktur,* Uelzen, Germany, Med. Lit. Verlagsanstalt, 3 Bände, 1973–1976.

Walther, David S., D.C., *Applied Kinesiology Synopsis,* Pueblo, Colorado, Systems DC, 1988.

Walther, David S., D.C., *Applied Kinesiology, Volume 1, Basic Procedures and Muscle Testing,* Pueblo, Colorado, Systems DC, 1981.

Wiener, N., *Kybernetik—Regelung und Nachrichtunübermittlung im Lebewesen und in der Maschine,* Düsseldorf, Econ-Verlag, 1963.

Yokochi, Rohen and Weinreb, *Photographische Anatomie des Menschen,* Stuttgart-New York, Schattauer Verlag, 1992.

Zerlauth, B., etc., "Histologie der Akupunkturpunkte," in: *Deutsche Zeitschrift für Akupunktur,* 35, 1992, pp. 34–38.

Zink, Christoph (Bearb.), *Pschyrembel Klinisches Wörterbuch,* Berlin-New York, Walter de Gruyter Verlag, 1990.

X. Contact Addresses

For Products, Services, and Information Used
and Recommended by ICAK Members

ORTHOMOLECULAR (NUTRITIONAL) PRODUCTS

Biotics Research Corp.
PO Box 36888
Houston, TX 77236
800-231-5777, 281-344-0725,
biotics@bioticsresearch.com
www.bioticsresearch.com

Their products include a series of neo-natal glandulars (as close as legally possible to live-cell glandulars in the US), vegetable-source minerals, and a line of digestive, proteolytic and systemic enzymes. They specialize in double-blind-tested delivery systems so nutrients really get absorbed well. They have produced products only for health professionals for 26 years.

Ecological Formulas and Cardiovascular Research
1061-B Shary Circle
Concord, CA 94518
925-827-2636, 800-351-9429, 800-888-4585,
Fax 925-676-9231
technical information 800-952-0432
ecologicalformulas@yahoo.com

Ecological Formulas is a 20-year-old company with 160 products. They have performed much groundbreaking medical research that has been used in formulating their products.

Generally, when a patient complains of a sore throat, a primary-care medical doctor doesn't attempt to distinguish between a viral or a bacterial infection. Since standard laboratory culture tests take time and are costly, he typically just prescribes an antibiotic. But by overusing a medicine that may not be indicated, the doctor contributes to the problem of antibacterial resistance. Therapists using AK can use Ecological Formula's Monolaurin (effective against viral infections) and Nutricillin (a natural antibiotic formula) to swiftly make a differential diagnosis and then prescribe the

correct one as indicated by muscle testing. This line of attack is recommended for cases of recurring sore throats or ear infections, etc.

In controlled studies, lauric acid has been found to solubilize the lipid envelope of capsid viral membranes, thus aiding in their destruction. Monolauren is a patented ester of lauric acid, found naturally in mother's milk, which help infants to have immunity to a wide range of viruses.

Ecological Formulas also formulates products to address many rare conditions including Meniere's syndrome. Their wide range of specific formulas may at last bring help to your patients when nothing else has.

Metagenics
100 Avenida La Pata
San Clemente, CA 92673
800-692-9400, 949-369-3355, Fax 949-366-2859
timkatke@metagenics.net
www.metagenics.com

Metagenics uses the results of its staff's original medical research to create efficacious nutraceutical formulations and "medical foods" for a wide variety of common health problems. Metagenics couples the best of traditional knowledge of the impact of nutrition and botanical medicines on health with the latest research in the nutrient modulation of gene expression, focused on healthy aging. They supply third-party assaying of purity and potency and third-party research data on their formulations plus excellent educational support material for patients.

Nutri-West Home Office, 307-358-5066
Fax 307-358-9208, 800-443-3333
marcia@nutri-west.net
www.nutri-west.com

The owner and operator is Dr. Paul White, an original ICAK diplomate. Call the home office for the nearest Nutri-West distributor.

Nutri-West products are known for their quality, purity, and efficacy. They won a FDA blue ribbon award for GMP (Good Manufacturing Practices). As a spokesman and formulator for Nutri-West, Dr. John

Brimhall has taught thousands of chiropractors and AK-inclined practitioners his successful protocol. He has developed a line of products that have passed rigorous muscle testing and field tests for efficacy, including the top-selling Nutri-West product, DSF (De-Stress Formula) which includes adrenal glandular.

Nutri-West South, 800-343-0754
South 99 White Bridge Rd, Ste. 202
Nashville, TN 37205-1450
615-352-4455, 615-352-4491
drobeone@mindspring.com

Ask for Mary for AK seminar information for the Southern US states of Alabama, Georgia, Tennessee, Louisiana, Mississippi and Arkansas.

Pure Encapsulations, Inc., 978-443-1999
490 Boston Post Rd.
Sudbury, MA 01776
http://www.pureencapsulations.com

PE is a trusted source of pure individual nutrients for AK testing. It is one of the only companies to provide complete disclosure of all ingredients. Their vitamins and amino acids are synthetically produced. They produce what are perhaps the most hypo-allergenic supplements available.

Standard Process Inc., 1200 W. Royal Lee Dr.,
Palmyra, WI 53156, 414-495-2122,
414-495-2512, 800-848-5061

Standard Process Inc. has made whole-food (animal and vegetable source) nutritional supplement products for over 70 years. They find foods that are high in naturally occurring nutrients and combine them and concentrate them. They have products that target specific organs and organ systems and specific nutritional compounds. Most of their ingredients are grown on their own 1000 acres of farms and carefully extracted in-house. Standard Process has long been a favorite of George Goodheart. Calcium Lactate, Immuplex and Catalyn are their most popular products with chiropractors.

Thorne Research, Inc., 25820 Highway 2 West,
Dover, ID 83825, 208-263-1337, 208-265-2488,
tia@thorne.com, http://www.thorne.com

Thorne products are known for their purity and good acceptance by hypersensitive patients. They now supply their products in vegetarian capsules.

TPCS, 660 W. Baker Street, Suite 229,
Costa Mesa, CA 92626, 800-838-8727,
714-760-1475, kimtpcs@aol.com, www.health-tpcs.com

This is John Thie's company, the makers of Iosol, a liquid organic iodine used especially for female problems.

Zenith Advanced Health Systems, International,
Inc., PO Box 1739,
Corvallis, OR 97339, 800-547-2741,
zah@proaxis.com, www.zenith4theplanet.com

Zenith offers complete nutritional systems, chelated minerals, unique oxygen-supplying products, and a line of cutting-edge adaptogens. They make Standard Formula, my personal favorite multi-vitamin-mineral-trace element-herbal complex. If you say you want to be a "member," you will get a 20% discount.

THE BEST SOURCES OF AK KITS IN EUROPE

Bio-Apotheque
Frauenstr. 17, 80469 München
Tel. 011 49 89-225630, Fax 011 49 89-2289300.

They supply AK Test sets with orthomolecular substances, Pure Encapsulations products, imported nutritional supplements and medicines. The small-sized bottles make this set good for travel.

Fa. Centropa
Waltherstr. 27, 80337 München
Tel 089 544229-0, Fax 089 54422988.

They provide AK test sets with large size samples.

TABLES AND TOOLS

Foot Levelers, Inc.
518 Pocahontas Ave NE
Roanoke, VA 24027
800-553-4860.
They do shoe inserts, etc. Goodheart uses them.

Impac
PO Box 535, Salem, OR 97308
503-581-3239, 503-364-7754
www.impacinc.net
Impac makes adjusting tools (the "Arthrostem" and various percussors) for osteopaths.

Hessco/Wessco
2344 Hwy 33/POB 170
Saukville, WI 53080
909-676-8116.
They distribute therapy tables.

MANUFACTURERS OF TABLES

Lloyd, Zenith, Hill, Kyro.
Kyro's DC101
A good, strong AK table with variable height.

DIAGNOSTIC LABS

Metametrix, Inc.
5000 Peachtree Ind. Blvd., Ste. 110
Norcross, GA 30071
770-446-5483 ext. 325.

Great Smokies Diagnostic Lab, Inc.
63 Zillicoa St.
Asheville, NC 28801-1074
828-253-0621.

Diagnostechs
6620 S. 192nd Place, Ste. J104

Kent, WA 98032-1948
425-251-0596.

ICAK CHAPTER CONTACTS

http://www.akse.de (German and English)
This site was initiated by Wolfgang Gerz, MD, ICAK diplomate and former president of the ICAK-D. The author is the webmaster for the English side of this site. Here may be found charts, graphics, articles by leading AK authors, links to other AK sites, an AK "chat room," sources of AK books, upcoming AK courses and other useful tools. This is a place to learn of the advancements in AK made by diplomates and other members of European and world-wide ICAK groups.

In many European countries, chiropractic is not a recognized profession. Those who practice AK there are mostly medical doctors, dentists and other licensed therapists. The medical doctors there have critically analyzed AK and developed methods of using AK muscle testing for accurate medical diagnosis.

Although these and other breakthroughs made in Europe have so far been ignored by the ICAK in America, it is highly recommended that those interested in AK make themselves aware of these advancements to the field through this site. ICAK members, world-wide, are invited to submit their papers with abstracts for addition to this site.

http://www.icakusa.com
The official web site of the International College of Applied Kinesiology for North America. This is the central source for information about AK.

www.icak.com
A semi-official site of the ICAK-USA.

ICAK CHAPTER CONTACTS 2000-2001
(CONTACT THE USA CENTRAL OFFICE FOR CURRENT UPDATES)

For meeting, membership and publication
information, please contact:

ICAK-USA, Central Office
Terry Kay Underwood, executive director
6405 Metcalf Ave., Suite 503
Shawnee Mission, KS 66202-3929
Phone: 913-384-5336, Fax: 913-384-5112
Email: ICAK@dci-kansascity.com
(Andria Dibbern, membership services /
publications coordinator)
Website: http://www.icakusa.com

ICAK-AUSTRALASIA
Richard P. Cheyne, D.C.
2 Champion St., Porirua East
Wellington, New Zealand
Phone: 6442377711, Fax: 6442377711
Email: richard.cheyne@clear.net.nz

ICAK-BENELUX
Geert Drenth, D.O.
Heuveneindewig 6
Zonhoven, 3520, Belgium
Phone: 32 11812075, Fax: 32 11812075
Email: geert.drenth@pandora.be

ICAK-CANADA
Zeya Alikhan
241 Hastings St. N, Box 417
Bancroft, Ontario KOL 1 CO, Canada
Phone: 613-332-3030, Fax: 613-332-1937
Email: zeya@bancom.net

ICAK-DAGAK
Hans Garten, MED, DIBAK
Nederlingerstr. 35, München, 80638, Germany
Phone: 49 891595951, Fax: 49 891596161
Email: vkmakpg@aol.com

ICAK-DEUTSCHLAND
Karl Kienle, M.D., DIBAK
Munzstr. 17, Schongau, D-86956, Germany
Phone: 49 8861 900583, Fax: 49 8861 900584
Email: karlkienle@gmx.net

IMAK Büro Deutschland,
International Medical Society
for Applied Kinesiology, German office
Lanzenhaarerstr. 2, 82041 Oberhaching, Germany
Phone: 49 89-66665389
Fax: 49 89-66665388

IMAK, International Medical Society
for Applied Kinesiology
Harald Stossier, MED
St.-Vieter-Str. 34, Klagenfurt, A-9020, Austria
Phone: 43 463 585635, Fax: 43 463 514222
Email: golfhotel@het4you.com.at

ICAK-FRANCE (non-official),
Richard Meldener, D.C., DIBAK
49 Rue Des Mathurins, 75008 Paris, France
Phone: 33 142658720, Fax: 33 142663767

ICAK-ITALY
Marcello Caso, D.C.
Centro Chiropractico, Salus Via Clara, Maffei, 14A
Bergamo 24121 Italy
Phone: 39 035 222 959, Fax: 39 035 222 959
Email: castedit@tin.it (Antonio Gil, D.C.)

ICAK-RUSSIA
Lyudmila Vasilyeva
Stroiteley 98, Novokuznetsk, 654006, Russia
Fax: 7 3843469821
Email: root@drenagkemerovo.su

ICAK-SCANDINAVIA
Patrick Wennergren, D.C., DIBAK
Kirropracetur Centrum, Kungsgatan 1 OB
Goteberg, 41119, Sweden
Phone: 46 317116600
Email: oddny@algonet.se

ICAK-SWITZERLAND
Michel Barras, D.C.
Ch. De Mornex 7, Lausanne CH-1003, Switzerland

Phone: 41 213232325,
Fax: 41 213232509
Email: mbar@pingnet.ch

ICAK-UK
Tracy S. Gates, D.O., M.R.O., DIBAK
Doneechka Clinic, Mill Straight, Southwater
West Sussex, RHI 3 7EY, England
Phone: 44 1403 734321
Fax: 44 1403 732689
Email: tracy@tsgates.demon.co.uk

FRACTALS

The Julia set fractals in this book were created with the formula: NEW z = OLD $z^2 + c$ where $c = -0.69000 + 0,32000i$ and $i = \sqrt{-1}$

Everyone who has a computer and an internet connection can make their own fractal diagrams. The site I used to make these fractals is no longer on line. Those who want to learn more about fractals or make their own are advised to do an internet search on fractals.

INDEX

O

Ocular lock 72, 85–88, 90–92, 233, 252, 266, 289, 298
Organ neurolymphatic reflex points 258
Origin 4, 17
Origin-insertion technique 4, 99, 100, 111, 278, 289
Osmosis 289, 307
Osmotic pressure 104, 289
Osteopathy 5, 67, 68, 71, 289, 290

P

Palmer, D. 94
Palpation 6, 9, 26, 178, 236, 237, 271, 289, 301, 302, 309
Paralysis 122
Phasic muscles 16, 23, 24, 125, 126, 130, 289
Phobias 265, 274
Physiology 3, 6, 12, 15, 17, 19, 43, 51, 56, 68, 71, 84, 102, 106, 113, 132, 289
Pischinger, Alfred 40, 56, 57, 59, 60, 65, 66, 313, 314
Popp, Fritz 55, 314
Postural analysis 134, 289, 302
Primary muscle 28, 30, 32, 131–138, 166, 200, 209, 231, 289, 290, 299, 300, 310, 311
Prime mover—See Agonist.
Proprioceptive neuromuscular facilitation 254, 278
Proprioceptors 22, 29, 31, 32, 34, 72, 74, 80, 83, 84, 132–134, 215, 236, 250, 254, 255, 277, 286, 288, 289, 290
Protein 27, 31, 49, 51, 52, 58, 59, 104, 108, 120, 216, 290, 305

Q

Quantum theory 43–50

R

Ragland sign 38
Reactive muscles 3, 26, 28, 30, 32, 35, 94, 122, 131–138, 142, 153, 173, 179, 193, 197, 200, 209, 216, 235, 278, 279, 290, 299, 300, 303, 309
Rebound challenge—See Challenge, rebound.

Recruiting 198, 208, 290, 309
Repeated muscle testing 109, 122–125, 197, 290, 296, 309, 310
Retrograde lymphatic technique 259–262
Reversals and conflicts 268–271, 274, 275
242, 247, 257, 258

S

Sabotage programs 268, 269, 274
Schmidt, Walter 250, 314
Sensory nerve – See also afferent nerve 21, 32, 53, 54, 64, 288, 290
Selye, Hans 35–39, 56, 73, 105, 314
Slow fibers 15, 16, 17, 124, 125, 290, 291
Spindle cell—See Neuromuscular spindle cell.
Stabilize 17, 80, 81, 90, 91, 240, 290
Stabilizer 17, 24, 25, 29, 133, 164, 178, 186, 204, 286, 290
Strabismus 230, 290
Strain counterstrain 235–237
Structure 233
Structural balance 4, 6, 17, 289, 290
Structural screening 278
Subclinical 94, 278, 301, 303
Subluxation 68, 69, 71, 74, 75, 90, 210, 235, 237, 252, 290, 304
Substance testing 257–259
Switching—See Neurologic disorganization.
Synergist 17, 24, 25, 29, 30, 63, 133, 136, 198, 236, 238, 241, 258, 286, 290
System of ground regulation 40, 51, 52, 54, 56, 57, 59, 61, 65, 66, 290, 291

T

Temporal tapping 271–274
Temporalis muscle 272
Temporomandibular joint 36, 291
Tendon 1, 4, 15, 17, 18, 21, 22, 29–32, 52, 56, 58, 60, 64, 84, 96, 99, 100, 111, 134, 143, 153, 248, 250, 283, 284, 285, 289, 291, 299, 309
Therapy localization 2, 8, 11, 26, 30, 32, 61, 66, 73–76, 79, 89, 90, 94, 105, 106, 109, 111, 121–126, 133, 156, 170, 186, 233, 234, 245, 253, 272, 273, 275, 286, 287, 291, 299, 302, 310, 311

INDEX OF THE MAIN MUSCLES DISCUSSED IN THIS TEXT

ABOUT THE AUTHOR

Robert Frost, PhD, received degrees in psychology, biology, and physics from the University of California, Santa Cruz. He has extensive training in both popular kinesiology and Applied Kinesiology, and is an independent trainer for alternative therapeutic techniques including the Alexander Technique and Neurolinguistic Programming. He also studied biomechanics as applied to dance with Andres Bernard at New York University. In Basel, Switzerland he worked in a medical clinic where patients who did not respond adequately to standard medical treatment were sent to him for physiological and psychological therapies. Through this practical training and experience with often extreme medical cases, he became an expert at reducing or eliminating back pain.

To learn more, please visit his websites at www.drrobertfrost.com and www.learnappliedkinesiology.com